Craig's
Care of the Newly Born Infant

A. J. KEAY
M.B., CH.B., F.R.C.P.(Edin.), D.C.H.(Lond.)
Consultant Paediatrician,
Western General Hospital,
Edinburgh

D. M. MORGAN
M.B., CH.B.(Leeds), F.R.C.P.(Edin.), D.C.H.(Lond.)
Consultant Paediatrician,
Airedale General Hospital,
Keighley

NORAH J. STEPHEN
RGN, RSCN, SCM, MTD
Principal Nursing Officer, Midwifery Division,
North Edinburgh School of Midwifery

Craig's

Care of the Newly Born Infant

A. J. KEAY and D. M. MORGAN

in collaboration with
Miss Norah J. Stephen

Fifth Edition

CHURCHILL LIVINGSTONE
Edinburgh and London 1974

CHURCHILL LIVINGSTONE
Medical Division of Longman Group Limited

Represented in the United States of America by Longman Inc., New York, and by associated companies, branches and representatives throughout the world.

First edition	1956
Second edition	1962
Third edition	1966
Fourth edition	1969
Fifth edition	1974

ISBN 0 443 01081 1

Printed in Great Britain
by R. & R. Clark, Ltd., Edinburgh

Foreword

The authors are to be congratulated on the results of their painstaking work. There is no more exasperating task than modernizing the past endeavours of another. Doctors Keay and Morgan have belied their initial hesitancy by proving themselves to be past-masters in literary resuscitation and intensive care. Would that they had retained the etymologically and aesthetically preferable spelling 'foetus'! Nevertheless there is solace in the total absence of the word 'neonatologist' despite the authors' advocacy of a subgroup of paediatricians who will devote their time solely to care of the newly born baby.

Perspective has been ably preserved throughout the text. The place of biochemical and other aids in diagnosis, treatment and monitoring is admirably described. An understanding indication is given of the bearing of procedures in special and intensive care units on the relationships between mother and baby, and on the clinical approach of the newly born by nursing staff. These are considerations of crucial importance. Only time will determine the extent to which skill in clinical observation simply interpreted, will be further displaced under hospital conditions by expertise in applying scientific advances. Must it be accepted that domiciliary care of the newly born baby is a thing of the past, and that instruction of the student nurse and medical student must be irrevocably based on that assumption?

To forecast is not possible. This was amply borne out in reverse fashion when an architecture student was heard to dilate on systematic lectures he had been required to attend. The subject of the lectures was Pavlov's Reflexes!

There is reason for personal gratification in the continued association of *Care of the Newly Born Infant* with Edinburgh. Deeply buried in the text, maybe unknown to the authors, there are teachings of the late Professor Charles McNeil, whose pioneer achievements included the initial development of the unit in the Western General Hospital of which Dr Keay is senior paediatrician. Nor can it be forgotten that the first edition would never have seen daylight had the famous Edinburgh publishing firm of E. & S. Livingstone not taken a gamble some twenty years ago.

East Lothian, 1974 W. S. CRAIG

Preface

The invitation to prepare the fifth edition of this book was both flattering and stimulating to the authors and gave us great pleasure. We were conscious of our obligation to continue the general theme of earlier editions but we were also aware that the rapidity with which advances are being made in the care of the newborn indicated the need for a considerable revision of the text and illustrations. With the intention of providing information for the team caring for the newborn in the maternity departments of district general hospitals of the 1970s, we have rewritten the greater part of this book. In so doing, we hope that we have not departed too widely from the spirit of earlier editions.

Both authors work in the paediatric departments of general hospitals and have a particular interest in the care of the newborn. The two departments concerned differ in many aspects. One is part of a Scottish teaching hospital and is housed in a Victorian building; the other is in a modern district general hospital in the Yorkshire dales. We have been fortunate to have the collaboration of Miss Norah J. Stephen, formerly Nursery Sister at the Western General Hospital, Edinburgh and at the British Hospital for Mothers and Babies, Woolwich and now Principal Nursing Officer, North Edinburgh School of Midwifery.

Where appropriate, an outline is given of those aspects of physiological function which have a bearing on clinical assessment and management. The spelling 'fetus' has been adopted. The classification of 'premature' has been dropped in favour of the more cumbersome but more precise subdivisions of low birth-weight infants which are in current use. All measurements are given in the metric system only. Much of the subject matter, including drug doses, previously included in appendices has been incorporated in the text.

An attempt has been made to present the subject in a logical sequence and to avoid undue repetition by free use of cross-references to other chapters in the book. The index has been simplified to assist the reader in tracing the principal reference to the subject sought, and only paragraph headings have been indexed. Further reading suggestions have been confined to review articles of books published in the 1970s which are likely to be available to most of our readers.

The additional cost of colour reproduction was considered to outweigh the relatively small advantage which it confers, and all illustrations are in black and white. Only those illustrations from previous editions for which the original prints were available could be considered for this edition; 104 of the original illustrations are reproduced and 155 new figures have been added. We thank those authors and publishers whose material has been used again. Most of the new illustrations were photographed in colour by one of the authors and converted to black and white prints by Mr J. Paul of the University of Edinburgh Medical Illustration Department to whom we are greatly indebted for his skill. We are grateful to Mr W. Croasdale of Airedale General Hospital for several prints. The source of other new prints is acknowledged in the captions.

Invaluable help has been received from many nursing and medical colleagues to whom we wish to express our gratitude. In particular, we should like to mention Dr J. Syme, Dr D. G. D. Barr, Mr I. S. Kirkland, Dr N. Boyle and Dr I. Mitchell. Miss E. M. Scott, Senior Nursing Officer, provided the figures shown in Tables 2.2 and 2.3; Miss S. J. Young, Unit Nursing Officer, provided the figures shown in Table 8.4. Our secretaries, Miss Yvonne Fraser, Mrs Dorothy White and Mrs Yvette Verner, have accepted our frequent requests for fresh drafts and modifications with an amazing tolerance and courtesy which was most encouraging to us. We also thank Miss Brenda Rice, Medical Librarian, Airedale General Hospital for checking the references. Finally, we are grateful to the staff of Churchill Livingstone who have guided us painlessly through the preparations for publication.

Without the encouragement, understanding and practical help of our wives this edition would never have been prepared. To them and our families we offer our apologies for the disruption of family life which they tolerated cheerfully and our heartfelt thanks for their continuing love and support.

A.J.K.
D.M.M.

Contents

1

The Challenge

In the whole field of child life and health there is no greater clinical challenge than that presented by the fetus and newly born infant. The magnitude of the challenge is a measure of the limits of our knowledge. Although recent years have seen great advances in our understanding of the physiology and pathology of this all-important period of our lives, new discoveries often only serve to reveal our ignorance in other respects. Great care therefore has to be taken in applying advances in scientific knowledge to the clinical situation. At the same time the clinician has to be prepared to sacrifice treasured concepts of management which are shown in the long term to be harmful in spite of apparent short-term advantage. Perspective is fundamental to successful clinical care.

CHANGING EMPHASIS

Inevitably the development of care of the newborn has been subject to the same influences which have conditioned progress in medicine as a whole. The influence of the anatomist was followed by that of the pathologist. A new but complementary approach resulted from the growth of bacteriology, later to be extended with the advent of virology. Physiology as applied to the newborn was slow in coming to the fore but together with the newer and rapidly developing disciplines of biophysics and biochemistry, physiology now provides the basis of most current subjects of neonatal research.

HISTORICAL BACKGROUND

Some knowledge of the history of the development of health services for the newborn helps to place our present situation in perspective and to point the way to likely future developments.

Prior to the Reformation any semblance of organized care was limited to that provided by the religious orders and monastic hospitals. For many years after the Reformation provision was of the scantiest and was dependent upon private philanthropy. In 1740 the first Foundling Hospital was established in London to be followed by others in Yorkshire, Kent, Shropshire and Buckinghamshire. The purpose of these 'hospitals' was to provide for unwanted infants. It is on record that on one single day in 1753, 163 mothers came to the London Foundling Hospital with the object of leaving their infants and that over a period of less than four years 15 000 infants were admitted from all over England; 10 000 of these died. Many if not most of the infants were only days or a few weeks old, but it has to be remembered that at the time in question the deliberate desertion or starvation of unwanted newly born babies was a common practice. Indirectly the foundling hospitals were instrumental in stimulating a new interest in the care of the newborn, and doctors associated with them were responsible for many improvements. At the Ackworth Hospital, William Buchan introduced mothercraft training along lines suggested some years previously by William Smellie. In the London Foundling Hospital, William Cadogan dispensed with swaddling clothes and condemned feeding with pap, advocating that the baby should be put to the breast within hours of birth. Richard Conyers discredited public belief in the value of charms. Faith in traditional folklore still prevailed. It was regarded as evidence of progress when bathing the newly born infant in warm beer displaced salting as a means of conferring 'some degree of civilization' on the baby. Until the end of the eighteenth century, gross congenital malformations continued to be attributed to emotional disturbance of the mother during pregnancy. Most doctors professed little or no knowledge of the newborn, and a mother's natural inclination was to look to elderly women for advice and help.

The Midwife

From the obstetric point of view the nineteenth century has been described as the great era of the family doctor. As man-midwife he contributed to a decline in status of the midwife who, in families able to afford a doctor, was employed in the capacity of ladies' nurse or monthly nurse to attend to mother and infant. Deliveries of mothers in poor economic circumstances were attended by those historically referred to as handy women, with little or no experience of the needs of the newly born baby. In reality the great era of the family doctor was the dark age of the midwife.

Confidence in women attending confinements had been lacking since the early seventeenth century when a public petition, supported by obstetricians including the two Chamberlens and submitted in 1616 to the Courts, attributed the high incidence of stillbirths and maternal deaths to the incompetence of midwives. Credit is due to Robert Manningham and William Smellie for independent attempts to remedy the situation. Manningham opened a small school for midwives and medical students in a workhouse infirmary in Westminster in 1739; and Smellie in 1741 organized a scheme combining free domiciliary attendance on women in labour with instruction of students in midwifery. Some years previously (1726) the University of Edinburgh, on the recommendation of the City Council, appointed a Professor of Midwifery with the instruction of midwives as his primary commitment.

Registration of midwives. Other petitions were made, largely at the instigation of the Society of Apothecaries and the Obstetrical Society of London, with the common objectives of the registration and control of midwives. No fewer than seven Bills were presented to Parliament between 1890 and 1902 without success and it was not until 1902 that an Act was eventually placed on the Statute Book. Meanwhile the Midwives Institute had been founded in 1881, the Obstetric Society having previously established a voluntary examination for the award of a certificate of proficiency which had become the hallmark of trained midwives. Responsibility for the awarding of this certificate was assumed in 1905 by the Central Midwives Board which had been established in accordance with the terms of the Act of 1902. The name of the Midwives Institute was changed to that of College of Midwives in 1941 and six years later was designated by Charter the Royal College of Midwives.

Subsequent regulations pertaining to legal entitlement to practice reduced the number of midwives on the Roll of the Central Midwives Board. Despite this the combined effect of a fall in the birth rate and of the official policy to expand institutional midwifery resulted in there being a surplus of domiciliary midwives. The Midwives Act 1936 established the municipal midwife, employed by the local supervising authority or by a voluntary organization acting for the local supervising authority. She was available to act as maternity nurse in a doctor's case but frequently took complete responsibility for the confinement and worked in close co-operation with the local health authority antenatal clinic. In many parts of the country municipal midwives requiring a medical opinion tended to refer to general practitioners with a particular interest in midwifery and subsequent regulations relating to the National Health Service encouraged the custom. One result was the development of a body of general practitioner obstetricians, many of whom held the Diploma of the Royal College of Obstetricians and Gynaecologists.

The Obstetrician

Obstetrics was a recognized special interest among consultants prior to the beginning of the nineteenth century and was practised in the larger cities by a limited number, some of whom were primarily physicians and others primarily surgeons. With the association of gynaecology with obstetrics those practising obstetrics became more closely linked with surgery. The College of Obstetricians and Gynaecologists was founded in 1929 and granted a Royal Charter in 1946.

Of successive advances in obstetrics many have had some bearing on perinatal care. The introduction in 1847 of chloroform anaesthesia by James Young Simpson and the trial many years later of scopolamine-morphine narcosis ('twilight sleep') were primarily in the interests of the mother. Both involved possible interference with normal respiratory function of the newly born baby. It is, however, probably correct to say that the most significant obstetric contribution to perinatal care was made by J. W. Ballantyne. His thesis for the degree of Doctorate of Medicine in 1889 at the University of Edinburgh was entitled 'Some Anatomical and Pathological Conditions of the Newborn Infant in their relation to Obstetrics'. Later he published books on *Diseases of the Foetus* and *Antenatal Pathology and Hygiene*. His enthusiastic advocacy of antenatal care led to the endowment of an antenatal bed in the Simpson Memorial Maternity Hospital, Edinburgh in 1901, and in 1915 he established the first clinic in this country for expectant mothers. His approach was dominated by perinatal considerations.

The Paediatrician

Study of disease and health in the newborn was slow to begin and slow to develop despite the fact that the first book on paediatrics written in English, *The Boke of Chyldren* by a general physician, Thomas Phaire (1544), referred to the newborn and gave advice on breast feeding. Early in the eighteenth century the obstetrician William Smellie related moulding of the head to the duration and nature of labour; and a physician, John Burton, described breast engorgement in the newborn. Burton, with other physicians of his time, was perplexed by the vagaries of neonatal jaundice but it remained for Michael Underwood in 1784 to demonstrate hereditary influences. Underwood also gave the first description of postnatal apnoeic attacks. The term haemorrhagic disease of the newborn was first coined by an obstetrician in 1891 but a number of years were to elapse before the relative aetiological significance of infection, trauma, asphyxia and coagulation defects was unravelled. Surprisingly it took even longer to recognize that swallowed maternal blood was a misleading occurrence.

Prior to the 1914–18 World War Henry Ashby of Manchester, John Thomson of Edinburgh and George Frederick Still of London were the only physicians who confined their practice to children. At the same time many general physicians dealt with sick children in the course of their routine consultant activities. In this they were continuing the practice of their predecessors. Their work among the newborn was limited and to a considerable extent shared with their obstetric colleagues.

What may be termed concentrated paediatric study of the newborn dates back no further than 1930, although St Thomas's Hospital, London was unique in establishing a paediatric unit in 1919 which incorporated the work of a mothercraft centre and supervision of healthy and ailing babies in the maternity department of the hospital.

Social Legislation

In 1915 the notification of births, an adoptive measure since 1907, was made compulsory and contributed to a decline in deaths amongst infants only a few weeks old. More recent legislation has made further major contributions to the welfare of the newborn by providing assistance for families in need, and for such contingencies as unemployment and sickness. Other important provisions include family allowances, maternity grants, maternity allowances and the home confinement grant. The trend of modern advances in curative and more especially preventive care of the newborn has been largely determined by administrative improvements based on social legislation.

Recent Advances

Improvement in the care of the fetus and newborn infant since the beginning of this century is reflected in the progressive decline in perinatal mortality rates (Chap. 2). Much of this improvement is secondary to the socioeconomic advances which have occurred with a resulting rise in the standard of living and higher standards of health and education generally. More recently the increasing volume of basic research into the physiology of pregnancy and delivery has led to a better understanding of the changes occurring. Some of the instruments involved in this research have been adapted for clinical use and many investigations until recently considered as research projects are now accepted as standard clinical practice.

TEAMWORK

The complexity of the physiological problems being investigated is generally beyond the ability of a single research worker and most work is carried out by teams of workers each with his or her own particular skill to contribute. Similarly in clinical work co-operation between several branches of the nursing, midwifery, medical and paramedical services is necessary to provide the optimum service for the fetus and the newborn. Delivery is no longer the time at which the obstetrician's interest ceases and the paediatrician's begins. The paediatrician is as interested in the progress of the fetus as is the obstetrician in the progress of the baby in the nursery. Although much of the care of the newborn will continue to be in the hands of general paediatricians, the most highly specialized units will require the full-time services of paediatricians confining their attention to the newborn period. Such neonatal paediatricians will on occasions, however, require the support of paediatric systems specialists such as paediatric cardiologists.

SPECIAL CARE NURSERIES

The success of special care nurseries depends more on the quality of the nursing care provided than on the equipment available. Training schemes in the nursing of the newborn are available at many centres but no national programme of subjects to be covered is recognized and there is no national standard established. It is to be hoped that this highly specialized branch of nursing will be given the recognition which it deserves. The shortage of nursing staff generally has in this, as in other areas, led to the production of monitoring instruments which are said to reduce the nursing load. Such instruments while allowing one nurse to supervise several consoles of instruments do not provide that individuality of care on which so many infants' lives have relied in the past. At the same time sitting before a bank of flashing lights does not give the attendant nurse the same feeling of providing a service and in some cases seems to be positively distressing. Time will tell whether the partial replacement of nursing by the electronic monitor will prove to be of any advantage as far as the newborn period is concerned. The use of electronic gadgetry has, however, greatly improved the ability to monitor the infant's environment. In this as in other aspects of care of the newborn the distinction between nursing and medical functions becomes blurred. The concept of working as a team is again evident to the advantage of all concerned.

INTENSIVE THERAPY

Intensive therapy involving a high concentration of nursing and medical skills is essential for the survival of the most seriously ill newborn infants and particularly for those who require surgical treatment in the first hours or days of life. In addition to advances in surgical technique advances in anaesthesia, fluid and electrolyte control and parenteral nutrition have greatly improved the chances of survival of the infant born with certain types of congenital abnormality including cardiac abnormalities. The paediatric neonatal surgeon and anaesthetist have become essential members of the specialist neonatal team.

SUPPORTING SERVICES

No clinical team of nurses, physicians and surgeons can work efficiently without support from the radiology and laboratory services. Most of the advances at present being made depend on the rapid provision of detailed investigational services. In many cases it has been advances in these departments that have paved the way for subsequent advances in therapy. It must also be recognized that advances in the paramedical services provided by physiotherapists, social workers, health visitors, etc. have been essential components of the general advance in the services provided for the newborn.

THE MOTHER

With such a plethora of staff and services the danger is that mother's place is forgotten and degraded. What may prove to be the most significant recent advance is the recognition of the need of a mother to make contact with her baby from birth onward. Her baby belongs to her, and she has need of her baby as much as her baby will later need her continuing love and care. Artificial separation of mother and infant makes the establishment of a permanent emotional bond more difficult. Involvement of mother in the care of her infant helps to maintain the link and prevents the feeling of detachment and uselessness which distresses so many mothers whose infants are being cared for in special care nurseries.

UNSOLVED PROBLEMS

Grateful as we must be for the advances which have taken place and which are still taking place in the care of the newly born infant we must at the same time recognize those areas in which little advance has been made or is likely to be made. This applies particularly to those congenital abnormalities which are compatible with a period of survival but for which no fully corrective treatment is available. Included in this group are the relatively large group with abnormalities of the central nervous system. At present the only means of prevention would appear to be the avoidance of further pregnancy in high-risk families or the selective abortion of fetuses which can be demonstrated to be abnormal or at very high risk. This involves close co-operation between obstetricians, paediatricians and human geneticists. A small number of congenital abnormalities may be prevented by a better understanding of the pharmacology of drugs given to pregnant women.

Peripheral Influences

The successful rearing of a healthy, intelligent infant and child has always been subject to influences over which medical and nursing staff have had little control. Many of these are related to the social and economic circumstances of the community concerned and include such factors as nutrition, housing and education. Much of the present improvement in the health of our newborn population is related as much to the rise in the general standard of living as to advances in medical and nursing skill. In some parts of the world religion or local folklore may have a major influence on ideas about the upbringing of children. Some aspects of management appear to be fashionable at one time but not at another. Breast feeding provides a good example of this. Fashions can be created and interest in breast feeding corresponds with the amount of effort expended in advocating its use. The current policy of encouraging hospital delivery has the secondary effect of reducing the length of stay in the maternity department for many infants. This in turn is establishing a new fashion which may no longer be required if the present fall in the birth rate continues. Although the doctor and midwife may have little control over such influences it is important that they should know that they exist.

The Continuing Challenge

Complacency is the enemy of progress and unless we can accept that there is a continuing challenge to provide the best possible care for the newborn infant further progress will not be made. As will be shown in the next chapter it is safer for infants to be delivered in some other countries than it is for them to be born in England or Scotland. Further improvement in the standard of obstetric, midwifery and paediatric care is therefore called for. This requires co-operative work by legislators, administrators, research scientists, doctors, midwives, teachers and parents. The training of the midwife and the doctor must strike a successful balance between instruction in clinical observation and the use of laboratory aids. Much of the knowledge of normal behaviour in the newborn has followed many hours of diligent observation of individual infants. At the same time other major advances in management have only been made possible by the examination of blood or other body tissues in the laboratory. Clinical and laboratory medicine are complementary. Students must be taught the merits of each. The clinician must respect the contribution of the research scientist, and the laboratory worker must understand the problems facing the clinician. Team work is essential and further advance will not be made without full co-operation between all those working to the same end.

There is a risk that as the team caring for the infant increases in size the infant's parents feel remote from their baby and deprived of their joy in welcoming a newcomer to their family. Parents and particularly mothers must be closely involved in the care of their infants even when they are very small or ill. Weeks of work in a special care nursery are of no avail if by the time an infant is ready for discharge home his mother feels that he is no longer her infant and that she cannot give him the love and care which he needs. Such aspects of the mother–infant relationship have received too little attention in the past and are a significant part of the continuing clinical challenge now presented to us.

2

Health Services for the Newborn

Measurement of Success

At the beginning of the twentieth century maternal mortality due to childbirth was a major cause for concern and efforts at improving maternity services were aimed at reducing the risk to the mother. In 1970 in England 109 mothers died from child-bearing, a rate of 15 deaths per 100 000 deliveries. This compares with rates of the order of 500 per 100 000 deliveries at the beginning of the century. The maternal mortality rate is no longer a useful parameter by which to assess the success of maternity services and attention is now focused on the infant. A successful pregnancy is one which results in an infant who is fully capable of developing his inherited powers of physical and mental development. Measurement of success is, however, not possible at birth. Our assessment still has to rely on measurement of failure as with maternal mortality. When an infant is stillborn or is alive at birth but dies within a few days the pregnancy cannot be considered to have had a successful outcome. Many infant deaths in the first few weeks of life are due to causes directly or closely related to factors occurring during fetal life or during delivery. Stillbirths and deaths during the first seven days of life have therefore many causes in common to both. Perinatal mortality rates are now generally accepted as the most useful means of assessing the success of health services for the newborn. Before discussing this matter further it is important to state the definitions of the terms involved.

LEGAL AND STATISTICAL DEFINITIONS

For the requirements of the law a child is regarded as *liveborn* if at any stage of pregnancy he breathes or shows other signs of life after complete expulsion from the mother. A child who, after the 28th week of pregnancy, has not at any time after being completely expelled from his mother breathed or shown any other sign of life is considered to be *stillborn*.

The birth rate is the number of births (live and still) registered per 1000 of the population.

The stillbirth rate is the number of still births registered per 1000 live and stillbirths.

The neonatal mortality rate is the number of deaths registered of infants dying under the age of 28 days per 1000 registered live births in the same year.

The perinatal mortality rate is the number of stillbirths and deaths occurring in the first week of life per 1000 live and still births.

The infant mortality rate is the number of deaths registered of infants dying under 1 year of age per 1000 registered live births in the same year.

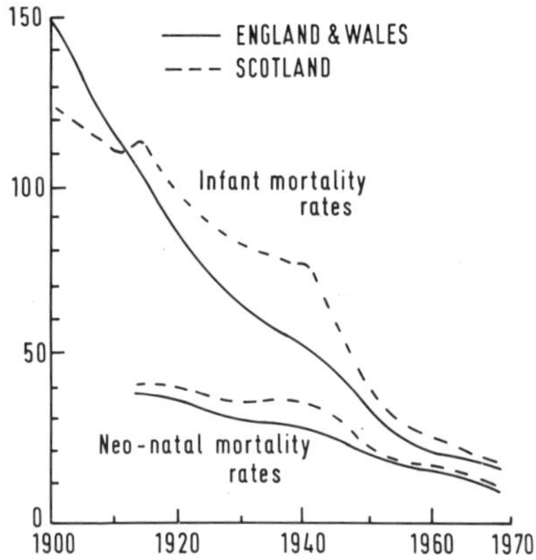

Figure 2.1 Comparison of the fall in infant mortality and neonatal mortality rates in England and Wales and in Scotland.

Perinatal Mortality

As will be seen from Figure 2.1 the extent of the fall in the infant mortality rates during this century greatly exceeds the fall in the neonatal mortality rate. This is largely due to improvement in living standards and in particular to higher standards of nutrition and hygiene. The improvement began before the introduction of the sulphonamides and antibiotics which helped to increase the rate of fall by reduction of mortality from non-viral infections. Notification of stillbirths was not required by law until 1928 in England and

Table 2.1 Perinatal mortality rates per 1000 total births

Year	England and Wales	Scotland
1950	37.4	42.7
1955	37.4	38.0
1960	32.8	35.4
1965	26.9	31.5
1970	23.5	24.8

Wales and 1939 in Scotland. Perinatal mortality rates could not therefore be calculated on a national basis before 1928 in England and Wales or 1939 in Scotland. Comparison of the rates for these two parts of the United Kingdom is shown in Table 2.1. In each country there has been a steady fall but Scotland has always lagged behind England and Wales. Such comparisons between countries can be extended both by widening the net so that comparisons are made with countries outside the United Kingdom and by narrowing the net to make comparisons between regions within a country. Figure 2.2 shows that we cannot be satisfied with our own situation

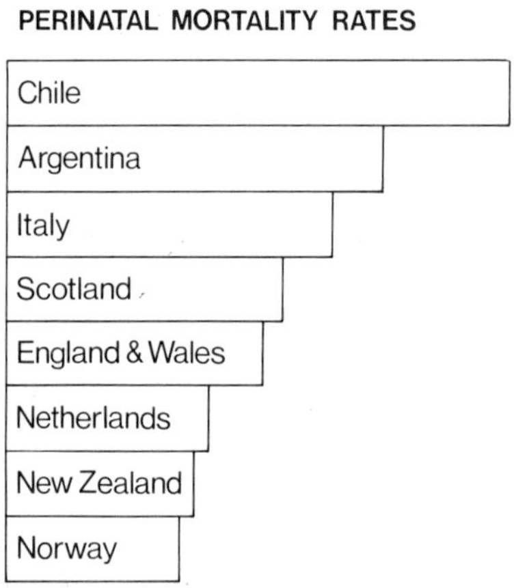

Figure 2.2 Comparative perinatal mortality rates in 1965. (Based on *WHO Technical Report Series*, no. 457.)

when it is clear that we are in a worse position than the Scandinavian countries and the Netherlands. The reason for this is equally well demonstrated by a study of regional differences within one country such as Scotland. Briefly the perinatal mortality rises as the socio-economic position declines.

SOCIAL FACTORS

Neonatal mortality rates are twice as high in social class V as they are in social class I. Mortality rates are higher in illegitimate than in legitimate births in all social classes. The infant mortality rate for illegitimate infants of mothers in social class V (1966–68) was six times greater than the rate for legitimately born infants of social class I mothers. Comparison between countries similarly shows that it is those with the highest standard of living which have the lowest infant, neonatal and perinatal mortality rates. The improvements which have occurred in individual countries during this century are in line with their rate of socioeconomic progress. The factors involved are many but include better nutrition resulting in better physique, improved hygiene and housing conditions resulting in fewer infectious illnesses, better education resulting in a better understanding of the need for antenatal care and, more recently, planned parenthood limiting the size of families and forestalling the birth of an unwanted or a deformed infant. The improvements made are largely the result of activity at national government level. This does not mean that further improvement cannot be achieved by improvement of the services at the level of the maternity unit.

HOSPITAL STATISTICS

The use of statistical evidence can equally well be applied to the local situation. It should be the duty of every maternity unit to keep under review not only individual failures in the form of stillbirth or neonatal death but also total performance over a period of one or more years. By comparison with earlier periods in the same unit, with the same period in other similar units or with national figures the success or failure of the unit can be assessed.

Of the two units in which the authors serve one has only recently opened its doors and figures are available for one year only. In the other unit statistical data are available from the mid-1950s and Table 2.2 shows a comparison of mortality for two periods at an interval of

Table 2.2 Showing the improvement in fetal loss associated with a lower incidence of low birth-weight infants. (Figures from the Maternity Department, Western General Hospital, Edinburgh)

	1956–57	1969–70
Total births	2869	2862
Stillbirths	73	37
Neonatal deaths	64	37
Perinatal mortality rate/1000 total births	47	25
Birth weight 2500 g and under		
Liveborn	222	173
Percentage of all liveborn	9%	7%
Neonatal deaths	44	25
Mortality percentage	20%	14%
Birth weight 2000 g and under		
Liveborn	116	70
Percentage of all liveborn	4%	2.5%
Neonatal deaths	55	33
Mortality percentage	47%	47%

13 years. The improvement demonstrated might at first glance appear satisfactory but comparison with figures from units in other countries shows that there is room for further improvement. On making a more detailed analysis it is clear that there has been a large fall in the absolute number of deaths in low birth-weight babies and this might be attributed to better neonatal care. Re-examination of the same figures by subdivision of birth weights shows that the improvement is very largely due to a reduction in the number of low birth-weight infants delivered and for infants weighing 2000 g or less at birth the percentage mortality has not altered. Figures such as these indicate the importance of factors reducing the overall incidence of delivery before fetal maturity is reached. These are in many respects those socioeconomic factors in which improvement has led to reduction in infant neonatal and perinatal mortality and to which reference will be made frequently in later chapters. Credit must also be given to changes in obstetric policy which have resulted from study of causes of perinatal mortality and in particular of major surveys such as that carried out in

Table 2.3 Showing changes in factors associated with delivery in the Maternity Department, Western General Hospital, Edinburgh

Type of delivery	1956 (%)	1970 (%)
Unbooked	10.4	0.7
Induced	3.3	36.4
Breech	3.9	2.7
Forceps	8.8	18.3
Caesarian section	4.9	5.5

1958 under the auspices of the National Birthday Trust Fund. The second report on this survey entitled 'Perinatal Problems' was concerned with the biological, sociological and obstetric factors involved. Table 2.3 shows some changes in obstetric practice at the Western General Hospital, Edinburgh over the period covered by the figures shown in Table 2.2. The increase in attendance at antenatal clinics, the higher incidence of induction of labour and the greater number of assisted deliveries have each helped to improve the situation. It is the improvement in both environmental influences and obstetric factors which has been responsible for the decrease in perinatal mortality rather than either aspect on its own.

Quality of survival. Further reduction in mortality rates presents us with a new problem—the quality of life for those who survive. This is not easy to present in the same manner as rates for perinatal mortality. Quality of life can be estimated for an individual but national figures can only be assessed indirectly by noting changes in such factors as school performance and admission rates to schools for the physically or mentally handicapped. Should an increased number of admissions to such schools be evident five to ten years after the introduction of a new method of management of the newborn, suspicion should be aroused and the efficacy of the method reassessed. As an example one may quote the harmful effect of delay in feeding of small infants practised during the 1950s which has led to impaired school performance and cerebral palsy in many of the children so treated. This was not evident or easy to foresee at the time the practice was in vogue. Close co-operation between all branches of the health services dealing with infants and children is essential to ensure that the long-term effects of changes in management of the newborn are communicated to those responsible for making and applying policy decisions in nurseries for the newborn.

Organization of Services for the Newborn

Experience in this country and elsewhere has shown that the services provided for the newborn vary in efficiency from one region to another. This can be demonstrated by comparing perinatal mortality rates for regions with similar socioeconomical and demographic patterns. Differences existing between such similar areas are frequently due to factors which are capable of correction by bringing the standard of perinatal care up to the standard practised in better areas. The most dramatic improvements are likely to occur in under-developed countries but in such situations it may well be more effective to use those monies available for the improvement of hygiene and nutrition before large sums are spent on services for the newborn. In countries with a high socioeconomical standard, however, services for the newborn may not reach standards available elsewhere and it is useful to consider how standards can be improved.

Administration. Within the health services of any country or region of a country there are a number of variable factors responsible for success or failure. These include efficiency of the organization of the services and its responsiveness to changing circumstances, the provision and maintenance of suitable buildings and equipment, the supply of well-trained nursing, medical and paramedical staff but above all the willingness of patients to use the facilities available and their confidence in the staff and in the methods employed. Satisfactory provision will not be identical throughout the world but in any area it is essential that the service be self critical and be prepared to keep under frequent review its effectiveness in providing the best service at an economic rate.

THE NATIONAL HEALTH SERVICE

At the time of the introduction of the National Health Service this country had seen the benefit of the introduction of set standards of practice for doctors, nurses and midwives but was only beginning to accept the need for organized health services on a wide basis. The service was introduced as a tripartite system based on the hospitals, the general practitioners and the local authority health services. Maternity services including those for the newborn were divided between the three branches and it took some time before satisfactory co-operation between these branches was achieved. The proposed integration of the health services promises a new era of co-ordination on a closer basis with the hope that the infant among others will benefit. At the same time the erection of new hospitals, many of them serving a district and replacing one or more older buildings, offers a further opportunity to improve our maternity services. This period of change in administrative structure and hospital building corresponds to a period in which mothers are increasingly aware of the advantages of delivery in a properly staffed and equipped hospital. In many parts of this country 95 per cent or more of deliveries already take place in hospital and it is clear that planning has to allow for 100 per cent hospital deliveries. Changing attitudes toward contraception and abortion make it difficult to assess the numbers of infants likely to be delivered in the years ahead but there is some evidence that the recent fall in the birth rate may not continue.

SPECIAL CARE NURSERIES

Changes have also been taking place in methods of management of newborn infants within special care nurseries in hospitals. In 1969 the Chief Medical Officer of the Department of Health and Social Security appointed an expert medical and nursing group to prepare a report which was published in 1971 on special care for babies. As this report presents the most recent assessment of our present requirements it will be quoted at some length. The report indicates the likely form of future organization. Special care services would be based on the special maternity and children's department of the district general hospital. A consultant paediatrician would have primary responsibility for the service and would work closely with the obstetric team. Planning would be in the hands of a maternity liasion committee. Two types of nurseries would be provided. All specialist maternity departments of district general hospitals would have special care nurseries and in addition there would be some intensive care nurseries.

INTENSIVE CARE NURSERIES

Intensive care for very low birth-weight infants, for those with severe respiratory distress and other problems requiring intensive care would be provided in combined special care and intensive care nurseries, the numbers of which would be limited. According to the report of the expert group such intensive care nurseries should be provided for half of infants weighing less than 1500 g at birth and for an equal number of infants weighing over 1500 g. It is estimated that 320 such cots will be required in England and Wales, their distribution depending on geographical and other circumstances. These intensive care nurseries would require substantial numbers of medical, nursing and supporting staff with specialized equipment and resources beyond those available in other district general hospitals. Where possible, intensive care nurseries would be associated with a neonatal surgical unit. If an infant were required to be transferred to another hospital for intensive care the mother would, if she wished, also be transferred. Where problems are forecast antenatally the mother would be transferred to the hospital with the intensive care nursery before delivery.

Domiciliary midwifery has virtually ceased in some areas but persists in others in small numbers. In order to provide an adequate service for the infant delivered at home great care must be taken in selection of those mothers who are to be delivered at home, and situations which signal danger to the infant should be an indication to arrange further antenatal supervision and delivery in hospital. Although the baby at risk travels most safely *in utero* it has to be recognized that situations may still arise where infants are born away from special care nurseries. Arrangements have to be made and kept under review for the provision of adequate transport facilities. This implies the provision of an ambulance which is adequately lit, ventilated and heated and which contains a portable incubator and resuscitation apparatus. Provision to prevent heat loss is extremely important. Drugs likely to be required should be available. These requirements are most easily met by a special ambulance constructed for the purpose and not used for other duties. As such a vehicle is costly, numbers may have to be limited but at least one for each intensive care nursery would appear to be justified.

STAFFING

The staffing of special care and intensive care nurseries is of paramount importance to the service they provide. In order to maintain a continuous day and night service by competent nursing and medical staff special care nurseries would only be provided in those district hospitals which have specialist departments staffed by at least two consultant paediatricians. Suitable training posts for medical and nursing staff are essential to provide the number of trained personnel which are likely to be required. The staffing ratio in intensive care nurseries would be at a high level to allow for training of junior staff and for research.

In special care nurseries 1 to 1.5 nurses per cot would be required and in combined special care and intensive care nurseries 3 nurses per cot are recommended for the intensive care cots. If a nurse with two or more months of experience in special care of newborn infants is classified as experienced, it is recommended that at least two experienced nurses who are able to resuscitate an infant should be on duty in each shift. For special care nurseries this would imply a minimum of nine experienced nurses as it requires an allocation of four to five nurses to keep one constantly on duty. On this basis a 24-cot special care nursery would require nine experienced and 15 other nurses to staff it at a ratio of one nurse per cot. A nursery of 24 special cots including eight for intensive care would need 24 experienced nurses and 16 others. Delegation of non-nursing duties to a ward clerk together with an adequate domestic and portering service are essential. A national standard for courses in training for special care nursing of the newborn is required.

Number of cots. It has been recommended that six special care cots are required per 1000 live births and that a unit should consist of at least 20 cots. This would imply that special care facilities would be available only where the deliveries exceeded about 3000 a year. The report recommends that only one nursery with a minimum size of 24 cots should normally be provided for a population of 250,000. As many maternity units in this country serve a smaller population and as not all are associated with a paediatric department in the same hospital it is probable that special care facilities will not be provided in every maternity hospital and that infants requiring special care will have to be transferred to another hospital. This raises problems of availability of staff to accompany such infants and allowance for this must be made in establishing staffing ratios.

DESIGN OF NURSERIES

The architectural design of nurseries has a very important bearing on the successful function of a unit. This is not the place for any detailed discussion of the relative merits of different architectural solutions to the problems presented but it is useful for those who work in nurseries to have some idea of the basic principles involved in the design of a special care or intensive care nursery. Adequate space must be provided to allow easy access to an infant by more than one member of staff and for positioning of any special apparatus required. At the same time cots or incubators must not be so widely spread that observation of more than one infant by one nurse is not practical. In order to use nursery staff and equipment in the most economical manner at least two rooms per unit should be capable of holding six to eight cots or incubators with an allocation of floor area of 4 square metres (m^2) per cot. In smaller rooms the floor area should be $5m^2$ per cot. In a special care unit there should be at least two single isolation cubicles. The remaining cots should be in rooms containing four to six cots each. Panelling between rooms should be glazed from a level below cot height to a sufficient height to allow ready observation between rooms and of each room from the nurse's station. The grouping of rooms and the circulation areas must be aimed at allowing ready access with the minimum amount of movement. Separation of clean and dirty lines of communication is an advantage. Careful planning of air movement will do much to prevent cross-infection and this may mean that artificial ventilation systems are essential. Similarly, good design, choice of material and good workmanship will eliminate unnecessary dust-traps and make cleaning easier. The temperature of each room should be controlled by the staff within the range 20° to 30°C. Double glazing is advisable, and if there are large areas of window facing the sun suitable means of preventing overheating of the rooms has to be provided. In all rooms there should be ample power points. Piped oxygen, compressed air and suction prevent the rooms being cluttered up by unnecessary equipment. Lighting must be of a high standard and capable of variation in intensity. Each room should have an intercommunication system linked with the nursing station.

Mothers' rooms. A number of ancillary rooms will be necessary but these will not all be listed here. They should include single rooms for mothers with day-room facilities. Since mothers will take an increasing part in the care of their infant as the time for discharge home is approached, allowance for the presence of mothers (and fathers) must be made in planning space and facilities in nurseries. One or more rooms will be required for the training of parents and for the education of staff. Other provision for staff will depend upon the relationship of the unit to the remainder of the hospital. In some situations a bedroom for medical staff on call will be necessary.

EQUIPMENT

Both intensive care and special care nurseries will require specialized equipment appropriate to the type of work being undertaken.

This will include both monitoring equipment and equipment necessary for special procedures being used. No attempt will be made to list such equipment here as requirements will vary from unit to unit. Future developments in techniques both of investigation and treatment together with the inventiveness of the instrument makers are likely to make any list out of date in a year or two's time. Special care work requires effective support from laboratories equipped to use micro methods. Blood gas analysis may be required at short notice at any time of the day or night and suitable staffing to provide such a service must be available.

Follow-up

The value of improved special care services for infants can only be assessed by the long-term follow-up of infants treated in such units. Arrangement for such follow-up requires co-operation with other branches of the health services. It is important that adequate records be kept of each stage in the progress of an individual infant and also of the performance of a special care nursery as a unit. To this end many units have evolved their own coding systems and it is to be hoped that before long a standard code for the newborn can be provided at national level so that statistical evidence on morbidity as well as mortality can be calculated readily. Such information would be invaluable to those engaged in research in this field.

Services for the newborn are not yet uniformly well developed in all parts of Great Britain. It is to be hoped that improvements in organization, the provision of physical facilities and in staffing will soon allow those parts of the country with the highest perinatal mortality rates to bring their results into line with the areas which have already achieved as high a standard as appears possible in the light of present-day knowledge.

FURTHER READING

Butler, N. R., Goldstein, A. & Ross, E. M. (1972). Cigarette smoking in pregnancy. Its influence on birth weight and perinatal mortality. *British Medical Journal*, ii, 127–130.

Department of Health and Social Security (1971). *On the State of the Public Health. The Annual Report of the Chief Medical Officer of the Department of Health and Social Security for the Year* 1970. London: HMSO.

Expert Group on Special Care for Babies (1971). *Report of the Expert Group on Special Care for Babies*. London: HMSO.

Naeye, R. L., Burt, L. S., Wright, D. L., Blanc, W. A., Tatter, D. (1971). Neonatal mortality. The male disadvantage. *Pediatrics*, **48**, 902–906.

Richards, I. D. G. (1971). *Infant Mortality in Scotland*. Edinburgh: Scottish Home and Health Department.

SCOTT, K. E. (1970). Report of the Committee on Maternal and Perinatal Health of the Province of Nova Scotia. *Nova Scotia Medical Bulletin*, **49,** 81.

SEYER, P. R. (1970). The regional organization of special care for the neonate. *Pediatric Clinics of North America*, **17**, 761–776.

WORLD HEALTH ORGANIZATION (1970). The prevention of perinatal mortality and morbidity. *WHO Technical Report Series*, no. 457.

3

The Parents

An addition to the family is always a great event to which all relatives look forward. The arrival of the newborn infant must therefore always be seen in the context of the family to which he or she will belong. That family is of interest to the obstetrician, midwife and paediatrician before their infant arrives. The parents may have come to seek advice before even embarking on a pregnancy. In some situations advice may be requested, before marriage is contemplated, about possible difficulties in producing a normal infant. Others, after marriage, may seek advice about the spacing of pregnancies. Such problems of planning of parenthood are much more readily discussed in present-day society than was the case earlier in this century. This change in attitude is chiefly due to advance in our knowledge of hereditary factors. Parents are mainly concerned about possible abnormal development of their child before birth. Further discussion of the significance of heredity will be found in Chapter 4, which is concerned with the fetus.

Planned Parenthood

Apart from their concern as to possible congenital abnormality, parents are also anxious to make sure that they are in a satisfactory position to look after a new infant properly. Problems may arise because of poor housing, an inadequate income, ill health or the presence of previous children. Many such factors tend to deter parents from having children when they are young and newly married. Perinatal mortality, however, is at its lowest in mothers who are between 20 and 30 years of age and who have had less than four pregnancies. Close spacing of pregnancies adds to the burden on mother's health and to the calls on her energy and purse. A prolonged interval between pregnancies may cause problems to some families. Careful planning of parenthood may obviate some of these difficulties and dangers and to this end doctors and midwives should be prepared to give advice about contraception or arrange for parents to visit a family planning clinic.

SOCIAL PROBLEMS

A social worker is an essential member of the team in the antenatal clinic and expectant mothers should be encouraged to discuss their social problems with her. This service should be extended to fathers-to-be. The prospect of the responsibility of having to look after their first infant may present some young couples with problems of management of their lives and financial resources beyond their unaided capacity. Understanding help and education at this stage may help them to establish a happy family and to prevent much unnecessary misery.

CONTRACEPTION

Whereas inability to have children may be a major problem for some couples, other parents may be principally concerned with how to prevent additions to their present family. Throughout the world limitation of family size is being widely encouraged in order to curb the population explosion. Vasectomy is the method of choice in many countries and is now available under the National Health Service (NHS) in this country. The 'pill' is a more popular method of contraception in some developed countries. Attitudes towards the use of induced abortion also vary from country to country and are dependent upon a number of religious and other factors. In general, however, there is at present a much greater understanding than hitherto of the need for limitation of family size and for planned parenthood.

Preparation for Parenthood

During the past ten to 15 years there has been a radical change in the outlook of husband and wife towards pregnancy and the care of the baby. The role of the expectant father has changed completely. He is no longer a passive observer in a women's world. He takes an active interest in the progress of the pregnancy and in many instances is with his wife throughout labour and delivery. In the post partum period he actively shares in the physical care of the baby and helps with the household chores. There must therefore be provision for both parents in an antenatal education programme.

AT SCHOOL

Preparation for parenthood begins at school. With the school leaving age now being 16 years more time could be devoted to this subject in education programmes. Education authorities should be encouraged to add instruction in parentcraft to lessons on home management and sex education. Involvement of midwives, health visitors, social workers and doctors in some classes might help to enlarge experience on both sides.

A programme for education in parenthood to be used in school could cover the following subjects.

Choosing a partner. This difficult subject might be used to open a discussion on what a boy or girl expects from a partner in marriage and how they see their own role as parents. From this they could be led to discuss the role of their partner, what attributes they would expect of each other and whether they consider that each other's demands are reasonable. An introduction should be made to the concept of family responsibility particularly with regard to children.

Home management. The importance of budgeting the family income should be stressed, showing how money can be allocated to cover the necessities of life such as food, fuel, clothing and rent. Basic instruction in dietary values and the planning of meals can be given. Planning of housework and its relation to work outside the home should be discussed. The need for relaxation and leisure enjoyment should not be forgotten.

Health education. The basic concepts of positive health as opposed to treatment of disease can be used as an introduction to the higher chance of a successful pregnancy with healthy parents. The particular risks of smoking during pregnancy can be underlined. Avoidance of accidents and poisoning in the home can be discussed. Special attention should be paid to the effect of parental habits on children and the responsibilities of parenthood. The value of health visitors should be stressed.

Social services. An outline of the social services available and of the particular help given to parents and their children should be given. Examples of the type of problems which young parents experience can be presented. The social benefits available should be explained.

Planning parenthood. On the presumption that sex education has already been given, the concept of spacing of a family and limitation of the number of children should be introduced. This leads into a description of contraceptive methods which might be given by a representative of the Family Planning Association.

Bringing up children. A general discussion on the pleasures and responsibilities of bringing up a family could round off this series. A couple with young children might be willing to take part or the pupils might visit a day nursery.

Films, slides and other visual aids may be used to make the parentcraft programme as attractive as possible. A variety of books, leaflets and magazines could be available for further study.

Parentcraft in the Maternity Unit

Not all young couples will have received any parentcraft instruction at school and the majority will welcome further information and the chance to talk over problems with others in the same situation.

Expectant mothers are a delightful class to teach as they are uniquely receptive and every opportunity should be taken to exploit this willingness for health education.

ANTENATAL CLASSES

In the first instance classes directly concerned with the pregnancy should be conducted by one of the midwives from the hospital where the expectant mother is booked for her confinement. Attractive environment for the classes is important with a friendly and relaxed atmosphere. Later in the programme the obstetrician, paediatrician, health visitor and physiotherapist can be involved. It must be remembered, however, that the majority of patients are working in early pregnancy, and classes should be arranged in conjunction with clinic attendances. Later in pregnancy they can be linked with physiotherapy classes. Special evening sessions for husband and wife should be arranged with opportunity and time for questions and discussion. Parentcraft classes must be continued in the early post-natal period.

CONFIDENT PARENTHOOD

Parentcraft classes in the antenatal period must concentrate on giving young couples confidence in their ability to be good parents. Facilities for classes will vary from hospital to hospital according to the availability of staff and accommodation for this purpose. The following outline of a suggested programme may be beyond the capacity of some maternity departments but is an indication of what can be done under favourable circumstances.

General care during pregnancy. This session is an introduction to the facilities available to help a mother-to-be during her pregnancy. The value of regular attendance for antenatal examination must be stressed and the routine of antenatal clinics explained. General advice about care during pregancy can be given together with reference to minor ailments which may arise and how these can be managed. The maternity benefits available should be explained and instructions given as to how they can be obtained.

Normal pregnancy. This will involve a simplified cxplanation of the course of pregnancy and the changes which take place in mother and fetus. Further explanation of the need for antenatal care can touch on some of the problems which may occur and how these can be avoided. An introduction to breast feeding can be given.

Educating both parents. Both parents are given an opportunity to meet some of the maternity department staff. Husbands can be advised about the effect of pregnancy on their wives. A film of a delivery may be shown. This is a useful opportunity for questions and answers and a discussion group.

Health education. Advice as to diet and weight control during pregnancy can be given by a dietician. The dangers of smoking particularly during pregnancy are emphasized (Fig. 3.1). Warning is given of potential dangers in the home which might cause accidents and the risk of children taking poisonous substances is stressed. The role of the health visitor during pregnancy and after delivery is explained.

Preparing for baby's arrival. This is a practical session at which advice is given about the purchase of a layette, cot, pram and other items which will be required. Samples should be available for display.

Baby's arrival. The labour ward sister gives a simple explanation of the process of labour and demonstrates how pain is relieved. Advice is given about recognizing the onset of labour and admission procedure explained. The role of the father during labour can be discussed. This session can be concluded by a visit to the labour suite.

Arrangements in hospital. In this final session both parents are introduced to hospital routine. They are told how members of the staff can be identified and what functions they perform. Arrangements for visitors and for receiving and making telephone calls are explained. The hospital policy with regard to smoking is stated. Finally a tour of the hospital can be made pointing out where the various facilities are available.

The first five classes could be given at weekly intervals in early pregnancy and the remainder in the last month of pregnancy.

As many visual aids as possible should be used to make the classes more attractive. Coloured slides of the unit and of the equipment used are very helpful as an introduction before a visit. Posters covering a wide range of subjects are readily available. The Birth Atlas from the Maternity Center, New York, has excellent anatomical illustrations which are particularly useful in the talk dealing with labour.

The requirements for bathing baby are shown using a doll. This demonstration is helpful to stress the importance of various items of equipment but the actual technique of bathing is best taught in the puerperium with mother's own baby.

A layette can be demonstrated using actual garments. Maternity fashions can be discussed including advice on suitable girdles and brassieres. Samples or leaflets describing articles can be obtained from the firms supplying such articles or from local shops.

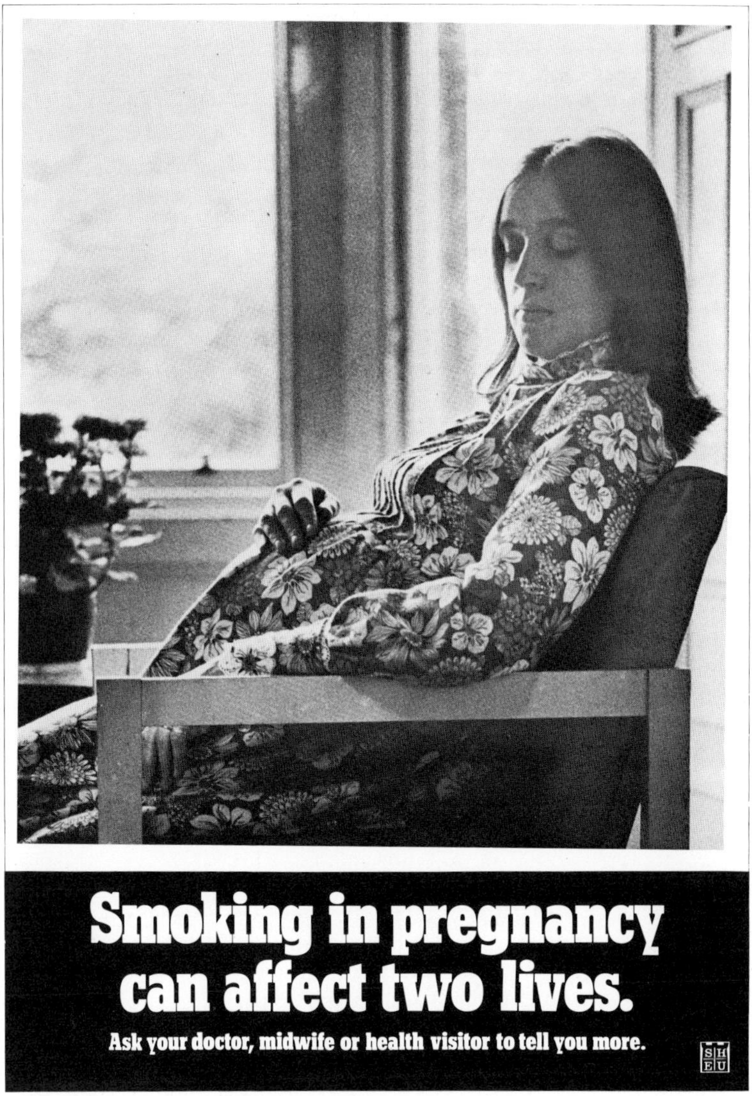
Smoking in pregnancy
can affect two lives.
Ask your doctor, midwife or health visitor to tell you more.

Figure 3.1 Poster for display in antenatal clinic. (By courtesy of the Scottish Health Education Unit.)

Breast feeding. Publicity for the advantages of breast feeding can readily be included in such a programme. As mentioned in Chapter 1 fashions vary with regard to the popularity of breast feeding. This subject will be discussed in Chapter 8, where the importance of antenatal advice and instruction is stressed as a most important factor affecting the mother's decision about breast feeding. Unless a mother has thought about breast feeding before delivery it is unlikely that she will be persuaded to give her baby this advantage.

In planning such a programme it must be remembered that the expectant mother has to travel to and from the hospital, and care must be taken not to overtax her unduly. At the same time it is essential to provide sufficient information to allay her fears and give her confidence in hospital and in the hospital team before she comes in to have her baby.

Parentcraft in the puerperium is discussed at the end of this chapter.

ANTENATAL CARE

The marked improvement in the standard of antenatal care which has occurred during this century has been one of the greatest factors in reducing maternal mortality, neonatal deaths and stillbirths. Antenatal care may be carried out by the general practitioner and domicilary midwife in the surgery or by the obstetrician and midwife in a hospital clinic. In hospitals the physiotherapist and medical social worker have a major role to play and their services are available in many health centres. The paediatrician and the geneticist may also on occasions be invited to join the team when particular problems are involved (see Chap. 4).

FAMILY HISTORY

At the first visit to the antenatal clinic the mother's history is carefully recorded paying particular attention to her own previous history and the history of both her own and her husband's family. Reference may have to be made to her family doctor for details of which the mother may not be aware. This applies particularly to the occurrence in either parent's family of conditions which are known to be inherited. It may be possible to reassure the mother that conditions which have occurred in other members of the family are not inherited.

MOTHER'S MEDICAL HISTORY

Any period of admission to hospital must be carefully recorded and enquiry made about any blood transfusion received following a road accident or operation. It is important to note the name and address of the hospital and the patient's name and address at that time so that further enquiries can be made. Specific enquiry must be made into a history of acute rheumatism, chest infections, jaundice and urinary tract infections as the extra burden of pregnancy may reveal diminished reserves of function which are the residual effect upon the heart, lungs, liver and renal system of such illnesses.

OBSTETRIC HISTORY

It is essential to find out the mother's normal menstrual pattern so that the expected date of delivery can be calculated as accurately as possible from the date of the last menstrual period. This becomes of great importance if the maturity of the fetus is in doubt. A full summary of all previous pregnancies and abortions must be recorded with the following points being noted:

Duration of pregnancy and whether labour was spontaneous or induced
Complications of pregnancy
Type of labour
Delivery—spontaneous, forceps, breech, caesarean section
Liveborn or stillborn
Birth weight of baby and type of feeding—breast or artificially fed
Complications of the puerperium. Duration of hospital stay is helpful in assessing the severity of the complication.

THE SOCIAL HISTORY

In order to assess the patient's social conditions it is necessary to make enquiries into the employment of her husband and details of the house in which she is living.

Medical Examination

A full medical examination is carried out with particular reference to the heart, blood pressure and lungs. The urine is tested for protein and sugar. If indicated a specialist physician is called in to advise on the management of any abnormality detected. Height is recorded carefully as a woman of small stature might have a contracted pelvis (150 cm or under may be significant). Weight is recorded. An obese patient at the beginning of pregnancy will be a bad obstetric risk during the pregnancy. Dietary advice and weight control must be achieved as early in pregnancy as possible. Blood is examined for ABO blood group, rhesus factor, V.D.R.L. slide test or Wassermann reaction and haemoglobin estimation. The rhesus-negative woman will need special monitoring during pregnancy and this will be intensified if antibodies are demonstrated (Chap. 14). The possibility of congenital syphilis in the fetus can be avoided by treating the mother in early pregnancy.

The size of the uterus must be checked with the period of amenorrhoea. A bimanual examination of the uterus gives a most accurate estimation of the gestation period.

ANTENATAL VISITS

Regular visits to the clinic are arranged monthly until the 28th week of pregnancy, fortnightly till the 36th week, and weekly until delivery. At each of these visits the blood pressure and weight are recorded and the urine tested for sugar and protein. The abdomen is examined to ensure normal progress and growth of the uterus and later, lie and presentation of the fetus. The haemoglobin estimation is repeated at the 28th, 32nd and 36th week of pregnancy, more frequently if the readings are not satisfactory. Regular antenatal examination can detect early signs of abnormality of pregnancy and appropriate advice or treatment can be given.

The midwife helps the mother to lead a healthy life during pregnancy by advice and by encouraging her to attend the parentcraft talks which have already been detailed. These talks help to dispel the fears many women have of childbirth by enabling them to understand how the fetus develops and how the body functions during labour. The physiotherapist contributes to the confidence of the woman by teaching exercises to aid posture during the later weeks of pregnancy and to encourage relaxation when in labour. The medical social worker may require to advise about arrangements for the care of the rest of the family while mother is in hospital. She may assist in providing for the new baby and in cases of hardship may even have to ensure that there is a suitable home for him to return to with his mother. The careful supervision of the mother during pregnancy is one of the chief factors in the reduction of maternal and perinatal mortality.

High-risk Mothers

The following patients are at greater risk during pregnancy and require frequent careful antenatal supervision. Every effort must be made to help them to understand the need for regular attendance at the antenatal clinic.

OLDER PRIMIGRAVIDAE

Patients coming into this classification are women going through their first pregnancy from the age of 30 years onwards. There may be a history of infertility. The maximum fertility in a woman is at about the age of 24 years and there is a gradual decline with increasing age. There is a greater tendency for preeclampsia and hypertension to develop in older mothers. These could precipitate accidental haemorrhage or the premature onset of labour, In labour such patients tend to become anxious and labour may be prolonged and the functional activity of the uterus poor. There is a higher ratio of operative deliveries in older primigravidae and consequently the baby is at greater risk.

BAD OBSTETRIC HISTORY

The patients who come under this category are those who have had previous pregnancies with unsuccessful outcomes such as abortion, stillbirth, neonatal death and abnormal children. Information regarding the previous pregnancies must be obtained from the hospital where she was previously confined including a report of any postmortem examination carried out. Certain factors may recur such as cervical incompetence, preeclampsia, hypertension. If the size of the pelvis is in doubt previous X-rays must be studied and the weight of previous babies taken into consideration. The possibility of chronic ill-health of the mother as a causative factor must be considered and such conditions as chronic pyelonephritis or diabetes mellitus excluded.

THE GRAND MULTIPARA

This term is generally applied to women who have had five babies or more. With increasing age these patients have a greater tendency to obesity. In many cases social conditions are poor and they are overworked and tired out. Dietary deficiencies may be present as they tend to feed their children and neglect themselves. There is a greater tendency to the complications of pregnancy particularly anaemia, preeclampsia and hypertension with their attendant risks of antepartum haemorrhage and preterm delivery. The grand multipara has a greater chance of multiple pregnancy, of placenta praevia and of antepartum haemorrhage. Malpresentations and malpositions are more common due to the laxity of the muscles of the abdominal wall and a pendulous abdomen. In labour complications are more liable to occur for reasons already mentioned and the stillbirth and neonatal death rate is greatly increased.

THE UNSUPPORTED MOTHER

The unmarried or unsupported mother is at greater risk as she may be living in poor social conditions. She may try to conceal her pregnancy and continue working and therefore will get little antenatal care. The unmarried mother requires very tactful and sympathetic consideration and the medical social worker can give most valuable advice and support to her.

Delivery

Delivery is the climax of a pregnancy to which parents look forward with both excitement and fear. Most maternity hospitals recognize the great significance of this event to both parents and allow or encourage fathers to be beside their wives during delivery. This can give great pleasure to both, and fathers can be a source of comfort and strength to their wives. Not all husbands behave well in the role and some may require help and guidance. This is best given in the antenatal period by attendance at the type of classes already outlined.

The Puerperium

As stated earlier the puerperium is a most important learning time when teaching is more meaningful because of the presence of the newly born baby. The policy of rooming-in increases the opportunities for mother to learn about her baby.

PARENTCRAFT IN THE PUERPERIUM

Informal classes can be held while mother is in the postnatal wards. The puerperium is a most important 'learning time'. With the present tendency for shorter periods in hospital after delivery the opportunity for postnatal education is limited and advantage must be taken of every opportunity offered.

The following subjects can be covered.

Care of breasts and nipples. A simple explanation of the physiology of lactation is given stressing that lactation is a natural function which is favoured by rest, a tranquil outlook and a good diet.

Bottle feeding. For mothers who choose not to breast feed instruction is given on the sterilization of bottles and teats and the preparation of feeds. The types of milk on sale can be discussed.

Caring for baby at home. A health visitor can usefully introduce education about the management of baby at home with particular reference to maintenance of temperature. Further care can be discussed introducing the advantage of regular attendance with baby at a clinic for periodic checks and for immunization procedures.

Family planning. This is a useful time to talk to mothers about contraception. Some mothers are more willing to discuss this subject with their midwife after delivery. Excellent leaflets are prepared by the Family Planning Association and can be distributed to parents (Fig. 3.2).

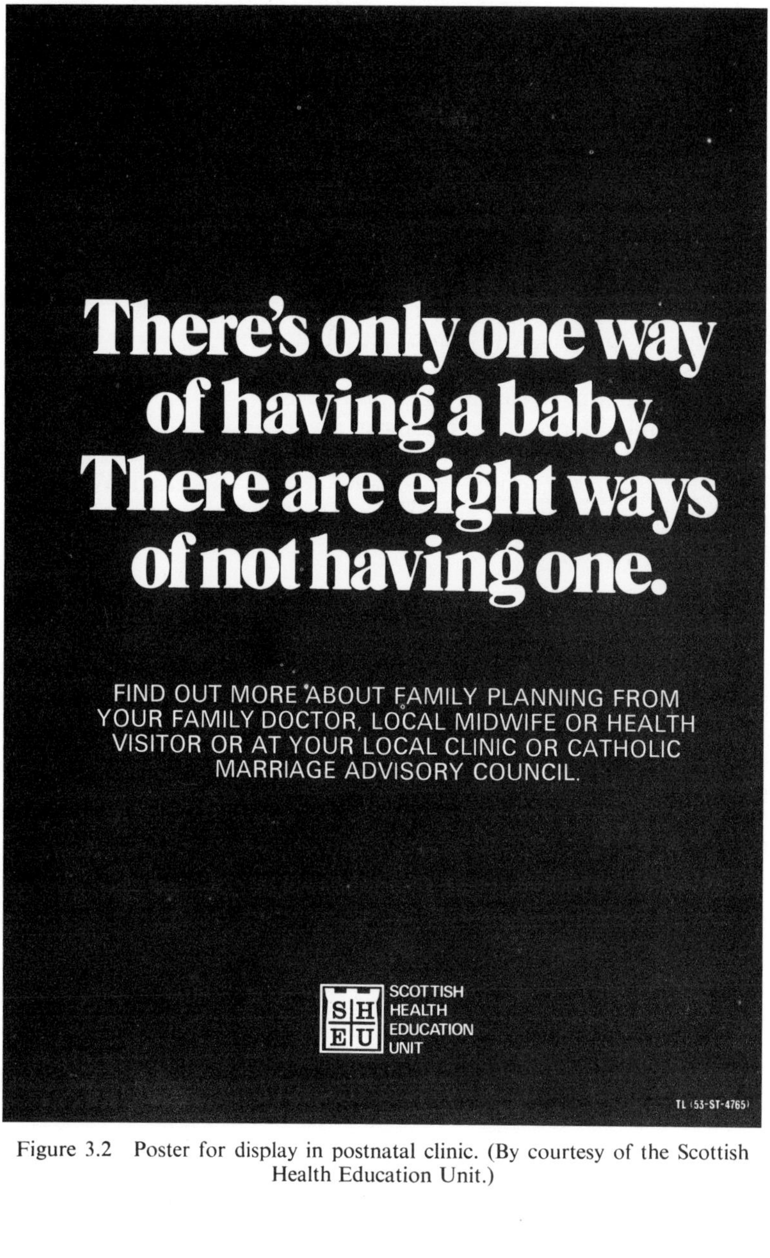
There's only one way
of having a baby.
There are eight ways
of not having one.
FIND OUT MORE ABOUT FAMILY PLANNING FROM YOUR FAMILY DOCTOR, LOCAL MIDWIFE OR HEALTH VISITOR OR AT YOUR LOCAL CLINIC OR CATHOLIC MARRIAGE ADVISORY COUNCIL.
SHEU
SCOTTISH HEALTH EDUCATION UNIT

Figure 3.2 Poster for display in postnatal clinic. (By courtesy of the Scottish Health Education Unit.)

Adoptive parents. Special parentcraft classes covering some of these subjects can be given to prospective adoptive parents.

The Father

The role of the father in supporting his wife and the rest of the family during his wife's pregnancy and delivery is often overlooked not least by fathers themselves. Many of the problems which arise during pregnancy could be prevented or diminished by more sympathetic understanding of the situation by the father-to-be. Ignorance of his wife's needs is the most common cause of this apparent neglect of duty and many fathers-to-be are very upset when their lack of support for their wives is pointed out to them. They commonly reply, 'I never realized. . . .' This unawareness on the part of fathers is more often due to lack of education than to lack of will and underlines the importance of the comments made earlier in this chapter on education in parentcraft at school and in the antenatal clinic. It takes two parents to act in unison before a child is conceived. We must make sure that both parents understand the responsibilities which follow their action.

4

The Fetus

Study of the factors involved in perinatal mortality and morbidity (Chap. 2) clearly indicates that the majority of these exert their efforts before the onset of labour and many are associated with the mother's general health and upbringing before conception occurred. It is therefore appropriate that consideration of the care of the newly born infant should not ignore the antenatal period. Knowledge of fetal development is essential to the proper understanding and management of the newborn infant. This chapter deals with subjects which are more directly the concern of the obstetrician and which are dealt with in more detail in textbooks of obstetrics. Prenatal medicine is nevertheless equally of interest to all who deal with the infant following delivery, and the recent developments in knowledge about fetal medicine serve only to indicate how much more we still have to learn about this relatively short period of our lives which shapes our future.

HEREDITY

VARIABILITY AND ABNORMALITY

The fertilization of the maternal ovum by the paternal sperm is the starting point of a new and eventually independent life. Before emergence as a newborn infant the fertilized ovum has to pass through an intrauterine stage of growth and development of such complexity that it is amazing how relatively alike one human being is to another.

Capacity for variability. Fortunately for us differences do exist and we are not produced as identical copies of either parent. It is this capacity for variability which allows for evolutionary forces to act over long periods of time and this has been to the advantage of the human in relation to other species.

Limitation of variability. The capacity for variability within an individual is limited by the genetic factors inherited equally from both parents. These may act either to his benefit or his detriment. Where the result is sufficiently detrimental, conception may not be successful or the fertilized ovum may die at an early stage.

Abnormality. With progressively less serious forms of abnormality intrauterine growth may proceed for longer periods resulting in abortion, stillbirth or the live birth of an abnormal infant. The progress of development may be disturbed by genetic disorder at the time of conception or by subsequent damage to the growing embryo and fetus by external influences. These subjects are considered further in Chapter 11.

Normality. The tendency for most major abnormalities of conception to cause death before development is well advanced ensures a high degree of normality and viability in surviving fetuses. In this chapter consideration will be given to the development of the normal fetus but mention will also be made of factors which can interfere with the normal development of a fetus which begins life without inherited abnormality. The absence of abnormality does not make us all identical and it is clear that we inherit characteristic features of physique and possibly behaviour from our parents which make us different from our siblings without being abnormal.

GENES AND CHROMOSOMES

Inherited characteristics are carried in deoxyribonucleic acid (DNA) as genes on chromosomes contained in the nucleus of body cells. In humans there are 22 pairs of somatic (body) chromosomes and 2 sex chromosomes giving a total of 46 chromosomes. This is known as the diploid number. The ovum and the spermatozoon each contain half that number, 22 somatic and 1 sex chromosome, and this is known as the haploid number. At fertilization the somatic chromosomes of the spermatozoon pair up with the somatic chromosomes of the ovum to form the 22 pairs of somatic chromosomes. A female has two X chromosomes, and a male has an X and a Y chromosome. These are known as the sex chromosomes. Every fetus receives one X chromosome from the mother and either an X or a Y chromosome from the father. The fetal sex chromosome constitution therefore depends upon which sex chromosome is received from the father (Fig. 4.1).

INHERITANCE

Each chromosome carries very large numbers of genes which are the ultimate factors governing inheritance. With the pairing of somatic chromosomes at conception the fetus receives pairs of genes, one from each parent.

Dominant. Some inherited abnormalities are carried on a single gene. In some conditions the presence of abnormality in one only of the gene pair is sufficient to produce its effect on the fetus. Such conditions are termed dominant.

Recessive. In other situations both genes in the pair must have the same abnormality before the fetus is affected. This type of inheritance is termed recessive.

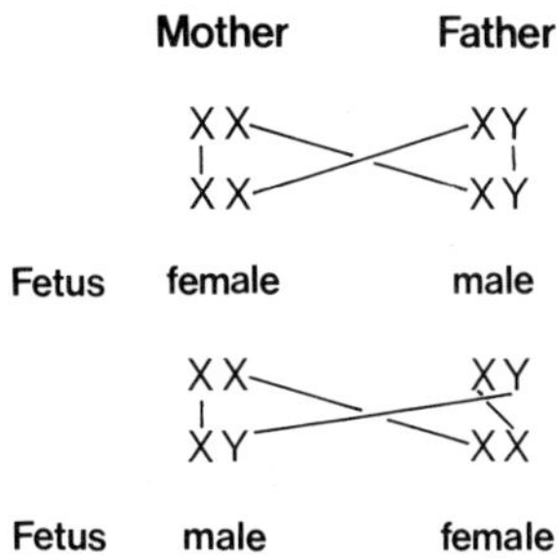

Figure 4.1 Inheritance of sex chromosomes indicating that it is the sex chromosome received from the father which determines the sex of the fetus.

Zygosity. If a person has only one gene carrying such a recessively inherited condition and the other gene of the pair is normal that person is not affected by the single abnormal gene but is a carrier of that gene. Where only one gene of a pair is abnormal the subject is heterozygous for that gene. If both genes are the same the subject is homozygous for that gene. If both genes are normal the subject is normal for that trait. If both are abnormal so is the subject.

Risk. If a male and a female carrier (heterozygotes) of a recessively inherited gene marry there is a 1 in 4 chance that each infant will be a homozygote and affected. There is also a 1 in 4 chance that he will be an unaffected homozygote. The remaining 2 of the 4 chances will be heterozygotes and therefore unaffected but carriers.

Sex linked. Certain inherited traits such as haemophilia are carried on the X chromosome as a recessive character. In the male with a single X chromosome the trait will be manifest. The female with two X chromosomes will generally be heterozygous. The trait will not be manifest but the female is a carrier. Her sons have a 1 in 2 chance of being affected. Her daughters have a 1 in 2 chance of being carriers. This is called sex-linked recessive inheritance.

EUGENICS

While some inherited disorders (Chap. 11) fall into these relatively simple patterns of dominant, recessive and sex-linked inheritance originally described by Mendel much more complicated patterns of inheritance govern the majority of normal variations which constitute our individuality. Our genetic inheritance is at present a sequel to the mutual attraction between our parents. Some scientists foresee the time when chance will be given a less free hand and artificial selection of genetic characteristics will be possible by eugenically planned mating, whether this be physiological or in the test tube. Others look forward to the possibility of altering genes. Many authors have warned of the potential risks of such concepts. Fortunately at present the human race remains dependent on chance to select the maternal and paternal genes of a fetus. This haphazard method has served us well in the past and it is difficult to believe that more organized control would result in a benefit which outweighed the dangers inherent in such proposals.

The Ovum

A detailed study of the development of the fertilized ovum is not called for in a book which is chiefly concerned with the newborn infant. It is helpful, however, to have some knowledge of intrauterine development as a preparation for the study of the infant at birth and it is hoped that the following outline will suffice.

BEFORE IMPLANTATION

Fertilization almost invariably takes place while the ovum is in the ampulla of the Fallopian tube. After fertilization the ovum is propelled along the tube to the uterus and at the same time undergoes repeated cell division. As a result the ovum assumes the form of a ball of cells (morula) in which a cavity (blastocele) appears—at which stage the ovum is known as a blastocyst. The multiplying cells of the blastocyst undergo a patterned distribution, some cells being gathered together to form what is called the inner cell mass and others remaining on the surface as a covering layer (trophoblast). At one point the trophoblast and the inner cell mass remain connected by a stalk of cells known as the body stalk. Arrived at this stage of development the ovum comes in contact with the uterine endometrium (Fig. 4.2).

IMPLANTATION

During the secretory phase of the menstrual cycle the endometrium undergoes changes intended to prepare it for reception of a fertilized ovum. If a fertilized ovum becomes embedded in it the endometrium undergoes further development, becoming greatly increased in thickness, vascularity and softness. The ovum or blastocyst penetrates and eventually becomes completely embedded in the endometrium, which is now known as the decidua.

The Embryo

Two cavities develop in the inner cell mass of the blastocyst. One is known as the amniotic sac and the other as the yolk sac. Between them there is a cellular area called the embryonic area or plate because it is from this plate that the embryo grows. In the embryonic area the cells become grouped into three primitive layers known as

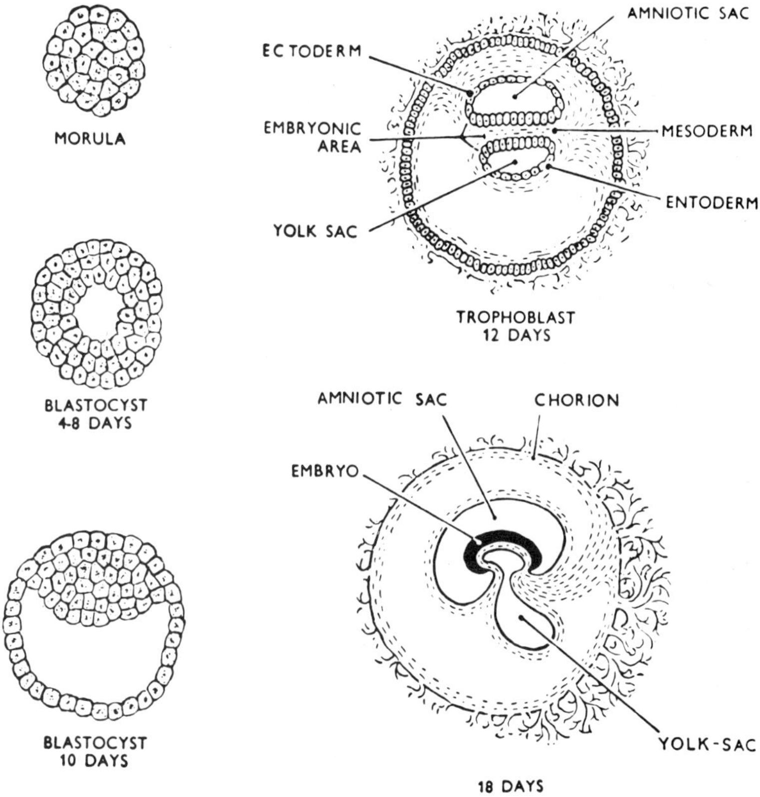

Figure 4.2 Diagrammatic representation of the development of the fertilized ovum.

the ectoderm, the mesoderm and the entoderm. In the course of subsequent growth the skin, certain mucous membranes and the central nervous system develop from the ectoderm; the blood, muscle, bones and certain organs from the mesoderm; and the lungs, alimentary mucosa, bladder, pancreas and parts of the liver from the entoderm.

The amniotic sac is filled with fluid and serves to protect the growing embryo, which derives its nourishment from the yolk sac pending the development of a rudimentary placenta. The yolk sac is connected by a duct (vitelline duct) with the embryonic gut. With expansion the amniotic cavity gradually envelops the embryo at each end and along the flanks, and at the same time brings the yolk sac and the vitelline duct into contact with the body stalk to form the umbilical cord. Development of the cord is usually complete by the sixth week.

Development of the Placenta

Buds of multiplying cells sprout out from the trophoblast where it comes into contact with the decidua. These buds or villi multiply in number and cover the entire ovum by the time it has been completely embedded in the implantation cavity. At the same time some of the villi become attached to the deep layer of the decidua (decidua basalis) and serve to anchor the ovum to the decidua. Other villi grow rapidly, penetrate the decidual blood vessels, and as a result are continuously bathed by circulating maternal blood. This stage of development is reached about the third week of pregnancy (Fig. 4.3).

UMBILICAL CORD

Thereafter the persisting chorionic villi multiply in number and increase in complexity. Each villus consists of a central core of fetal mesoderm and embryonic vessels in which fetal blood circulates and two cellular layers: an inner—Langhan's layer—and an outer—the syncytium. Fetal and maternal blood do not come into contact with one another, but Langhan's layer selects and absorbs substances necessary for the nourishment of the embryo from the maternal blood. Absorbed substances are conveyed to the embryo from the vessels of the developing umbilical cord, which is continuous at one end with the chorion and attached to the embryo at the other.

CHORIONIC VILLI

In contrast with those in the uterine decidua the chorionic villi which cover the capsule of the trophoblast and which are nearest the uterine cavity degenerate and undergo atrophy. By the end of the third month the placenta acquires a discoidal shape consisting of some 15 to 20 clumps (cotyledons) of chorionic villi anchored to the decidua basalis and bathed in the maternal blood flowing through the spaces separating the chorion and decidua. Occasionally failure to disappear of a collection of chorionic villi in relation to the capsule of the trophoblast gives rise to an accessory placenta.

Twinning. In the great majority of instances of twin pregnancy resulting from fertilization of a single ovum there are one placenta, one chorion and two amniotic sacs. Exceptionally, however, two placentae may develop. Where in a twin pregnancy fertilization of two ova has taken place, there are always two placentae which may, however, fuse and have the macroscopic appearance of a single placenta. Decision as to whether twins are identical or non-identical

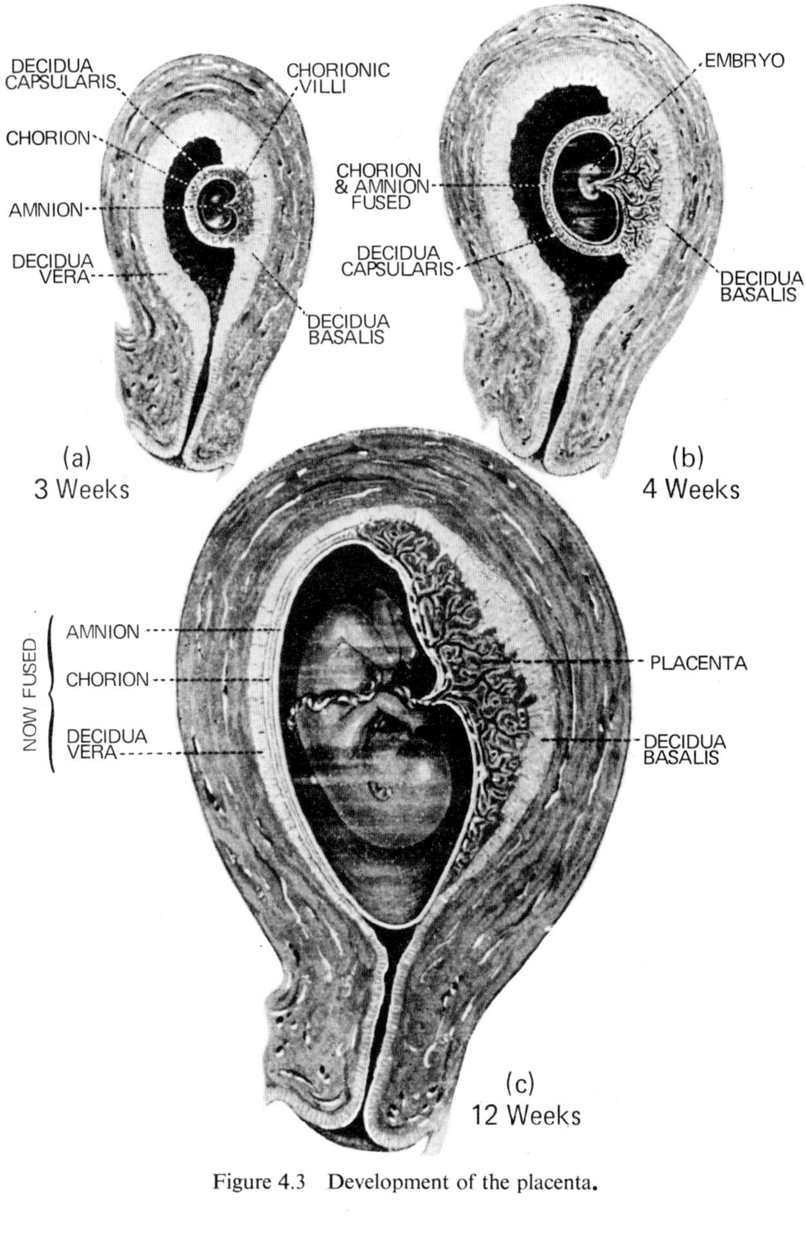

Figure 4.3 Development of the placenta.

cannot therefore always be made on a cursory examination of the placenta(e).

FUNCTIONS OF THE PLACENTA

Knowledge concerning the functions of the placenta is incomplete but growing.

Fetal lung. The placenta acts as a fetal lung. In the placenta carbon dioxide is transferred from the fetal to the maternal circulation. Simultaneously the fetus obtains oxygen from the mother's haemoglobin.

Nutrition. The fetus derives its nourishment from the mother's blood. It is believed that Langhan's layer of the chorionic villi is capable of selective absorption of substances necessary for growth of the embryo and later of the fetus. Substances passing from the maternal blood into the fetal circulation include: amino acids, necessary for tissue development; glucose, needed for energy and growth; and calcium, phosphorus, iron and other minerals necessary for the formation of the skeleton, teeth and blood. It is unlikely that fatty acids pass through the placenta. Glucose is converted into fat by the fetus as required. In the early months of fetal growth, prior to normal liver function being established, glucose is stored as glycogen in the placenta where it is converted into glucose when required.

Excretion. Waste products of fetal metabolism are transferred across the placenta to the mother's blood.

Protective barrier. The placenta acts as a protective barrier to the fetus by preventing the passage of certain but by no means all potentially harmful substances from the maternal to the fetal circulation. Very few infecting organisms can pass the placental barrier. Known exceptions are the virus of rubella, the virus of cytomegalic inclusion body disease and the spirochaete of syphilis. The bacillus of tuberculosis and the protozoon of toxoplasmosis are very rare exceptions. Recently it has been suggested that the virus of mumps should be added to these.

The newly born baby frequently possesses a temporary passive immunity to such infections as diphtheria and measles. The immunity is acquired from the mother, and although the exact mechanism is not known it is generally accepted that transmission takes place across the placenta. Transfer of fetal antigens in a reverse direction can take place. Rhesus positive cells from a fetus may enter the circulation of the rhesus-negative mother and may stimulate the formation of antibodies. Other substances which may penetrate the placental barrier include sedative, anaesthetic, antibiotic and antisyphilitic drugs.

Endocrine. The placenta functions as an endocrine gland secreting oestrogenic and other hormones. Maternal hormones can pass through the placenta to enter the blood of the fetus.

Disturbance of normal placental function can result in interference with healthy fetal development. Contributory factors include abnormal structure and size, degenerative changes and premature separation of the placenta.

THE FETUS

The first recognizable human characteristics appear about four weeks after conception. They consist of the rudimentary eyes and ears, and projecting buds representing the beginnings of limb formation. At this stage the embryo consists of a large head and a rather tapering body ending in a tail, weighs approximately 1 to 1.3 g and measures 9 to 12 mm in length. The head and tail almost meet because the embryo is markedly curved.

By the eighth week the hands and feet are recognizable; the external genitalia are developing, but differentiation of sex is not possible for a further three or four weeks; the tail has almost completely disappeared, and the head has assumed a normal human shape (Fig. 4.4). At twelve weeks the placenta is well developed, the umbilical cord shows normal spiral characteristics and the fingers and toes are distinguishable (Fig. 4.5).

It is customary to apply the term 'fetus' to the results of conception

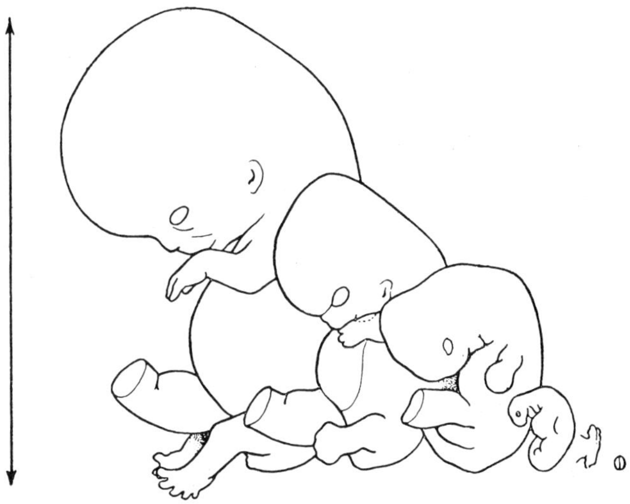

Figure 4.4 The stages of growth from the end of the third week to the end of the eighth week *in utero*.

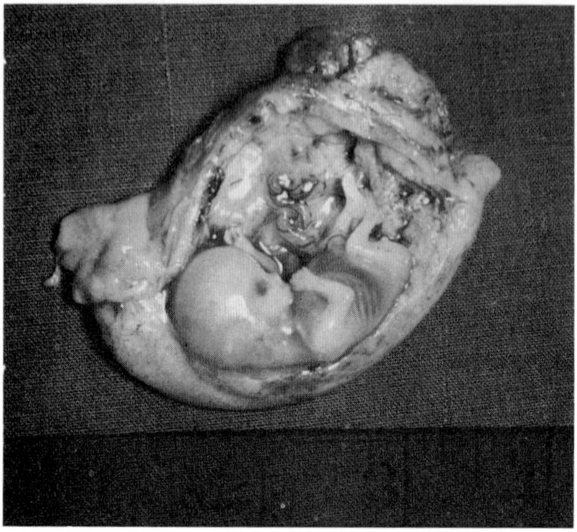

Figure 4.5 Fetus of 12 weeks gestation.

which have undergone progressive development for some 12 weeks. By this time the growing organism measures about 9 cm in length and weighs about 29 g. A uterus is present in the female. Centres of ossification are present in many bones. Lanugo first appears about the sixteenth week of gestation, and in a further four weeks vernix caseosa is present. Within some 24 weeks of conception hair appears on the head and the deposit of subcutaneous fat begins. During the subsequent 16 weeks of pregnancy the hair on the scalp increases in amount, the nails grow in length and the vernix caseosa becomes more plentiful. As the subcutaneous fat is laid down in increasing amount the face and forehead lose their creases, the skin acquires a smooth texture and pink colour, and the body as a whole becomes more rotund.

After a gestation period of 40 weeks the fetus measures approximately 51 cm in length and weighs about 3200 g, but wide variations occur. In general, male infants tend to be slightly heavier than female infants, and where the mother's age is under 30 years the weights of successive babies tend to increase.

Differentiation of Certain Special Structures

THE BRAIN, CORD AND RELATED STRUCTURES

Mention has been made of the embryonic cell mass or plate. At one end of the upper surface of the plate a thickened prominence of ectodermal cells develops. The edges of the prominence rise up to form two elevations which extend forwards and backwards and eventually fuse to form a tube. This is known as the neural tube and the brain and spinal cord develop from it (Fig. 4.6). Simultaneously cells from the mesodermic layer of the embryonic plate

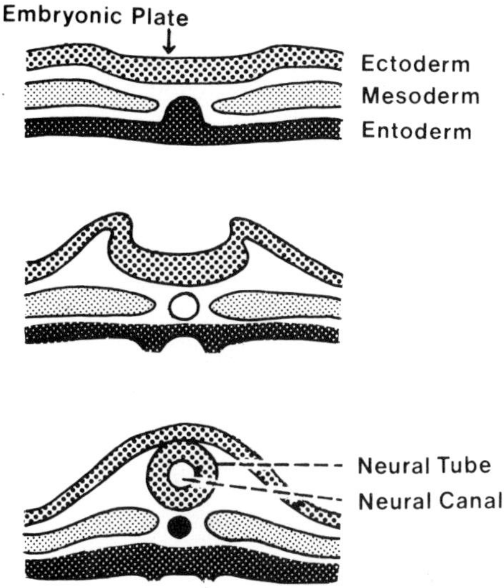

Figure 4.6 Early development of the spinal cord.

arrange themselves alongside the neural tube. These cells assume a segmental distribution, and each segment (somite) represents the commencing development of a vertebra with its related muscle structures. Closure of the neural tube involves separation of ectodermal cells forming the future central nervous system from the remainder of the ectoderm, which expands and extends to form the covering of the growing embryo.

THE ALIMENTARY SYSTEM

The envelopment of the embryo by the enlarging amniotic cavity has been described. As it folds over them the amniotic cavity presses on the sides of the embryo, bending them over until they meet to form a tube on the under (or ventral) side of the embryo. The tube is closed at its head and tail ends by the simultaneous enveloping processes of the amnion anteriorly and posteriorly. In this way a portion of the yolk sac becomes enclosed within the embryo as a primitive gut and communicates at one point with the remaining extraembryonic part of the yolk sac by means of the vitelline duct. The enclosed portion of yolk sac represents the rudiments of the alimentary tract.

In the course of time the fore end of the gut dilates to form the pharynx, in the walls of which several elevations (branchial arches) appear. These are related to the later development of the mandibular and maxillary bones among other structures. The stomach first appears as a local dilatation of the gut. By far the greatest part of the tract elongates to form the small and large intestines. From the sixth to the tenth week the abdominal cavity, together with loops of intestine, protrudes into the base of the umbilical cord (Fig. 4.7).

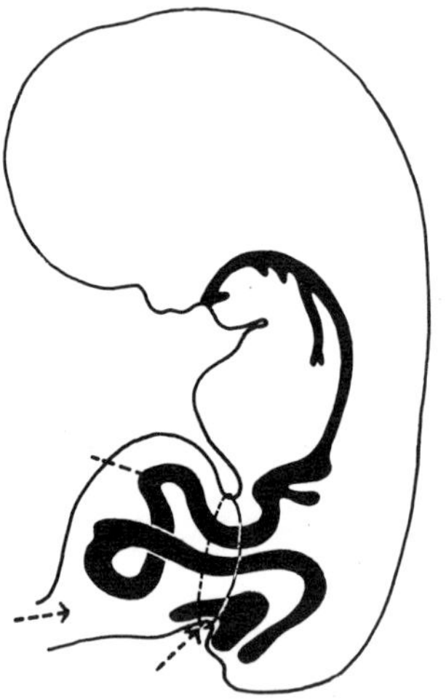

Figure 4.7 Protrusion of the gut into the base of the umbilical cord.

This is probably due to the abdominal viscera growing more rapidly than the perioneal cavity. The position is reversed after the tenth week, and the sac with its contents is withdrawn into the abdominal cavity.

Rotation of the gut. At first the small and large intestines lie respectively to the right and left of the midline. Later the gut rotates upon itself, the large intestine taking up a position in front of the small intestine, the caecum lying in proximity to the liver. Subsequently the caecum descends into the right iliac fossa (Fig. 4.8).

Cloaca. Meanwhile a local dilatation (the cloaca) develops in the hindend of the gut. The cloaca is closed to the exterior by a thin ectodermal layer known as the cloacal membrane, and is later divided by a septum into a narrow dorsal portion (the future rectum) and a wide ventral portion (the future bladder and urogenital sinus). The cloacal membrane shares in the division of the cloaca, becoming differentiated into an anterior urogenital membrane and a posterior anal membrane. Later openings develop in these membranes to

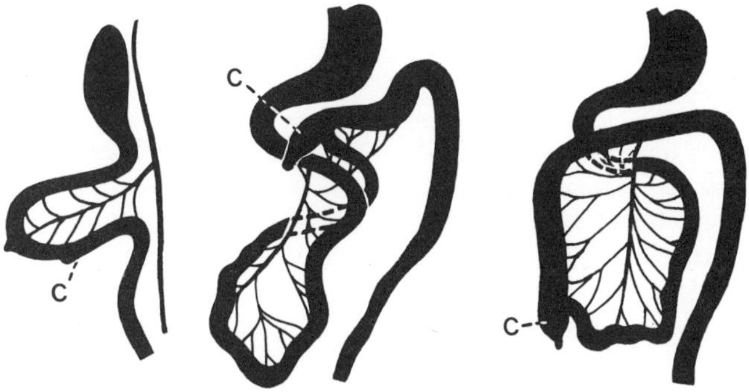

Figure 4.8 Rotation of the midgut. C = caecum.

form rudimentary urethral and anal orifices. In both sexes the external genitalia develop in the vicinity of the cloacal aperture (Fig. 4.9).

UROGENITAL ORGANS

Kidney. The rudimentary kidneys first appear about the fifth week and are not structurally complete until the 35th week. Embryologically each kidney consists of two parts—one giving rise to the rudiments of the renal pelvis, the calyces and the collecting tubules, and the other part giving rise to the glomeruli and secretory tubules. The first part is connected with the ureter, which by the sixth week opens into the part of the cloaca which later becomes the bladder.

Bladder. The greater part of the bladder develops from the cloaca (Fig. 4.9). In the small embryo the bladder extends to the level of the umbilicus. With growth of the embryo the bladder assumes a relatively lower position. In the course of descending migration the upper part of the bladder is extended and narrows until it consists of no more than a narrow tube—the urachus—which later becomes obliterated.

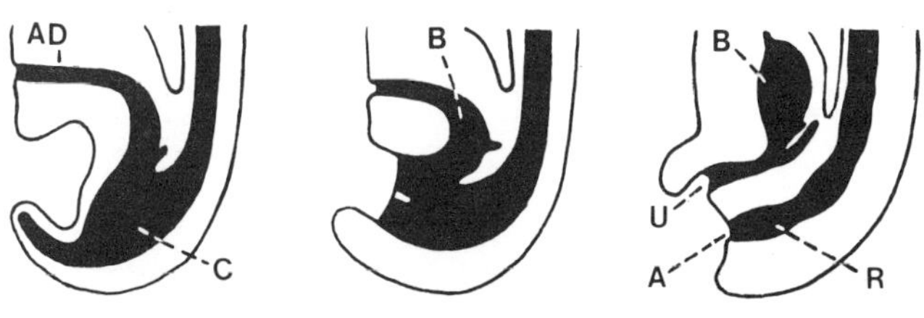

Figure 4.9 Development of the bladder and rectum. C = cloaca; B = bladder; A = anal membrane; AD = allantoic duct; U = urogenital sinus; R = rectum.

Genital tract. In the course of embryonic growth ducts develop in connection with the reproductive system. The Mullerian ducts, originating as invaginations from the embryonic abdominal cavity, extend to the cloaca into which they later open. They persist in the female, fusing in part of their length to form the uterus and extending to form the vagina. The Fallopian tubes develop from parts of the Mullerian ducts which do not undergo fusion. In the male these ducts atrophy. The other ducts, the Wolffian ducts, eventually atrophy in the female and persist in the male as ducts of the genital gland. The Wolffian ducts ultimately open into the urethra.

External genitalia develop in the region of the cloacal orifice. A swelling (the genital tubercle) appears in front of this orifice and eventually develops as the glans of the penis or clitoris. Folds extend back from the genital tubercle and flank either side of the cloacal orifice. In the male these folds meet to enclose the urethra which extends to the glans with growth of the penis. In the female these folds do not fuse and are the forerunners of the labia minora. There is another swelling on the lateral aspect of each fold. These additional swellings are the rudimentary halves of the scrotum in the male and form the labia majora in the female.

RESPIRATORY ORGANS

The beginnings of respiratory organs first appear (about the fourth week) as a groove in the ventral wall of the pharynx. Eventually the groove encloses on itself to form a tube which is completely separated from the alimentary tract except at a slitlike point of communication at the upper pharynx. This new tube represents the rudimentary trachea. Its upper end forms the larynx, and at its lower end buds protrude from which develop the bronchi and lungs (Fig. 4.10).

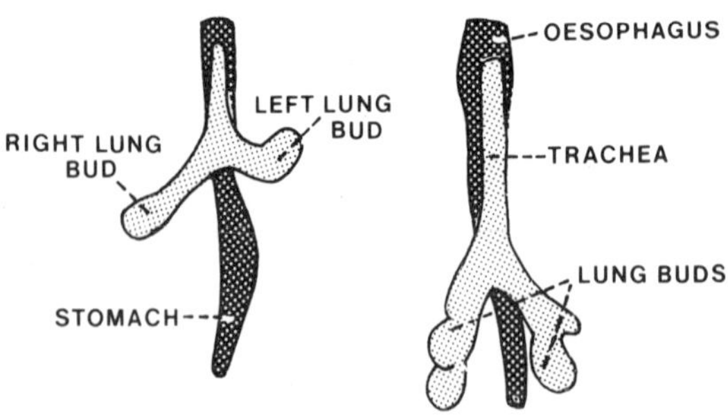

Figure 4.10 Development of the respiratory organs as buds from the pharynx.

HEART AND VESSELS

The fetus develops its own blood and the earliest vessels to appear are situated in the yolk sac, body stalk and chorion. The heart develops from a pair of tubular vessels (the primitive aortae) which form in the embryonic mesoderm and which become continuous with the umbilical arteries leading to the chorion. At one point the primitive aortae come in contact, the partition separating them disappears, and the resultant single tube represents the rudimentary heart. This simple tubular heart increases in length and becomes S-shaped. Constrictions then appear in the tube which gradually becomes differentiated into five parts, each of which subsequently becomes divided by a septum or septa. As a result there are formed the inferior and superior venae cavae, the two atria, the two ventricles, the aorta and the pulmonary artery. Projections in the walls of the cardiac chambers then develop to form valves at either end of each ventricle. This stage is reached by about the eighth week of intrauterine life, by which time the heart functions as an effective circulatory pump. Structurally the heart differs from the adult heart in that the foramen ovale is patent.

During the time that the single tubular heart is undergoing differentiation into parts, complicated adjustments of the relative position of the various parts, one to the other, and to developing arteries and veins are taking place. As the heart assumes its S-shape it is, as it were, twisted and rotated on itself with the primary object of securing true alignment with the great vessels entering and leaving it.

Circulation. Blood which has circulated in the fetus is pumped by the fetal heart through the two umbilical arteries into the placenta. There the blood transfers carbon dioxide to the mother's circulation, from which it acquires oxygen and substances necessary for fetal nutrition prior to returning to the fetus via the umbilical vein. This vein gives off two important branches before reaching the liver—a branch to the left lobe of the liver and another branch (the ductus venosus) which joins the inferior vena cava.

The recently oxygenated blood from the ductus venosus mixes with venous blood returning from the lower limbs and organs below the level of the diaphragm. After mixing in this way the blood passes to the right atrium of the heart, where a septum covers an opening, the foramen ovale (not present in later life), between the left and right auricles. The inferior edge of the septum faces the oncoming stream of blood, some of which passes to the right atrium but the greater part of which is diverted to the left and passes through the foramen ovale to enter the left auricle. From the left auricle it is pumped via the aorta to the vessels of the upper limbs, the neck and brain. In this way the brain is assured of adequate oxygen.

Blood which enters the right atrium mixes there with other blood, returning via the superior vena cava from the head and upper limbs. The contents of the right atrium pass to the right ventricle. Blood leaves this ventricle by the pulmonary artery. Only a small portion of the blood goes to the lungs (which do not function *in utero*), the great bulk being diverted along the ductus arteriosus to the descending aorta. Thence it eventually passes by the hypogastric (umbilical) arteries to the placenta once again (Fig. 4.11).

DIAPHRAGM

At first the embryonic heart, lungs and gut are contained in one body cavity. In the course of time a septum of mesodermal tissue develops and becomes attached to the anterior and posterior body walls. This septum is the forerunner of the diaphragm. It is pierced in the middle by the gut and is deficient laterally. Dorsally the septum gravitates in a caudal direction. Eventually the lateral openings in the diaphragm are closed by extension of new tissues. The structures of the diaphragm are derived developmentally from a number of sources.

TEETH

The development of the deciduous teeth begins about six weeks after conception. Ectodermal cells migrate below the surface to form the enamel organs which fit like caps over small collections of mesodermal cells lying in the primitive jaw. These groups of cells, partly ectodermal and partly mesodermal, form the teeth buds. The rudiments of all 20 teeth are present by the tenth week, and they begin to calcify by the fourth month. Dental germs consisting of the beginnings of the permanent teeth first appear about the eighteenth week of intrauterine life. By the time of birth the rudimentary buds of 24 permanent teeth have been laid down.

Prenatal Environmental Influences

One thousand years ago antenatal clinics were held in China to ensure tranquillity in the mother in order to promote mental health and tranquillity in their infants. The Chinese were more concerned with the mental than the physical progress of the fetus. We may be in danger of going to the opposite extreme. Recent investigations provide evidence in animals that environmental influences during pregnancy can affect the behaviour of that fetus in later development. In humans a relationship has been demonstrated between the activity of a fetus and his subsequent behaviour as an infant. The

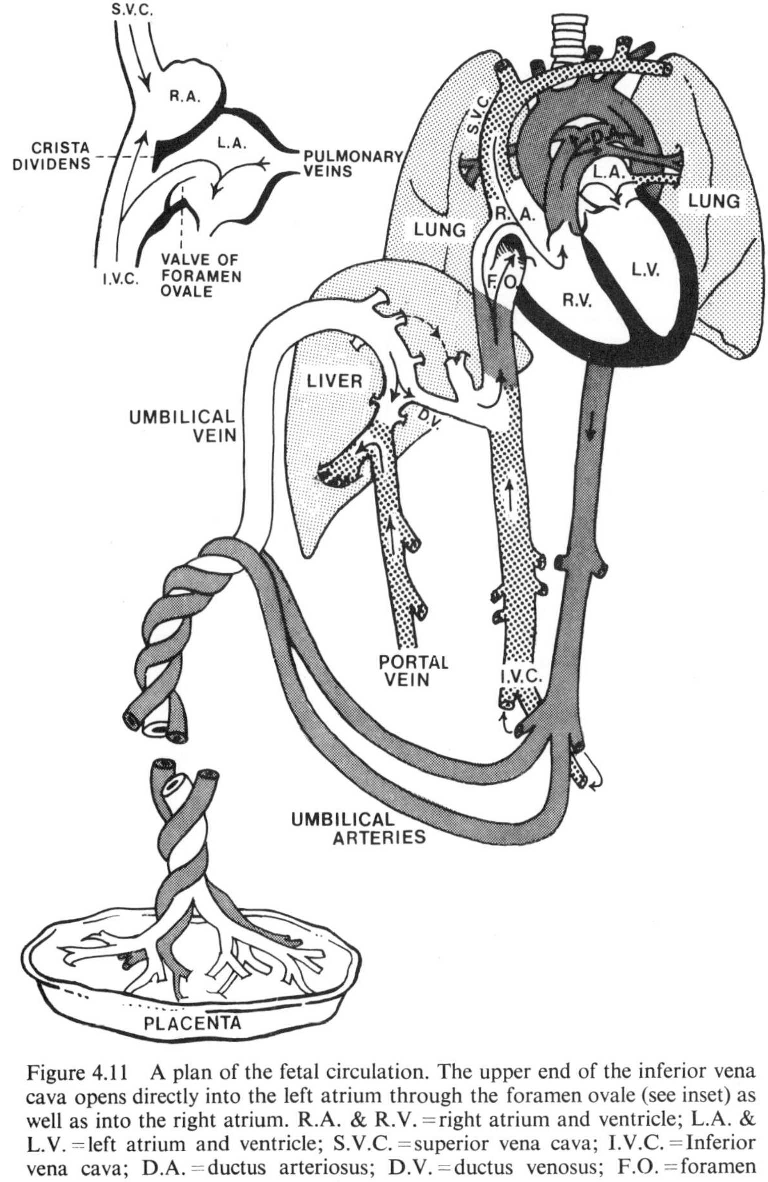

Figure 4.11 A plan of the fetal circulation. The upper end of the inferior vena cava opens directly into the left atrium through the foramen ovale (see inset) as well as into the right atrium. R.A. & R.V. = right atrium and ventricle; L.A. & L.V. = left atrium and ventricle; S.V.C. = superior vena cava; I.V.C. = Inferior vena cava; D.A. = ductus arteriosus; D.V. = ductus venosus; F.O. = foramen ovale. (By courtesy of G. S. Dawes.)

relative importance of intrauterine environment in shaping postnatal behaviour is, however, not clear and the need for appropriate management cannot therefore be assessed.

Assessment of the Fetus

Menstrual age. The recent years have seen many developments in clinical and laboratory methods of assessing fetal growth, development and well-being. An essential factor in this assessment is knowledge of the age of the fetus so that its development can be compared with the normal for that stage of development. Gestational age, that is age from conception, is generally calculated by reference to the date of the first day of the last menstrual period. Strictly this gives menstrual age and the relation to true gestational age depends on the interval between onset of menstruation and ovulation. Where this is known the mean interval between conception and delivery has been reported as 265 days. It is, however, more convenient to measure the duration of pregnancy as from the last menstrual period giving an average duration for a full-term pregnancy of 280 days. The first day of the last menstrual period is generally accepted as the date from which the gestational age is calculated to the nearest week. Although this method has the obvious merit of simplicity it has equally obvious fallacies. Mothers may not be sure of the date of their last period. Bleeding following the withdrawal of oral contraceptives may be mistaken for a true period. Early bleeding at the time of implantation of the ovum or due to a threatened abortion may similarly be accepted as menstruation. Other methods have been employed to measure the length of gestation.

Assessment by size. Bimanual assessment of the size of the uterus in the first trimester of pregnancy is a more reliable means of assessing fetal size and age than measurement of the height of the fundus at later stages of pregnancy when factors other than fetal size affect the fundal height. Radiographs of fetal bones can give information about the appearance of centres of ossification and bone length from which fetal age is often calculated. It has been shown, however, that there is poor correlation between the bone age of twins although they are presumably of the same gestational age.

Amniotic fluid. Examination of amniotic fluid following amniocentesis is a more promising method of assessment (Fig. 4.12). Studies of urea and creatinine concentration have shown these to rise steadily after 30 weeks gestation and the concentration reached is an index of gestational age. The cells contained in amniotic fluid alter with advancing pregnancy and this change can be recognized with suitable staining techniques. Investigation of amniotic fluid

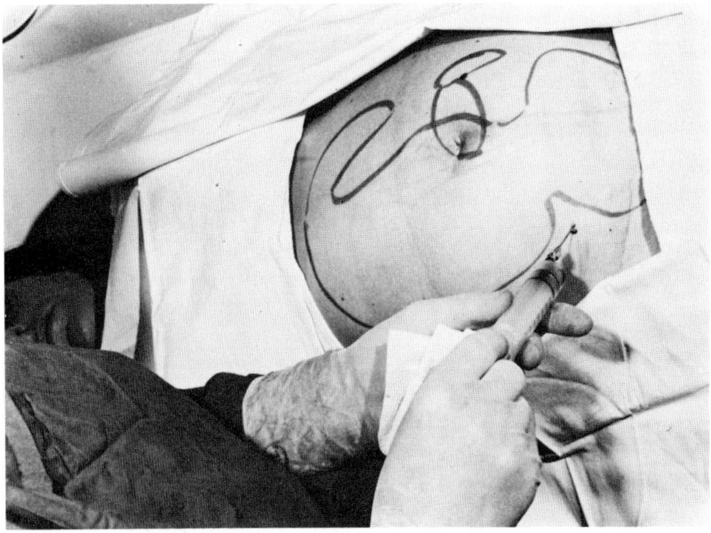

Figure 4.12 Amniocentesis. (Photograph by courtesy of Dr J. M. Monaghan.)

enzymes have shown that these too alter with gestational age. Examination of amniotic fluid by any of these methods does not yet give a precise measurement of fetal age but is sufficiently accurate to be of clinical value.

Ultrasound. Measurement of biparietal diameter of the fetus can be made with a considerable degree of accuracy by ultrasound (Fig. 4.13). This method can be used to assess fetal age but does not detect those situations where the fetus has a normal skull size but

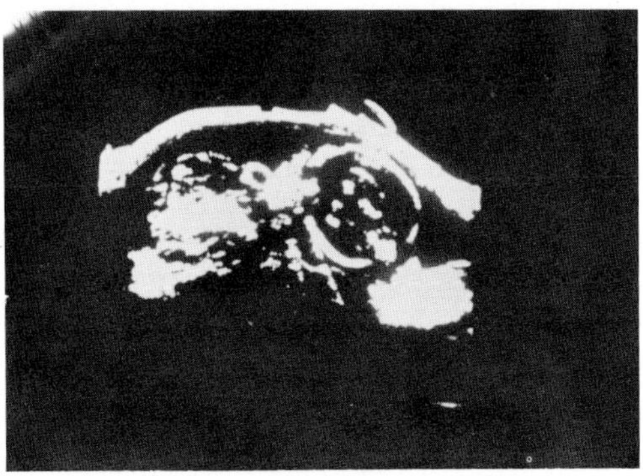

Figure 4.13 Ultrasonogram of 28 weeks fetus. (Photograph by courtesy of Dr J. M. Monaghan.)

is poorly nourished and small for dates. Repeated examinations will give an indication of the rate of fetal growth. Retarded ultrasonic growth rates have been shown to be associated with an increased incidence at birth of congenital abnormality, low Apgar score and perinatal mortality. The equipment involved in this technique is unfortunately too expensive to allow its universal application.

In spite of the development of newer laboratory methods of assessment the older clinical methods of measuring fetal age by menstrual age and size of the uterus remain the most universally applicable and acceptable in spite of their recognized limitations.

RATE OF GROWTH

With an estimate of fetal age an assessment can be made as to whether uterine size conforms with that expected for that stage of pregnancy. If the rate of growth of the uterus is smaller than that expected it is probable that this is due to slow intrauterine growth of the fetus, which is said to be 'small for dates'. This implies an increased risk to the fetus, and unless fetal growth improves the pregnancy may not end successfully. As there is a considerable variation in the rates of growth of normal fetuses it is most important to know whether the small-for-dates fetus is a healthy but small fetus or whether growth is being retarded by some abnormal process. Similarly, excessive rates of uterine enlargement indicate a possible abnormality which requires investigation. Other methods of assessing fetal well-being are available for use where there is evidence of departure from the normal range of intrauterine growth.

ASSESSMENT OF PLACENTAL FUNCTION

Urine oestriol. Placental function can be estimated by examination of the oestrogen content of maternal urine. Of the oestrogens present oestriol is the largest fraction, and as oestriol is produced by a combination of placental and fetal activity its ouput in the mother's urine is an indication of placento-fetal function. Levels of maternal urinary oestriol rise about the 32nd to 34th week of gestation. In about 90 per cent of cases of retarded fetal growth oestriol excretion is depressed. Serial measurements are more useful than single levels. A falling level is a danger sign as is absence of the expected rise at 32 to 34 weeks gestation. Oestriol levels below 5 mg in 24 hours indicate a high risk of early neonatal death.

AMNIOTIC FLUID

Rhesus incompatability. Amniocentesis which was discussed earlier as a means of assessing fetal maturity can also be used to provide other information about the fetus. Examination of amniotic fluid has been practised for many years in the antenatal diagnosis and management of rhesus incompatability in rhesus-negative mothers. By measuring the optical density (OD) of centrifuged amniotic fluid at a wavelength of 450 nm the concentration of bilirubin present can be calculated. This in turn gives an indication of the severity of the haemolytic process in the fetus. Repeat tests allow an assessment of the rate of deterioration and the risk of intrauterine death. Amniocentesis is not without risk, particularly of fetomaternal haemorrhage which may aggravate the maternal sensitisation to the Rh or other blood group. It is therefore only carried out where the previous history of severely affected infants or the demonstration of rising antiglobulin titre in maternal serum indicates that the fetus is at risk. Dependent upon the amniotic findings and the size of the fetus either premature induction of labour or intrauterine transfusion may be indicated.

Sexing. More recently amniotic fluid cells have been examined for sex chromatin after suitable staining. This is of value in families with a history of a disorder such as certain types of muscular dystrophy or of haemophilia which are inherited as sex-linked recessive conditions and males only are affected. If at an early stage of pregnancy it can be shown that the fetus is a male and therefore at risk the mother can be offered a therapeutic abortion.

Chromosomes. Tissue culture of fetal cells from the amniotic fluid is a slower process and often difficult to achieve. Where successful, abnormalities such as Down's syndrome can be diagnosed *in utero* but the result is not always available early enough in pregnancy to allow a therapeutic abortion by the vaginal route and a decision has to be taken as to whether hysterotomy is justified at the stage of pregnancy reached.

α-Fetoprotein. It has recently been reported that α-fetoprotein is raised in the amniotic fluid of pregnancies in which the fetus was later shown to have anencephaly or spina bifida. As this rise has been noted as early as 13 weeks gestation the possibility of antenatal recognition of these major abnormalities now appears feasible at a stage when therapeutic abortion is acceptable.

Lecithin-sphingomyelin ratio. Reference will be made in later chapters to the significance of phospholipid substances in the alveoli of the lungs which act as surface tension reducing agents. The principal substance involved is dipalmitoyl lecithin. Studies of the lecithin content of amniotic fluid have shown a slow rise in concentration from the 26th to the 33rd week of gestation followed by a marked rise particularly after the 35th week. As the amniotic fluid concentration of another phospholipid, sphingomyelin, remains fairly static throughout pregnancy the lecithin-sphingomyelin ratio is used as an index of fetal pulmonary maturity. When the ratio is less than 1.5 there is a high risk of pulmonary complications but little or no risk if the ratio exceeds 2.

As pregnancy nears term and particularly during labour the fetus may become increasingly at risk and continuous or frequently repeated means of assessment are indicated. These require different techniques from those used in the earlier stages of pregnancy although estimation of maternal urinary oestriol excretion remains of great value throughout the last trimester of pregnancy.

Fetal heart rate. Auscultation of the fetal heart by listening over the mother's abdomen is the time-honoured method of measuring fetal health particularly during labour. Intermittent examination is satisfactory when all is going well and the rate remains between 120 and 160 per minute. In situations where the rate alters with uterine contractions it is important to know the relationship between the fetal heart rate and contractions. Both of these can be recorded by instruments such as the cardiotocograph shown in Fig. 4.14. When

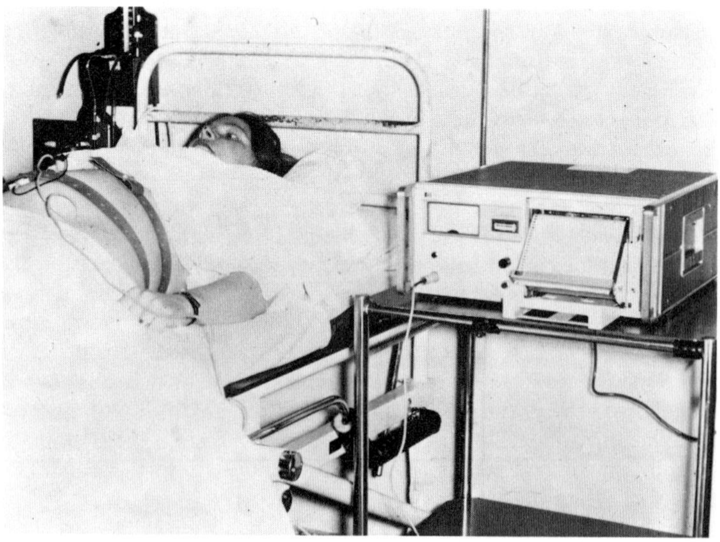

Figure 4.14 Cardiotocograph recording fetal heart rate and uterine contractions.

labour is sufficiently advanced a fetal electrocardiogram can be obtained with an electrode fixed to the presenting part of the fetus. Ultrasonic detectors employing the Doppler effect have also been used to record fetal heart rates.

Fetal blood pH. A different method of assessment involves measurement of fetal blood pH. Samples of capillary blood are taken after a small incision has been made in the fetal scalp. The fetal pH remains level until just before delivery when there is a fall to between 7.35 and 7.25. A fall to below 7.2 at this or an earlier stage of delivery indicates fetal acidosis due to accumulation of lactic acid. This occurs when the supply of oxygen to the fetus is inadequate and fetal pH can therefore be used as an indication of hypoxia provided that there is no cause for maternal acidosis. Repeated fetal scalp blood sampling gives an indication of the pattern of change in pH and aid in the decision as to immediate management. It is claimed that not only may the necessity for immediate caesarian section become clear but that more frequently it is shown that slowing of the fetal heart rate is not an indication of severe fetal distress.

Meconium staining. The other classical clinical sign of fetal distress is meconium staining in a vertex presentation. This sign can be used after rupture of the forewaters. Before the membranes rupture spontaneously or have been ruptured artificially meconium staining can be recognized by direct inspection with the amnioscope. In some centres particularly on the continent of Europe, amnioscopy is carried out routinely in mothers who are ten days past their expected date of delivery.

Fetal heart monitoring, scalp blood sampling and amnioscopy each have their proponents but insufficient time has elapsed to give a firm opinion as to which if any is the most dependable method of assessing fetal risk and the need for intervention in labour.

Disorders Affecting Fetal Growth

As indicated earlier in this chapter hereditary factors may produce abnormalities of the fetus and newborn infant and these are considered in Chapter 11 under the heading of Congenital Abnormalities. Consideration is also given in Chapter 11 to those acquired factors such as infection and drugs transmitted across the placenta which if occurring at the time of organogenesis may produce physical abnormality. Disorders of fetal growth can occur which interfere with the normal development of the fetus without producing abnormality of individual organs. These disorders will be considered here as their recognition and management may contribute to the birth of a healthy newborn infant.

MATERNAL FACTORS

The 1958 British Perinatal Mortality Survey has provided information about many of the antenatal factors which are likely to result in impaired fetal growth.

Socioeconomic factors. Many of these factors can be included under the general heading of socioeconomic and it is important to realize that improvement in the standard of living and of the health education of a community is of prime importance in maintaining fetal health and reducing perinatal mortality. This is a function of national and local government and is slow in producing an effect.

High-risk pregnancies. Of more immediate significance is the recognition of high-risk pregnancies in which the fetus is in greatest danger (Chap. 3). Such recognition requires an alertness to at-risk situations by doctors and midwives and a realization by pregnant women of the need for regular antenatal care. Such care can best be given by a team approach which in addition to doctors and midwives will involve medical social workers, dietitians and physiotherapists. The organization to achieve this is easier to arrange in large hospitals but these may be at a considerable distance from the patient's home. The amount of travelling involved may deter the mother from attending and the advantage of the improved service be lost. In high-risk pregnancies the importance of attendance at a fully staffed and equipped centre is such that the patient must be persuaded of this and given every help to encourage her to attend. Education in the advantages of antenatal care and the risks of avoiding it should begin at school age (Chap. 3).

The management of the fetus at risk is primarily in the hands of the obstetrician concerned but it is important that a close relationship be established between obstetric and paediatric teams so that each may be aware of the other's problems and the relative value of different possible means of management both antenatally and postnatally. Discussion about individual cases before and after delivery will help to evolve a common policy of action which should be kept under frequent review bearing in mind paediatric reports on the long-term follow-up of infants who have shown evidence of fetal growth disturbance or fetal distress. This subject is considered further in Chapter 21.

FURTHER READING

BATSTONE, G. F., BLAIR, A. W. & SLATER, J. M. (1971). *A Handbook of Prenatal Paediatrics.* Aylesbury: Medical and Technical Publishing Co.

BRITISH JOURNAL OF HOSPITAL MEDICINE (1971). Fetal Health. Special issue.

BRITISH MEDICAL JOURNAL (1973). Perinatal therapeutics and toxicology. Leading article, i, 5–6.

BRITISH MEDICAL JOURNAL (1973). Smoking hazard to the fetus, i, 369–370.

BROCK, D. J. H. & SUTCLIFFE, R. G. (1972). Alpha-fetoprotein in the antenatal diagnosis of anencephaly and spina bifida. *Lancet*, ii, 197–199.

CAMPBELL, S. (1972). Ultrasound in obstetrics. *British Journal of Hospital Medicine*, **8**, 541–555.

EMERY, A. E. H. (1974). *Elements of Medical Genetics*, 3rd edn. Edinburgh: Livingstone.

EMERY, A. E. H. (1973). *Antenatal Diagnosis of Genetic Disease*. Edinburgh: Churchill Livingstone.

GLUCK, L., KULOVICH, M. V., BORER, R. C., BRENNER, P. H., ANDERSON, G. C. & SPELLACY, W. H. (1971). Diagnosis of the respiratory distress syndrome by amniocentesis. *American Journal of Obstetrics and Gynaecology*, **109,** 440–445.

OUNSTED, M. & OUNSTED, C. (1973). *On Fetal Growth Rate* (*Its Variations and Their Consequences*). *Clinics in Developmental Medicine No. 46*. London: Heinemann for Spastics International Medical Publications.

SMITHELLS, R. W. & SPEIDEL, B. D. (1971), Prenatal influences and prenatal diagnosis. *British Medical Journal*, iv, 105–108.

STANDING MEDICAL ADVISORY COMMITTEE (1972). *Human Genetics*. Prepared by the Standing Medical Advisory Committee for the Central Health Services Council, the Secretary of State for Social Services and the Secretary of State for Wales.

5

The Newborn

ADAPTATION TO THE EXTERNAL ENVIRONMENT

The idyllic state of the fetus *in utero* with its complete dependence on the mother contrasts strongly with the degree of independence required of the newborn infant. Between these two stages of life the fetus is subject to a degree of physical trauma and deprivation which would cause us grave concern were it to occur under other circumstances. That the great majority of us have survived this shattering experience without harm is the best evidence available of the ability of the fetus to adapt successfully to the external environment.

Such adaptation is not without its problems and the ease with which the fetus achieves its conversion to an independent existence depends to a considerable extent on the intrauterine development of the fetus and the course of labour. The systems principally involved at birth are the respiratory, the cardiovascular and the nervous systems. Later, digestive, renal and hepatic function are of more importance.

A study of adaptation to the external environment should begin with a consideration of fetal function *in utero*. Some aspects of this have already been mentioned in Chapter 4. Further attention will be paid here to those aspects of fetal development which are related to the establishment of respiration after birth.

Respiration

FETAL RESPIRATION

Study of the respiratory pattern of the human fetus *in utero* is not generally possible and information has to be acquired by indirect means or by analogy from animal experiments.

Fetal lambs. A great deal of experimental work carried out on lambs has enlarged our knowledge but left many questions still unanswered. It is now clear that the fetal lamb has irregular rhythmic respiratory movements which may be very fast but only small volumes of fluid are moved by them. The fetal lung is constantly producing a fluid which differs from amniotic fluid. It is this pulmonary fluid which moves, and amniotic fluid only enters the fetal lung under situations of stress when deep respiratory movements may be provoked because of severe fetal hypoxia. It has to be noted that there is a wide range of fetal blood-gas values in which such deeper respiratory movements are not triggered.

Fetal blood-gas exchange takes place in the placenta and is dependent on a good blood flow on both the maternal and fetal sides of the placenta. Even with satisfactory blood flows and normal maternal health fetal blood oxygen levels are well below those in maternal blood. This is partly due to the large requirement of the placenta for oxygen and partly to the relative imbalance of fetal and maternal blood flow in differing parts of the placenta resulting in an uneven blood-gas exchange. There is, however, a sufficient safety margin achieved by variations in blood flow through the placenta without change in heart rate to compensate for small rapid changes in blood-gas levels.

Fetal distress. Larger changes in fetal blood gases may be reflected in fetal tachycardia which is the first true sign of fetal distress and which may be sufficient to compensate for a temporary period of difficulty as may occur during a uterine contraction. More prolonged or more severe difficulty with progressive hypoxaemia of the fetus is commonly manifest as bradycardia and results in acidaemia. This sign of fetal distress is an indication that the adaptive processes in the fetus have been stretched to their limit. Since the introduction of continuous recording of fetal heart rate and its relation to uterine contraction and the use of fetal scalp blood samples for measurement of pH more has been learned about the significance of change in fetal heart rate and its relation to intrauterine hypoxia. Further refinements of present techniques should help to unravel some of the remaining problems related to fetal respiration.

Oxygen conservation. The cardiovascular system of the fetus is clearly closely involved in the regulation of fetal blood gases. Further adaptation to hypoxia may be achieved by selectively shutting down the circulation in parts of the body which are less important to fetal well being. Thus by vasoconstriction of the vessels supplying the limbs, lungs and abdominal organs blood flow and therefore oxygen uptake in these areas is reduced allowing more of the oxygen present to be made available to the heart and brain. Some of the lactic acid produced in the underperfused areas, where anaerobic glycolysis is taking place, returns to the central circulation and produces a metabolic acidosis even in the absence of markedly lowered oxygen levels in scalp vein blood. This oxygen conserving adaptation mechanism is of significance in relation to the establishment of regular respiration after birth and will be discussed later.

INITIATION OF RESPIRATION

Nervous system. Normal activity of the central and peripheral nervous system is essential to the establishment and maintenance of respiration after birth but appears to take little part in the maintenance or control of fetal respiration.

Chemoreceptors. Such control is mediated through the cardiovascular system in utero and is probably regulated by chemoreceptors in the aorta. Similar chemoreceptors in the carotid arteries appear to exercise control of the respiratory system after birth. It is possible that the carotid chemoreceptors become more sensitive to oxygen lack after delivery and trigger regular respiratory movements. Other probable stimulating factors are temperature change and tactile stimuli.

Peripheral stimuli. The fetus who is uniformly supported in a fluid environment *in utero* becomes after birth a weighted object, and nervous stimuli are produced at the points where his body is supported. From a warm draught-free environment he is ejected into a colder atmosphere with air currents which evaporate moisture from his skin producing a fall in temperature and the sensation of cold. Hypoxaemia, touch and cold are three of the stimuli which reach the brain and which stimulate the respiratory centre to discharge nerve impulses initiating movement of the diaphragm and other muscles involved in respiration.

LUNGS AND HEART

Pulmonary fluid. During the passage down the birth canal some of the fluid contained in the fetal lungs is expelled by pressure on the chest. Following onset of respiration the remainder of the fluid is absorbed by the lymphatic system of the lung.

Chest expansion. The muscular movement of the first breath increases the capacity of the chest and allows air to flow into the lungs as they too begin to expand.

Pulmonary blood flow. Changes also take place in the blood vessels with reduction in pulmonary vascular resistance and increase in pulmonary blood flow. These changes do not take place instantaneously but the healthy newborn will expand his pulmonary circulation to a degree which allows an adequate exchange of oxygen and carbon dioxide within a few minutes of birth. Further adaptation continues over the next few days and includes closure of the foramen ovale and the ductus arteriosus. The infant's blood volume will be augmented by transfusion of up to 90 ml of blood from the fetal side of the placenta unless this is prevented by early clamping of the cord or holding the infant above the level of the placenta before the cord is clamped. With cessation of the placental circulation the infant's systemic blood pressure rises.

Surfactant. The muscular movement required to take the first few breaths is very much in excess of that required for later regular respiration. Newborn infants are capable of producing negative intrathoracic pressures of the order of 40 to 70 cm of water but most infants achieve primary expansion of their lungs with negative pressures of the order of 15 to 25 cm of water. The surface tension produced by the film of fluid lining the alveoli would naturally cause the alveoli to collapse completely when air is allowed to escape in expiration were it not for the presence of surfactant, a substance which reduces surface tension. Surfactant is a phospholipid produced in the fetal lung as part of the pulmonary fluid. Because of its presence alveoli do not collapse completely once expanded and the lung maintains a residual capacity of the order of 15 to 30 ml per kg of body weight. After the high negative pressures required to initiate respiration lower pressures of about 4 cm of water are sufficient to maintain respiration.

Respiratory centre. In the healthy newborn infant the sensory stimuli and blood-gas alterations are sufficient to arouse in the brain motor impulses which produce the initial muscle movements required and air enters the alveoli. The centre of this reaction is the brain and any factor which depresses central nervous function will interfere with the onset of respiration. Although a falling oxygen tension and a rise in carbon dioxide tension at first stimulate the respiratory centre persistence of these trends leads to depression of function. An infant who has been chronically hypoxic during labour may be delivered with a respiratory centre which is already non-responsive and further falls in oxygen have no stimulating effect. Similarly if the infant's brain has been depressed by sedative drugs given to the mother or by injury during delivery it will fail to react to the stimuli reaching it after birth.

The airway. Other difficulties in establishing normal respiration may occur if the infant's airway is not clear of fluid when the first breath is taken. Aspiration of amniotic fluid, mucus, blood or meconium may occur and these may prevent air reaching some or even all of the alveoli. Abnormality of the motor nerves, the muscles of respiration and the thoracic cage may also cause problems. Several of these factors may be combined particularly in low birth-weight babies in whom there may be the added problem of deficiency of surfactant.

Anaerobic metabolism. The newborn infant fortunately retains for a short period after birth some metabolic pathways which allow it to withstand postnatal hypoxia for longer periods than would be tolerated by an older infant or child. This period is reduced in those infants who have been hypoxic before delivery. Anaerobic metabolism releases lactic acid, and infants who have to rely on anaerobic metabolism will develop a metabolic acidosis. The brain is the organ which is most likely to suffer damage during periods of hypoxia. In order to preserve an infant's future chance of normal development and happiness respiration must be established before brain damage occurs. Knowledge of the condition of the fetus prior to delivery is as essential to those who are to care for the infant at birth as is the ability to assess the state of the infant at the time of delivery.

Resuscitation

Preparation. Whereas the majority of infants achieve respiration spontaneously after birth, midwives and doctors who attend deliveries must be trained and equipped to resuscitate the infant who does not start to breathe or who after a few gasps stops breathing. It is convenient to have a resuscitation trolley, which should be kept in an easily accessible place which is well heated, free from draughts and well lit. In many labour wards a special bay is set aside for this purpose. At any delivery one person must accept responsibility for resuscitating the infant with or without the help of others. Who the person is matters less than that he or she should be experienced, know what they are going to do, how to do it and the risks involved. They should be present before delivery, aware of the progress of labour and the state of the fetus. The equipment available including means for keeping the infant warm should be checked.

Clearing the airway. Once the infant has been delivered time is of supreme importance and it is very useful to have a large clock indicating seconds and minutes which is started when the cord is clamped or ceases to pulsate. The face and nose are wiped clean as soon as the head is delivered, and when the trunk has been delivered the infant is received into a warm towel and the head is kept lower than the body and turned to one side to allow the pharyngeal fluids to escape. This can be helped by gentle aspiration of the pharynx using a disposable mucus extractor. Overzealous suction or excessive movement of the tubing in the infant's mouth may cause local injury to mucous membrane and create new problems rather than aiding resuscitation. If suction is provided mechanically the negative pressure should not exceed 50 cm of water. The stimulus of aspiration together with the stimulus provided by changes in temperature and blood gases are generally sufficient to institute respiration.

Oxygen. If the initial movements are poor and if the heart rate is slowing, oxygen should be given to the infant through a suitably sized face-mask or funnel or through a catheter passed into a nostril.

APGAR SCORE

These simple resuscitative procedures should have been completed within one minute of birth and the opportunity should then be taken to assess the infant's state more completely. The assessment is made on examination of the infant's respiratory movements, pulse rate, muscle tone, reaction to stimuli and colour. The assessment score originally introduced by Apgar has proved its value and is commonly employed (Table 5.1). By adding the scores of 0, 1 or 2 for each individual assessment a total score ranging from 0 to 10 is made. This score together with the time from birth at which it was made should be recorded for comparison with subsequent scored assessments should these become necessary. Either one or two minutes after delivery is suitable for the initial assessment.

Table 5.1 Apgar score sheet

Name..................	Date............		Age........	(min)
	0	1	2	Score
Heart rate	Absent	Below 100	Over 100	
Respiratory effort	Absent	Slow, irregular	Good, crying	
Muscle tone	Limp	Some flexion of extremities	Active movement	
Response to catheter	No response	Grimace	Cough or sneeze	
Colour	Blue Pale	Body pink, extremities blue	Completely pink	
			TOTAL	

Repeat assessment. Infants with Apgar scores in excess of 7 at 2 minutes are breathing satisfactorily and no assistance is required. Where the score is in the range of 4 to 7 further action is dictated by the infant's general condition and particularly his heart rate. If the rate is over 100 per min and not falling the simple measures discussed above should be repeated. The Apgar score should be repeated and if the score is falling the procedures described in the next paragraph should be instituted. Many infants with Apgar scores of 4 to 7 at 1 minute will show improvement over the next 3 or 4 minutes, and if the score is 7 or more by 5 minutes no further action is required.

ARTIFICIAL RESPIRATION

An infant with an initial Apgar score of less than 4 or a score that is falling towards this number is very unlikely to improve without further resuscitative measures. Laryngoscopy should be carried out immediately and the posterior pharynx aspirated. If this does not produce an immediate response with onset of normal respiration an endotracheal tube should be passed and intermittent positive pressure respiration (IPPR) using oxygen at a pressure limited to 30 cm water applied. This procedure is described in greater detail in Chapter 19. When the heart rate is above 100 per min, the infant pink and spontaneous respiration established, the endotracheal tube can be withdrawn.

Alkali. If there is evidence of metabolic acidosis antenatally from scalp vein sampling and if the infant does not achieve spontaneous respiration within one or two minutes of IPPR an umbilical venous catheter should be inserted (Chap. 19) and 5 to 10 ml of 8.4 per cent sodium bicarbonate solution given slowly intravenously. Failure to establish respiration following this indicates severe cerebral depression or a major cardiorespiratory disorder. If the infant can be maintained in a satisfactory state on IPPR this must be continued using an artificial ventilator where available. Arterial blood-gas studies will be essential to monitor progress (Chap. 19). Other investigations such as X-ray of chest must be arranged to exclude the possibility of diaphragmatic hernia, possible pneumothorax and to assess pulmonary aeration and cardiac size (Chap. 11).

HEAT LOSS

The risk of an infant losing heat in any involved resuscitative procedure is high and a very careful watch should be kept on skin and rectal or oesophageal temperature. Keeping the room temperature at or above 25°C helps but it is not sufficient to prevent hypothermia. Wrapping baby's trunk in foil reduces heat loss. Extra local heat is generally required and can be given by an overhead infrared heater, an electrically heated pad or warm water-bottles. Care must be taken to prevent skin burns. Heat loss may also occur during the transfer from labour ward to a nursery. The infant should be well wrapped or transferred in a heated, portable incubator.

DOMICILIARY DELIVERY

Ideally mothers booked for domiciliary delivery should include only those in whom there is confident expectation of normal delivery without need for resuscitation. Abnormalities occurring during pregnancy or the first stage of labour are in general an indication for arranging hospital delivery rather than for planning major resuscitative procedures in the home. Midwives and doctors attending domiciliary deliveries must be equipped and trained to deal with unexpected problems of resuscitation. This can and should include the ability to pass an endotracheal tube, and those concerned with domiciliary midwifery should be strongly encouraged to undergo training in this technique. Intermittent positive pressure can be supplied from a hand pump or by blowing with the cheeks rather than the lungs. If an endotracheal tube has not been passed a Guedel airway can be used.

Emergency situations. Situations can and do arise when delivery occurs in places in which there are no facilities for resuscitation. Bearing in mind the general principles of the methods already discussed all but the most severly hypoxic infants can be resuscitated. Drainage of fluids from the mouth is encouraged by positioning the infant and holding open the lower angle of the mouth with a finger. If spontaneous respiration does not occur mouth to nose respiration should be started (Chap. 19). One finger of the hand supporting the infant's chest is used to feel the apex beat and to provide an indication as to the infant's response.

Chemical stimulants. No mention has been made so far of the use of chemical stimulants. This subject has been left to the end because it plays a very minor part in resuscitative procedures. Apart from the use of nalorphine hydrobromide (Lethidrone) 1 mg intravenously in infants who appear drowsy as the result of pethidine or morphine having been given to the mother, stimulant drugs have not proved useful mainly because the effective dose is very close to the dose which will provoke convulsions. For those infants in whom respiration ceases shortly after it has begun some advocate the use of vanillic acid diethylamide (Vandid) one drop of the solution on the infant's tongue. As many such infants have metabolic acidosis the use of a chemical CNS stimulant may cloud the necessity for correction of the biochemical abnormality and is not recommended.

PROGNOSIS

The prognosis of infants who require resuscitation at birth depends primarily on the underlying condition which has caused delay in onset of respiration. If this should be brain injury or chronic prenatal hypoxia the prognosis is not so satisfactory as in those infants where there has been short-term hypoxia or depression of a normal brain by drugs. It is therefore dangerous to generalize about prognosis but from what has been said it follows that a short episode of perinatal hypoxia is seldom a cause of neurological damage whereas neurological damage may well be a cause of delayed onset of respiration.

Temperature Control

Reference has already been made on many occasions to the liability of the newborn infant to lose heat. This applies particularly to those parts of the world where the air temperature is normally below 30°C. In climates where the temperature rises above 30°C much higher temperatures may occur indoors and under such circumstances newborn infants may become overheated and their body temperature rises. Recognition of the difficulty which infants have in maintaining a stable temperature is essential to understanding the management of the newborn and particularly of the preterm infant.

HEAT LOSS

Heat is lost from the skin by radiation, convection, evaporation and conduction. Evaporation of fluid on the skin is most marked where there is movement of air across the wet infant. Exposure of the infant increases all these channels of heat loss. The greater proportional surface area of the small infant and the relative absence of the insulating layer of fat in the preterm infant all contribute to heat loss. As skin temperature falls a gradient is established and heat will then be lost from the deeper tissues and the infant's central or core temperature will fall. The infant is capable of producing extra heat in response to an initial small fall in temperature but the capacity for heat production is quickly overtaken by the even greater liability to heat loss. A marked fall in core temperature is associated with a fall in metabolic activity, reduction of heat production and a further fall in body temperature. Thus a vicious circle is set up. Eventually a point of no return is reached and the infant will die.

HEAT PRODUCTION

The infant produces heat by metabolic activity in the muscles and elsewhere. The newborn, however, is not able to shiver and increase heat production by this method when chilling occurs.

Brown fat. An alternative source of heat is, however, available in the form of catabolism of brown fat. Brown fat is present in the newborn between the shoulder blades, behind the sternum, in the neck and around the kidneys and suprarenal glands. The chief function of these collections of fat is to supply a source of fuel which the infant can utilize quickly when extra heat is required.

Use of calories. It is important to remember that heat production is dependent on a regular source of calories. This is normally the diet. If any infant's temperature falls an increasing proportion of the calories contained in the diet will have to be used for heat production and the infant may not have sufficient calories left for normal growth. Failure to gain weight is therefore an effect of heat loss followed by the need for increased heat production.

NEUTRAL THERMAL ENVIRONMENT

There is a relatively narrow range of environmental temperature which will allow the exposed newborn infant to maintain a constant temperature without diverting extra calories to heat production. This range is called the neutral thermal environment. Clothing the infant or covering it with a heat reflecting shield will lower the neutral thermal environment but may reduce access and prevent full observation. In each individual situation a suitable compromise has to be reached. For the small preterm infant who requires constant observation a special environment such as an incubator is used. It must not be forgotten, however, that radiation loss continues in an incubator and that frequent opening of the side ports allows movement of air and cooling by convection and evaporation. The nursing aspects of this important subject are considered further in Chapters 6, 9 and 10.

Digestion

The newborn infant cannot thrive unless supplied with calories, essential amino acids, vitamins and certain trace elements. Whereas these were all supplied transplacentally *in utero* in a predigested form the newborn has to learn to cope with a diet which requires a considerable amount of digestion before its contents can be absorbed and utilized.

Maturation of enzymes. The enzyme systems required for this digestion have not been required *in utero* and are not all fully prepared in the baby at birth. Maturation of function occurs within the first few days but care has to be taken not to overload the infant's digestive capacity during the process. Different enzymes respond at different rates and in particular if would seem probable that the disaccharidases, the sugar-splitting enzymes, can be overloaded in the first week of life. The evidence with regard to fats is difficult to interpret. Infants appear to split fats satisfactorily but to have difficulty in absorbing split fats. Human milk fat causes the least difficulty. The result of overload is generally evident as diarrhoea and a sore bottom. Acid end products are often released in the bowel and may be absorbed producing a metabolic acidosis.

Control of diet. Human breast milk is least likely to produce these disturbances which occur more commonly with cow's milk preparations. The modifications of cow's milk discussed in Chapter 8 have reduced digestive disturbances considerably but problems are arising again with the proven advantage of feeding preterm infants early and with larger volumes than were previously used. Current feeding regimes tax the digestive systems of the newborn to or beyond their limit of endurance.

Elimination

The elimination of waste products involves the bowel, the liver, the kidneys and the lungs. In the absence of hypoxia, hypoglycaemia and hypothermia even the smallest newborn is capable of evacuating normal meconium, stool and urine provided that there is no mechanical obstruction. Elimination of CO_2 from the lungs is a function of the respiratory and cardiovascular systems which has already been discussed. The physiological changes occurring in the liver and kidney are of vital importance to the infant and to our care of the newborn.

HEPATIC FUNCTION

Apart from its importance as a biochemical factory in which new proteins and other substances necessary for tissue growth are prepared the liver has a major part to play in the elimination of toxic products of body metabolism. Several products may share the same detoxification process and may therefore compete with one another for priority in attention if the process is overloaded.

Conjugation. Several substances including some drugs can only be excreted by the liver after they have been joined to another substance such as glucuronic acid, a reaction called conjugation. Bilirubin is a typical toxic end product which can be rendered non-toxic by conjugation with glucuronic acid to form bilirubin diglucuronide. Conjugation of bilirubin which is only soluble in fat solvents produces the water soluble bilirubin diglucuronide which is not harmful to tissues and which can be excreted in the bile. The conjugation is catalysed by the enzyme glucuronyl transferase. For the first few days of life this enzyme is not present in adequate amounts and the liver is not capable of dealing with all the bilirubin presented to it and jaundice becomes evident (Chap. 14).

Synthesis. The ability of the liver to produce proteins may be stretched beyond its limits particularly in the presence of infection or other cause of increased tissue breakdown or protein loss in the newborn period. Should the serum protein level fall sufficiently oedema will occur. The production of some proteins such as prothrombin is dependent upon an adequate dietary supply of a precursor, in this case vitamin K. Hypoxia, hypoglycaemia or infection will all reduce liver activity and accentuate any of the problems mentioned.

Albumin. Substances such as bilirubin which are not water-soluble before conjugation have to be attached to albumin to allow their transport in plasma. Albumin binding sites are limited and other substances compete for the available sites. A fall in blood pH renders bilirubin less tightly bound to albumin and more liable to pass into tissues such as the brain where it can cause cell death. The ability of the liver to provide albumin is therefore of importance in the prehepatic stage of bilirubin metabolism.

RENAL FUNCTION

The lower rate of glomerular filtration found in the newborn is mainly due to high vascular resistance which reduces renal blood flow. A progressive decrease in intrarenal vascular resistance during the first few weeks of life allows greater blood flow and increased filtration.

Solute load. At birth the renal cortex is relatively underdeveloped and the juxtamedullary nephrons have a higher blood flow than the cortical nephrons. The reduction in glomerular filtration rate prevents overloading of the proximal tubules whose function is immature at birth. As a result of these differing aspects of renal function the newborn's kidney is poorly suited to excrete a saline load but is better able to conserve sodium and water although the capacity to concentrate the urine is limited. Difficulty in excretion of ammonium compounds and titrable acid impairs the capacity to correct metabolic acidosis which occurs readily in the newborn particularly in preterm infants.

Maturation. The capacity of the kidney to mature after birth does not appear to be influenced by preterm delivery and is related to the load presented to it. Ninety-five per cent of healthy infants will pass urine within 24 hours of delivery. Urine output is of the order of 20 to 35 ml per day in the first two or three days of life while fluid intake remains low and rises to 100 to 200 ml per day by the end of the first week.

Lack of reserve. In spite of the limitations of renal function discussed above the kidneys of the newborn are almost always able to maintain a satisfactory state of health and growth. It is under conditions of dietary overload, infection or other stresses that the lack of reserve renal function becomes of major significance.

ERYTHROPOIESIS

The high number of red blood cells (5.5×10^6 per mm^3) and the high level of haemoglobin (Hb) (17 g per 100 ml) necessary for adequate oxygenation of the fetus are not required after birth with the establishment of a more efficient mechanism of breathing using the lungs.

Physiological anaemia. After a temporary rise in the first day or two of life due to shift of plasma to the extravascular compartment there is a steady fall in both the red cell count and the haemoglobin. This is due to a sharp reduction in erythropoiesis during the first nine days of life followed by a slow gradual recovery which is not complete until the third month of life. The associated fall in haemoglobin (to 11 g per 100 ml) is described as physiological anaemia of the newborn. In preterm infants the fall is more marked and the haemoglobin may be only 7 g per 100 ml by the eighth or ninth week. Although sharing a common cause this is often called anaemia of prematurity. Such anaemias are not preventable by giving iron supplements from birth but added iron may be useful after the second month of life.

White blood cells. The white blood cells also undergo considerable change during the first few days of life and these changes make interpretation of white cell counts difficult at this age. In general neutrophils rise from about 8000 per mm^3 at birth to around 13 000 per mm^3 at 20 hours and then fall to about 4000 per mm^3 by 72 hours and remain at this level. Lymphocytes fall from about 6000 per mm^3 at birth to 3000 per mm^3 at 72 hours and then rise slowly to 6000 per mm^3 by 10 days.

FURTHER READING

AVERY, M. E. (1968). Normal development and physiology of the fetal and neonatal lung. In *The Lung and Its Disorders in the Newborn Infant*. Philadelphia: Saunders.

DAWES, G. S. (1971). Fetal and neonatal respiration. In *Recent Advances in Paediatrics*, 4th edn. Edited by D. Gairdner and D. Hull. London: Churchill.

HEY, E. (1971). The care of babies in incubators. The physics and physiology of temperature control. In *Recent Advances in Paediatrics*, 4th edn. Edited by D. Gairdner and D. Hull. London: Churchill.

SPITZER, A. (1971). Renal physiology—impact of recent developments on clinical nephrology. *Pediatric Clinics of North America*, **18**, 337.

6

Nursing Care of the Healthy Newborn

The newborn infant is entirely dependent on the nursing care provided by his mother or by the attendant midwife. Nursing staff have a difficult role to play as they must instruct and encourage the infant's mother to look after her infant herself. At the same time they must be ready to act as a substitute mother should the mother be too ill to look after her own infant or be inefficient at doing so. With their training and experience many midwives must feel superior in skill to the infant's own mother. They may feel that they are better qualified to care for a baby than is his own mother. This attitude may be resented by the mother and it is essential that midwives understand the situation and appreciate the mother's deep emotional attachment to her baby. Mothers of very small infants being nursed in incubators feel isolated and useless and this may affect their whole attitude to their child in the future. The special problems relating to the nursing of low birth-weight infants are discussed in Chapter 10.

THE MOTHERING INSTINCT

The mother–baby relationship must be considered before dealing with the physical needs of the newly born infant. The mothering instinct is part of all female make-up whether accepted or denied, and during the nine months of pregnancy and immediately following delivery it is dominant. All thought is centred around the baby's safety and physical requirements. Nearly all mothers have an intuitive knowledge about babies but they may 'mother' their babies in their own individual way. Separation of the mother and child at birth especially in hospital should be avoided as far as possible. The newly delivered mother must be given time to fondle and handle her baby shortly after birth in the delivery room.

The age-old practice of putting the newly born baby to the breast in the delivery room has unfortunately largely fallen into disuse. The sucking reflex at this time is very good and in fact may not be so good again for a few days. This early success encourages the mother and helps to establish an immediate vital relationship with her baby.

The rooming-in system of nursing the mother and baby side by side is practised widely especially in newly built hospitals. Mother and baby are not separated and the mother can watch over her baby, pick him up, nurse him and feed him when he demands it. It is, however, essential to ensure that the new mother has sufficient rest during the day and sleep at night. Nursery accommodation should be available so that the infant can be removed if he is disturbing his mother.

Nursery Staffing

Neonatal nursing demands a very high standard of nursing care. Those involved must have keen powers of observation, alertness and a readiness to make quick decisions. The neonatal nurse must have a high sense of responsibility and a devotion to her task. Not all nurses are suited for this type of work particularly as the attributes already mentioned must be coupled with gentleness and extreme patience. The use of monitors, respirators and other electrical equipment calls for a type of expertise which was not formerly expected of nurses. Training in midwifery or in general children's nursing or a combination of these is not sufficient in itself to qualify a nurse for work in special care nurseries or neonatal intensive therapy units, and further special training is required. Courses in neonatal nursing are available in many parts of the country but there is at present no national standard set and no national certificate is issued.

Midwives. Student midwives receive theoretical and practical education in the care of the newborn which is part of the curriculum in the midwifery training course. Midwives are therefore particularly well suited for further training in nursing in special-care baby units. Trained midwives in maternity departments often work in nurseries as part of their further postcertificate education. In order to maintain a continuing high standard of care it is essential that the senior nursing staff in a nursery should be appointed to posts in the nurseries and not be part of a circulating pool of trained staff. In each nursery there should be sufficient trained permanent staff to ensure that at least one senior member is on duty at all times of the day and night.

Nursery nurses. The recommendations of the expert group on special care for babies with regard to staffing ratios has already been quoted in Chapter 2. Difficulties may arise in achieving the high nurse-to-patient ratios advised if reliance is placed on employing only trained midwives to fill these places. The skills of nursery nurses are suitable for some of the duties in maternity department nurseries after in-service training.

Registered nurses, particularly those with a children's nursing certificate, can fill most of the posts in a special care nursery. The wider experience of the midwife is, however, required for the more senior posts.

STAFF–PATIENT RATIO

For administrative purposes within the NHS normal babies are not counted as occupying beds whereas babies who are classified as 'sick' do count as occupying beds. An allocation of beds for 'sick babies' is made in each maternity unit and such beds or cots generally form a special care nursery. Because of this difference in administrative attitude staff–patient ratios have to be considered in relation to special care nurseries separately from the care of well babies. In many hospitals the same nursing staff may be looking after both groups of babies and wide differences in staff-to-patient ratios therefore appear to occur. The report of the expert group on special care for babies comments that nurse staffing ratios should be flexible ranging between 1 to 1.5 nurses per cot in special care nurseries, rising to 3 nurses per cot in intensive care nurseries. These recommendations are based on the assumption that an allocation of 4.5 nurses is required to keep one nurse on duty throughout the 24 hours. As already mentioned in Chapter 2 the expert group also made recommendations about the ratio of experienced nurses to those still training in special care for babies.

LIAISON

The role of the family doctor and health visitor is of prime importance and with the integration of the Health Service under Area Health Boards in 1974 many of the remaining barriers of different employing authorities and regulations will be swept away. The liaison health visitor is now a fully established link between a hospital and the community. She is often attached to a local group practice and has a wide knowledge of her patients and their home problems. She may visit the mothers and babies herself in the wards and obtain additional information from the ward sister, house officer and the paediatrician. Any special problems are discussed and the health visitor imparts this information to her colleagues if this particular patient is outwith her own area. The family doctor also gains a great deal from this liaison through the group practice attachment. The health visitor and family doctor may also be invited to take part in case discussions within the obstetric department.

Nursing Function

As part of their training student midwives will spend some time working in a special care nursery but the majority of their training and experience will concern the well baby and his mother. Contact with mother may have been made first in the antenatal clinic and it is a pleasure for both the expectant mother and the midwife to know each other before mother is admitted to the labour ward.

Nursing care of the mother and baby in the puerperium is radically different from the role of the nurse in the general field. The vast majority of newly delivered mothers are not ill and within a few days are ambulant and independent. There is minimal patient dependency and sometimes the new student midwife finds this a situation which is difficult to accept and which requires a different attitude on her part. The new mother requires a great deal of support and advice in coping with her baby and adjusting her emotional feelings. She requires very deep human understanding, sympathy and professional skill. The value of an experienced sister midwife at this time is tremendous, working closely with the hospital and family doctor.

DELIVERY ROOM

The design and construction of delivery rooms often fail to take into account the special requirements of the newborn infant. In particular the air temperature may fluctuate and air currents occur. Movement of air over the wet skin of a newborn infant causes evaporation and loss of heat even when the air itself is warm. A cold draught is naturally even more likely to cool the baby. Placing a newborn infant under the warm-air intake of an air-conditioned room may cause as much heat loss from evaporation as heat gain from the warmth of the air. Delivery rooms must be kept warm and the temperature should never fall below 25°C and preferably should be nearer 30°C. Mothers and staff may feel uncomfortable in the higher range of temperature quoted, and if a temperature about 25°C is not tolerable it is essential that the area where the baby will be resuscitated has an extra source of heat such as an infrared heater. The heater can be a fixture or on a mobile trolley so that its position can be changed (Fig. 6.1).

Preparation for delivery. Before delivery takes place the cot and blankets into which baby is to be placed should be warmed and extra heat supplied if necessary. The resuscitation equipment is checked. This should include the following:

- A clock showing minutes and seconds
- Mucus extractors
- Source of suction
- Cotton-wool balls (sterile)
- Face-mask and bag
- Oxygen supply
- Endotracheal tubes
- Infant laryngoscope
- Syringe and needles
- Ampoules of 8.4 per cent sodium bicarbonate.

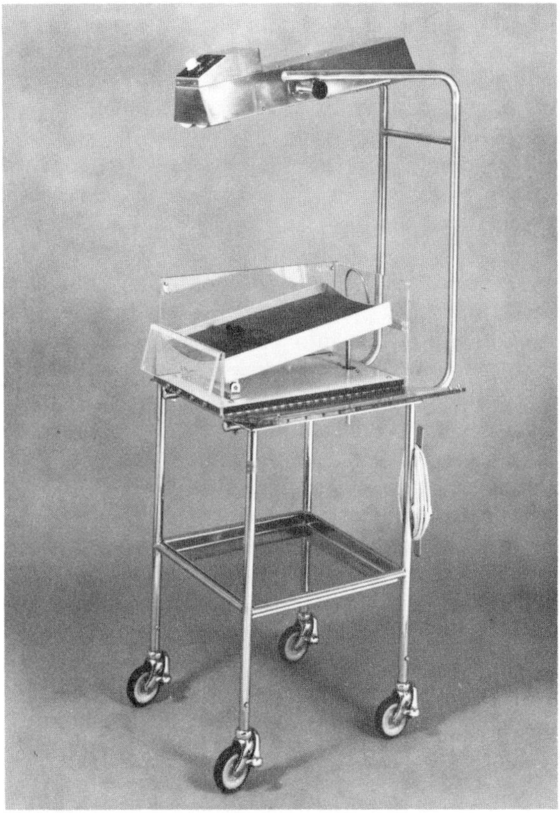

Figure 6.1 Infant resuscitation cot with warmer. (Photograph by courtesy of A. C. Daniels & Co.)

Delivery. When the baby's head is delivered the midwife should quickly feel for the umbilical cord which may be round the baby's neck. It may be possible to slip the loop of cord over the baby's head or down over the anterior shoulder as it is being delivered. The cord should only be clamped and cut before delivery if it is very thin, and thus liable to rupture, or very tight or looped more than once around the neck in which case it could strangulate the baby during birth. The baby's oxygen supply is completely cut off when the cord is prematurely cut and subsequent delay in delivery of the shoulders could result in anoxia and stillbirth. The midwife swabs the eyes using separate large, dry sterile cotton-wool balls to remove any secretions from the birth canal containing pathogenic organisms. There are different schools of thought regarding this procedure and some do not approve of wiping the eye-lids at birth at all. Others advocate the use of prophylactic eye drops such as silver nitrate 1 per cent or sulphacetamide drops 10 per cent (Albucid) immediately following birth. While waiting for rotation of the shoulders external mucus may be wiped from the nose and mouth with a sterile gauze swab.

Suction. When the baby is completely born he is held with the head tilted down for a few moments to allow drainage of fluid and mucus from the trachea and pharynx. This mucus should be aspirated by the midwife from the baby's mouth. The healthy baby cries at once and no further treatment is required. If the mouth still contains secretions further suction of mucus should be carried out to prevent mucus and liquor amnii being inhaled into the bronchi and causing alveolar collapse and pneumonia. Should the airway be completely obstructed serious hypoxia will result. Mucus extraction must therefore receive priority over other procedures at this time. A simple mouth-operated mucus extractor with a trap can be used and there are several disposable varieties on the market which are very effective (Fig. 6.2). Various types of mechanical suction apparatus are also available. The mucus extractor must be directed over the dorsum of the tongue into the pharynx for not more than 5 cm. Gentleness must be exercised to avoid trauma to the delicate lining of the nasopharynx.

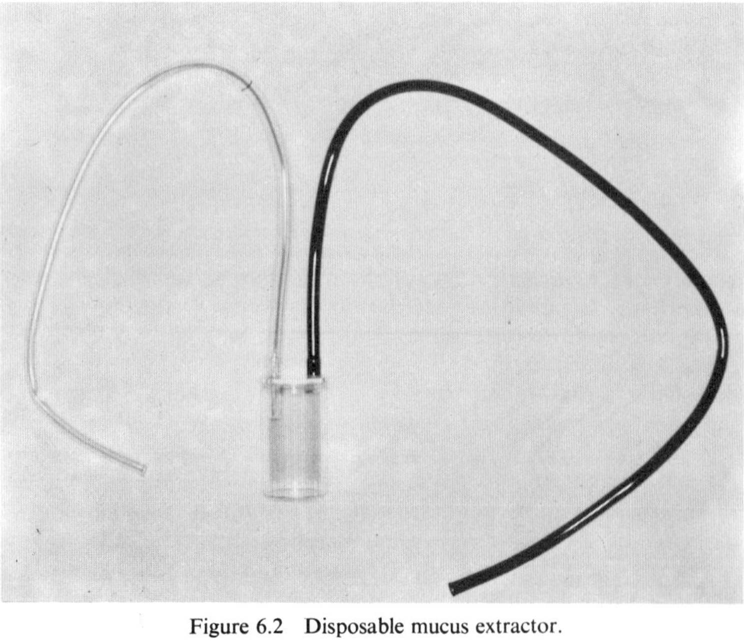

Figure 6.2 Disposable mucus extractor.

Resuscitation was discussed more fully in Chapter 5.

Assessment at birth. Once baby has been delivered an immediate assessment of his general condition should be carried out paying particular attention to the interval between delivery and the onset of regular respiration. A stop-watch or clock is essential equipment in a delivery room. This should be started as soon as the head and trunk have been delivered. The method of assessment originally devised by Apgar and named after her is widely used and has proved its value (Chap. 5). Each of five signs are given a score of 0, 1 or 2, as was shown in Table 5.1, and the scores for each sign added to give a possible total of 10. Where staffing permits, the score should be assessed at 1 minute and again at either 3 or 5 minutes depending on the condition of the infant. A score of 8 to 10 indicates satisfactory respiration. With a score of 4 to 7 a moderate degree of hypoxia or cerebral depression is likely to be present. When the score is 3 or lower a severe degree of hypoxia and/or cerebral depression is present and immediate action is called for.

Resuscitation. At every delivery, before the infant is born, one member of the team should be given responsibility for the resuscitation of the infant. If the person responsible is a midwife who has not been trained in the passage of an endotracheal tube she should know how to give air or oxygen by a bag and mask and understand the indications for calling for further help. These indications would be, an infant with an Apgar score of three or less at any stage, an infant in whom the Apgar score was falling in spite of oxygen administered by face mask and an infant where the Apgar score had not reached 8 by five minutes. Should delivery take place as an emergency in a place where no resuscitative equipment is available mouth to nose respiration should be used if artificial resuscitation is required (Chap. 19).

The cord. The time at which the cord is cut varies according to the practice of the obstetrician concerned. Delay in cutting the cord until pulsation has ceased allows the infant to receive a transfusion of placental blood provided that the infant is not held above the level of the placenta. The cord is clamped with Spencer Wells artery forceps 5 cm from the umbilicus. A second clamp is applied 6 cm from the umbilicus and the cord divided between the two forceps. The baby is received into a warm sterile towel and carefully dried. The towel is then discarded and the baby is wrapped in a fresh, warm towel and placed in the cot. The cord is finally occluded by one of three methods.

Sterile disposable plastic cord clamps are applied about 1 cm from the umbilical skin and closed by pressure with the fingers. The cord is then cut approximately 1 cm beyond the clamp to prevent it slipping off. The clamp may be removed after 48 hours but in many instances it is left on until the cord separates (Fig. 6.3).

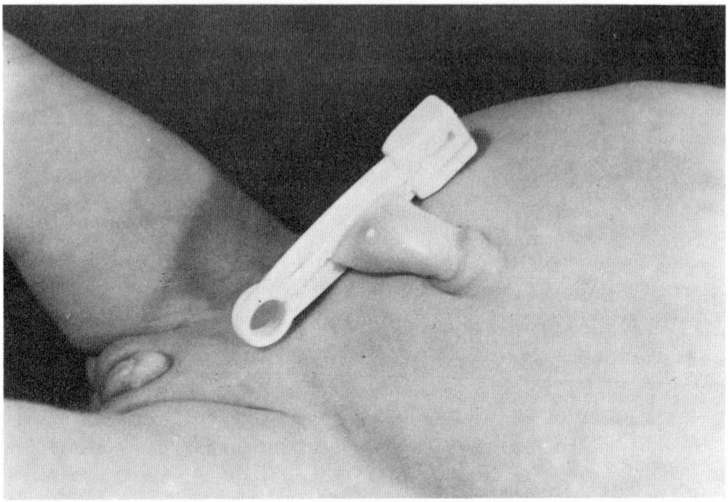

Figure 6.3 Disposable cord clamp.

Rubber bands which are placed around the cord by the use of forceps and tape. It is useful to have a sterile pack containing the following ready for use: rubber bands size 28, fine tape about 15 cm long, straight Spencer Wells forceps. The pack containing the above equipment is opened. The middle of the tape is clipped at the point of the forceps and one half laid along the length of the forceps. The rubber band is then looped round the tape and forceps four times just below the point of the forceps. The tape is then released from the end of the forceps and the ends approximated. The tape is now in position through the folds of rubber band. The forceps with the rubber band *in situ* are applied about 4 cm from the umbilicus. The forceps already on the cord are removed. Steady traction is applied to the tape and the rubber band is drawn over the cord stump to within 1 cm of the umbilical skin (Fig. 6.4). The excess cord is cut between the rubber bands and the forceps and the tape removed and the procedure is completed. As with the clamp, the rubber band may be removed after 48 hours if the cord has shrivelled satisfactorily.

Ligation. The cord is clamped and cut 5 cm from the umbilicus. Ligatures made of nylon material which is very strong and suitable are available. The first sterile ligature is placed 2.5 cm from the umbilicus and the second ligature between the umbilicus and the first

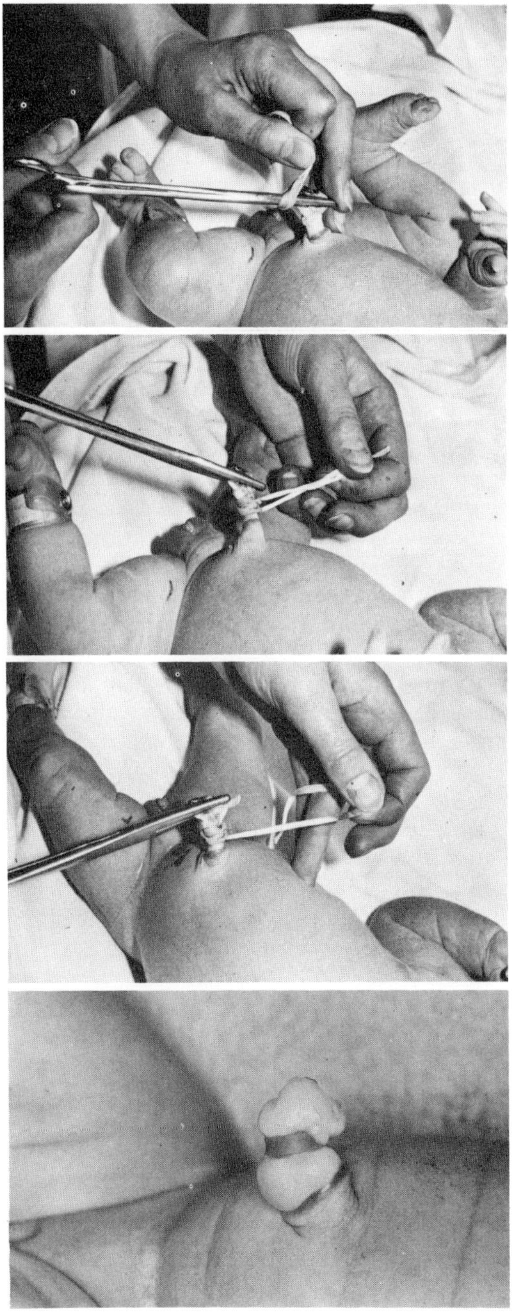

(a)

(b)

(c)

(d)

Figure 6.4 Stages in the application of a rubber band to the cord.

ligature. The excess cord is cut between the first ligature and the forceps and as a precaution against haemorrhage the forceps may be reapplied to the end of the cord.

Rubber bands and umbilical clamps provide continued pressure as the Wharton's jelly shrinks and thus reduce the possibility of haemorrhage. They are thus potentially safer than ligatures.

EXAMINATION OF THE BABY

A preliminary examination of the baby should be carried out in the delivery room to establish the infant's sex, to look for any congenital abnormality of form and to assess any abnormality of function which requires immediate treatment. The more detailed examination of the baby which takes place during the first 24 hours of life is described in Chapter 7.

In the delivery room the sex of the baby will be decided following an inspection of the external genitalia. Should the genitalia appear in any way abnormal no statement about the baby's sex should be given to the mother by the midwife until baby has been examined by an experienced doctor. Similarly should the midwife find any abnormality of form or function medical advice should be sought.

Identification of the baby. It is most important that an entirely dependable system of identifying each baby be operated in a maternity unit and that this be applied as soon as possible after birth in the presence of the baby's mother. It must be completed before the infant leaves the delivery room. One of the most commonly used methods is to write the infant's surname and date and time of birth on a small pink or blue card according to sex. The card is then inserted into a transparent bracelet which is clipped round the infant's wrist or ankle (Fig. 6.5). As the special press stud closing such bracelets cannot be opened the bracelet can only be removed by cutting it off.

Other methods of identification such as taking finger or footprints are popular in some parts of the world.

Apart from those who have been anaesthetized for operative deliveries most mothers are conscious and well enough to be shown their baby and check the identification label and sex prior to being transferred to the ward from the delivery room. The husband is very often now present with his wife and he can also participate in this. This is a most reassuring and satisfying experience for both parents. On discharge from hospital the label is removed on the doorstep of the nursery by the Nursery Sister, checked by the mother and given to her for safe keeping.

Records. It is essential that accurate records are made throughout labour, so that the complete record of antenatal care, labour and the immediate postdelivery phase can be passed on to staff of the

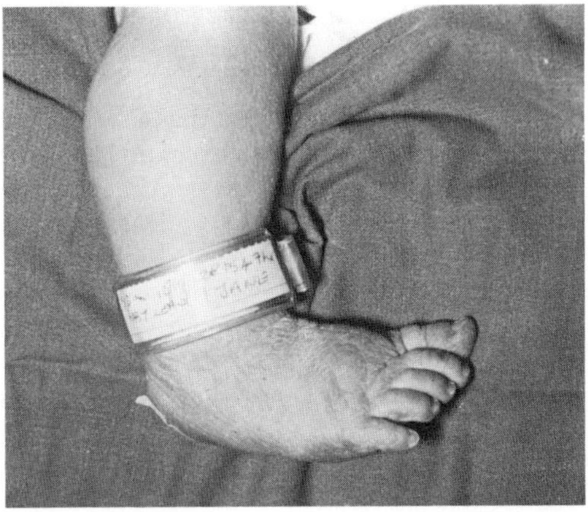

Figure 6.5 Name band.

neonatal nursery when the baby is transferred. In addition to details of identification the following are of special note:

Type of delivery
Drugs given to mother in labour
Condition of baby at birth, Apgar score, resuscitative measures and drugs given.

Care after resuscitation. Once respiration is satisfactorily established, the preliminary brief examination has been completed and the identification bracelet applied, mother, if well, should be given an opportunity to handle her infant. As will be mentioned in Chapter 7 mother may like to watch her baby being examined and wish to examine him herself. She will certainly wish to cuddle her baby and should be allowed to put him to the breast should she wish to do so. During this period of mothering a midwife should be present to make sure that the infant is not allowed to become cold and to remove him should mother fall asleep.

If the delivery room is not as warm as the recommended temperature of 25°C it is necessary to move the baby to a warmer environment as soon as possible. Baby is placed in a cot which has been prepared previously and kept warm. The cot is labelled and the record on the cot label checked with the record on baby's bracelet in the presence of another nurse. Cot and baby are then transferred to a specially heated admission area which should be kept at 30°C. Infants in this nursery should be observed closely with particular reference to possible aspiration of mucus. The umbilical cord must be carefully checked for bleeding at least $\frac{1}{2}$ hourly during the first 6 hours and hourly until the end of 12 hours. The baby is allowed to rest following delivery for approximately 1 to 2 hours prior to further examination, weighing and initial cleansing. The temperature must be checked with a low-reading thermometer per rectum and the skin temperature taken in the groin to ensure that the baby is maintaining his body heat. The rectal temperature should be 37.0°C. A skin temperature which is more than 0.5°C lower than the rectal temperature is a sign of heat loss. Additional heat should be applied to the baby if there is more than 1°C of difference between the two recordings. There is a risk of further reduction in temperature if the baby is exposed and handled and an additional source of heat should be available if the infant has to be undressed.

Weight and length. The baby's weight must be very carefully recorded and checked by a second midwife as great anxiety and distress can be caused by an error. Length must be measured accurately and again it is necessary to have a second midwife present to extend the baby's trunk and limbs fully and check the measurement (Chap. 7).

Initial cleansing. After birth the baby is frequently covered with vernix caseosa, patches of blood and possibly meconium or other natural discharges. If not cleaned these become smelly and it is therefore customary for social reasons to clean the newborn baby. Such cleansing, however, requires exposure and handling during which heat loss will readily occur unless suitable precautions are taken. The initial cleansing should not be carried out until the baby has settled after the upset of delivery and has a normal and stable temperature. An interval of at least 1 or 2 hours after birth should elapse before the initial cleansing. The room used must be at 30°C and free from draughts. Cleansing can be carried out in the cot and does not involve immersion of the baby in water as in subsequent bathing. Sterile cotton wool swabs are used to wipe off the vernix. If necessary the swabs can be moistened in sterile water or a diluted solution of an antiseptic detergent such as pHisoHex. After use the pHisoHex should be rinsed off the skin. Prolonged use of pHisoHex has potential dangers but the benefit of the short-term use in preventing staphylococcal skin infection far outweighs the theoretical risk. In the initial as in subsequent cleansing special attention should be paid to the skin creases.

After cleansing, the cord should be treated with an antiseptic such as 0.5 per cent hibitane in 70 per cent surgical spirit. The buttocks may be coated with an emollient cream to make subsequent removal of meconium easier. The temperature should be checked.

Clothing. The nurseries and wards should be maintained at a temperature of at least 20°C and, therefore clothing for baby can be kept to a minimum. Clothes should be simple and boilable. The baby at all times must be able to move freely without constriction of tight wrappings. There is now a complete range of disposable baby clothes but they are not yet entirely satisfactory and are expensive to use. Disposable napkins are probably the only disposable items which are widely used and proving to be satisfactory. Vests with envelope shoulders allow greater ease in dressing the baby. Gowns should be short and fasten with tape down the back. Terry towelling napkins if in plentiful supply are excellent but they must be properly laundered. Mitten and bootees must also be made of boilable material and have carefully finished inside seams. When the inside seam is left unstitched there is a danger of loose threads being wound round the fingers and toes. Cases of gangrene have been reported following constriction of fingers by loose threads. Although there is a complete range of disposable bed linen these items are expensive and it is doubtful if they will ever be as efficient as the conventional linen. Blankets made from cotton cellular material can be boiled and laundered easily. Pillows are not used in neonatal nurseries.

Cots. A variety of patterns of cots are now available. The more expensive have a metal supporting frame on castors with cupboard space for all baby's toilet requirements and shelves for use during nursing procedures. On top of these a transparent plastic bassinet can be placed flat or at preset angles of tilt. Such cots are designed to contain all the baby's linen and bathing requirements. A typical example is shown in Figure 6.6. Simpler cots may have a tubular metal frame supporting a perspex or canvas bassinet. Some such cots have a small storage box at one end. The main advantages of these cots are their relative cheapness and the smaller space which they occupy. When not in use the frame of some can be folded up. They are therefore easy to transport. Each type of cot will require a mattress which should be covered in a waterproof washable material. The cot and mattress should be thoroughly cleansed with an antiseptic solution between use by different babies. Cotton sheets and blankets can be autoclaved after washing.

Rooming-in is widely used so that the baby can be with his mother during the day. As rest and sleep is of prime importance in the postnatal period he should be taken into the nursery during the day if fretful and certainly during the night. The baby requires early morning and late evening feeds and his demands on the new mother are very great. The process of adjustment can produce extreme exhaustion and emotional stress which can be avoided if really sound sleep is ensured.

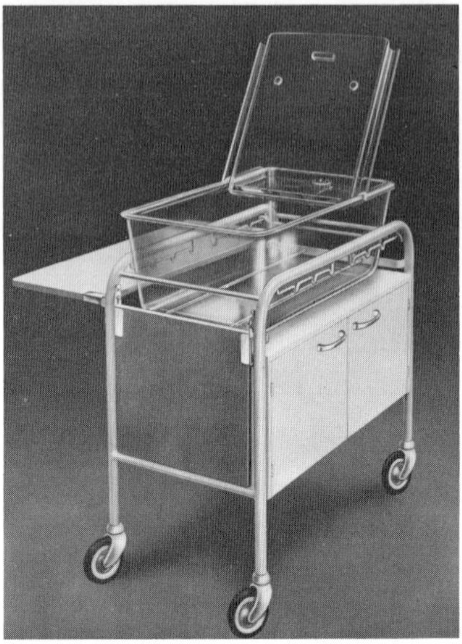

Figure 6.6 Cot suitable for special care nurseries. (Photograph by courtesy of Hoskins and Sewell Ltd.)

Routine Care in the Nursery

In the care of any infants after delivery the midwife has a major responsibility in making and recording observations about his health and progress. She must be quick to recognize early signs of deviation from normal and make sure that these are recorded and reported. The medical staff rely to a very great extent on nursing observations about the behaviour of infants in their clinical assessment of the need for investigation and treatment. While it is essential that midwives should understand the comparatively wide range of normal behaviour they must seek help if they are in doubt about an infant. Senior midwives and doctors should not be critical of a student midwife who reports what she believes to be abnormal but which is in fact a normal variant. It is better to be safe than to be sorry.

DAILY OBSERVATIONS

General well-being. A healthy thriving newborn has a clear pink skin, is active, has good muscle tone, cries lustily, feeds well and feels warm. Departure from this state indicates some abnormality.

Temperature. Rectal temperatures are recorded at least once daily. Low reading thermometers with a scale down to 25°C must be used. If the rectal temperature falls below 36.0°C the baby should be moved to a warmer room and a full medical examination carried out with the possibility of infection in mind. Rectal and skin temperatures should be recorded half hourly until the rectal temperature returns to 37°C.

Weight may be recorded daily or at birth, third day, fifth day and daily thereafter. The weight will be down on the third day due to deficient fluid intake and the passage of urine and meconium. It should have begun to rise from the initial fall by the fourth day. Great care must be taken not to allow the mother to become obsessed by the baby's weight pattern.

Stools. Meconium which has been present in the bowel from the 16th week of pregnancy and which is dark green in colour is generally passed within 24 hours of birth and for the first two or three days. When feeding is commenced the stool alters to a greenish brown colour, the changing stool. After the third or fourth day the stools of the breast-fed baby are yellow in colour, soft in consistency and about three or four per day are passed. The artificially fed baby has more formed grey-coloured stools with a slightly offensive odour. Green stools can occur in a healthy baby.

Other observations. Urine is normally passed during the first 24 hours of life if the bladder has not already been emptied during delivery. A record should be made of the time of passing of the first urine and the frequency of subsequent passage. Any abnormality of colour should be reported. The midwife must also record the onset of pallor, jaundice, cyanosis or purpura. Small mouthfuls of regurgitated milk should not be recorded as vomits but anything greater should be recorded and reported with particular note of the approximate volume, colour and consistency of the vomit and its relation to feeding. Difficulty in respiration particularly when feeding may indicate nasal obstruction particularly if accompanied by subcostal indrawing. Noisy respiration, if associated with frothy mucus, is an early sign of possible oesophageal atresia which requires immediate investigation.

It is not possible to mention all the conditions which may be observed. If doubts about a baby's condition or behaviour arise the opinion of a more experienced nurse or doctor should be sought.

FEEDING

It is interesting to note that in spite of all the great advances in preparing formulae for artificial feeds breast milk remains unsurpassed. Oliver Wendell Holmes said that a pair of good lactating breasts were of far more value than the two cerebral hemispheres of a learned professor's brain. It is the duty of all midwives to promote breast feeding but it is a very personal matter between the mother and her baby. Good antenatal preparation is essential (Chap. 8). The early feeds must always be carefully supervised. The normal healthy baby will suck eagerly and in order to protect the nipple from trauma the duration of sucking time should be increased slowly from 3 to 4 minutes each side on the first day reaching 10 minutes each side by the fifth or sixth day. Breast feeding should never be associated with pain.

Care of the nipples. The breasts and nipples must be carefully cleansed before feeding and carefully dried when feeding is completed. An ointment such as lanoline is applied to the nipples after each feed. A good supporting brassiere or binder is essential. Test weighing may be carried out after the fifth day if the baby is still losing weight or has had a large weight loss initially but it should never be done as a routine as it can undermine the mother's confidence and raise doubts about her ability to produce sufficient milk. If the baby is being fed by bottle a record must be kept of the type of feed, frequency of feeding and the amount taken. Records must be kept for all babies of vomiting and regurgitation of feeds.

DAILY CARE

The eyes must be carefully examined for signs of infection and wiped with a swab moistened in sterile water. The face should be washed in the same way.

The mouth may be examined daily for signs of thrush infection. The skin flexures must be carefully dried and inspected daily as moisture left in these areas can cause excoriation and subsequent infection.

The umbilical cord should be examined. It should dry and separate about the sixth or seventh day. The umbilical area must be carefully cleansed with 0.5 per cent hibitane in 70 per cent spirit and any inflammation, discharge or odour reported immediately.

The buttocks must be carefully washed with pHisoHex and water and gently dried each time the baby is changed. If they become excoriated ointment such as Savlon is applied and the rectal temperature recording is discontinued. The temperature is then recorded in the groin or axilla.

FURTHER READING

British Medical Journal (1972). Mothering the baby. ii, 419–420.

Expert Group on Special Care for Babies (1971). *Report of the Expert Group on Special Care for Babies*. London: HMSO.

Myles, M. F. (1971). *A Textbook for Midwives*, 7th edn. Edinburgh: Churchill Livingstone.

Stone, F. H. (1971). Psychological aspects of early mother–infant relationships. *British Medical Journal*, iv, 224–226.

7

Examination of the Healthy Newborn Infant

Once her baby has been delivered and respiration has been established mother's chief concern will be, 'Is my baby all right?' This question generally has a double significance implying concern not only for her baby's immediate survival but also her anxiety about possible abnormalities which might affect his future well-being.

PRELIMINARY EXAMINATION

Midwives and doctors must share mother's natural concern and prepare to answer her questions after a rapid examination of the infant to exclude major abnormalities and to establish sex (Chap. 6). This preliminary examination may be carried out in full view of the mother. Mothers gain great pleasure in handling their infants after delivery and may wish to examine them themselves. This should be encouraged provided that heat loss is prevented. A midwife or doctor should be close by to answer mother's questions about her baby particularly with reference to anything that is puzzling or worrying her.

Significant congenital abnormalities are discussed in Chapter 11.

In this chapter we shall describe the features of a healthy newborn infant and discuss some minor departures from normal which can be considered as variants of normal and which are not generally included under the title of congenital abnormalities.

FIRST DAY EXAMINATION

The rapid examination of the newborn infant carried out in the delivery room is insufficient for a full assessment of baby's state of health, and a more detailed examination should be carried out by a competent physician within the first 24 hours of life. In maternity hospitals this examination is commonly carried out by a paediatric house physician. Much help can be given to the doctor by the midwives or nurses caring for the infant, who should report any abnormalities of appearance or behaviour noted by them. Similarly any anxieties about her infant expressed by the mother should be made known to the doctor examining the infant. Before the examination is started the doctor concerned should also read the history of the mother's pregnancy and delivery and learn about any significant family history.

PLACE OF EXAMINATION

Warmth, freedom from draughts, space, good lighting and easy access are essential so that the infant can be fully exposed without risk of heat loss thus allowing a complete physical inspection. It is generally easier to examine an infant on a flat surface rather than in the depths of a cot. If a table is used it should be provided with a low rim to prevent baby rolling off. The surface should be covered with paper or other disposable material to prevent cross infection from one infant to another.

RECORDS

A detailed examination is of limited value unless an accurate record is kept of the findings. This record may be made on a standard form suitable for transfer of the information contained to an information retrieval system. Much of the value of the routine physical examination of infants in the past has been lost because adequate records have not been kept or the information has been recorded in such a manner that subsequent collation of data was difficult. At present no standard record is in general use but it is hoped that in Scotland a standard neonatal record related to the similar records kept for mother's pregnancy and delivery will be in use by 1973. This will allow information about all newborn infants and the preceding pregnancy to be stored in computer form. Ultimately it is planned that this record will form the basis for an ongoing record of that individual's health (Chap. 21).

OBJECT OF EXAMINATION

The first day examination is intended to provide an assessment of the infant's state of development and well-being and to detect any evidence of departures from normal in form or function which might require treatment immediately or at a later stage. It also provides a base line against which an assessment of progress can be made and with which comparisons can be made at subsequent examinations including the examination which will be made at the time of the infant's discharge from the maternity hospital.

Repeat Examinations

The physical examination will be essentially the same at the 24 hour and the discharge examination but certain features may be more appropriate at one of these examinations and these will be mentioned separately. One or both of these examinations may be conducted in mother's presence. Particularly in respect of the examination at the time of discharge mothers are happy to see that their infant has been thoroughly assessed. Should any finding indicate the advisability of further examination the reason for this should be discussed with mother. Her co-operation is more likely to be achieved if she appreciates why a further examination is being requested. At the same time it must be appreciated that undue anxiety can be caused by a request for a repeat examination for a trivial cause. It is essential that mothers can be given a chance to express their anxieties and that their questions be accepted and answered seriously although they may seem unreasonable to those with greater knowledge of the newborn.

IDENTIFICATION

At the outset of any examination of a newborn infant the examiner should check the identity and sex of the infant and verify that the record of the examination is labelled with the correct name, sex and reference number.

General Inspection

The inspection of the infant must include an overall appraisal of the infant's prenatal growth and nutrition with an assessment of the degree of maturity reached. Following this a more systematic examination of the regions of the body and of the various systems should be carried out. Assessments of maturity of development of low birth weight infants is dealt with in Chapter 9.

DEFINING THE NORMAL

In this chapter while discussing the routine examination of the normal healthy newborn infant we shall also describe some of the minor variations of normal which do not justify the term abnormality. To describe a 'normal' healthy newborn infant would be to describe a whole range of sizes, shapes, weights and colours depending on racial, familial and individual factors.

Length and weight. As far as length and weight are concerned measurements of large numbers of infants of different gestational ages provide material for statistical analysis, and for each gestational age the distribution curves of weights can be plotted. If it is then accepted that the smallest 10 per cent and the largest 10 per cent are excluded the intervening 80 per cent are said to be of appropriate weight for dates. This can also be expressed by saying that those infants lying between the 10th and 90th percentiles of weight for that gestational age are of appropriate weight for dates. Charts showing the range of weight, length and head circumference at each week of gestational age are readily available (Fig. 7.1). By international agreement an infant weighing 2500 g or less at birth is said to be of low birth weight (Chap. 9).

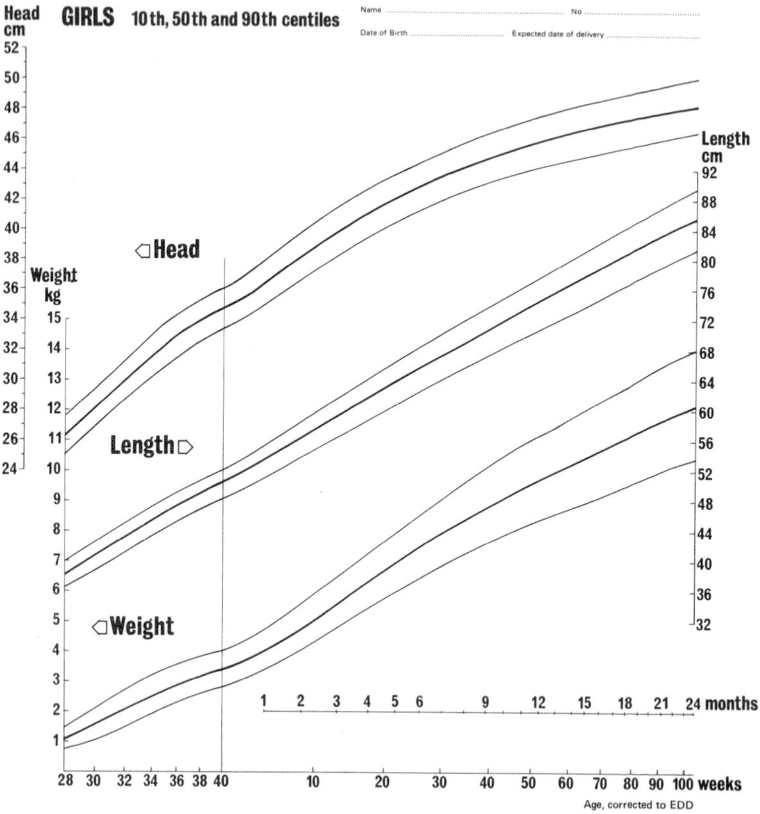

Figure 7.1 Chart prepared by Drs D. Gairdner and J. Pearson showing 10th, 50th and 90th centiles for head circumference, length and weight from 28 weeks gestation to 100 weeks after birth. (By courtesy of the authors and the Editor of *Archives of Disease in Childhood*.)

Gestational age. A full-term delivery is one which takes place between the 37th and 42nd weeks of gestation. Preterm and post-term infants are those who fall outwith this range.

MEASUREMENT

Examination of the infant includes the measurements required to assess that infant against the standard in use. Any standard is only useful if it is known to be significant with regard to the population being examined. Standards may require revision from time to time to keep them up to date.

Similarly the measurements taken on the infant must be accurate and reproducible. As far as possible the techniques used should correspond with the techniques used to measure the infants who formed the population used to establish the standards. As weight is the easiest to obtain it is unfortunately often the only measurement made. Crown–heel length or crown–rump length together with head

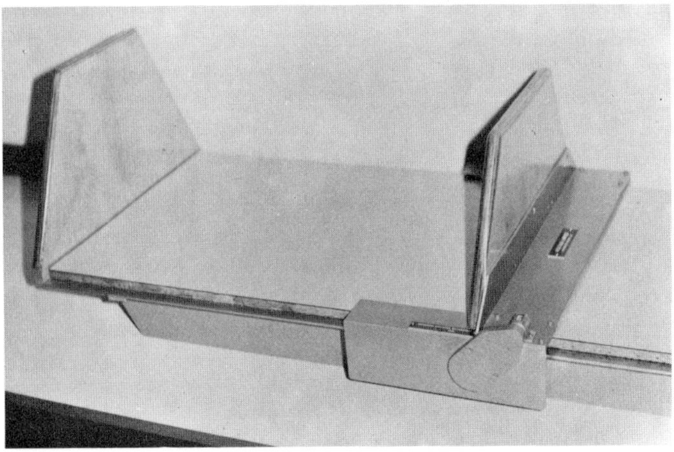

Figure 7.2 Measuring table.

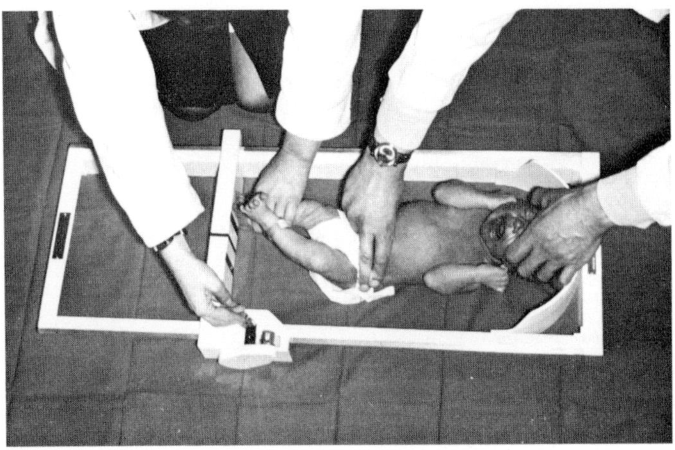

Figure 7.3 Neonatometer.

circumference are equally important but are more difficult to measure.

Length should be measured with the infant supine and the knees lightly pressed down to obtain maximum leg extension. The head, trunk and limbs must be in line. By using a measuring table (Fig. 7.2) with boards at the head and feet the crown–heel length can be measured as the distance between the boards. Similarly crown–rump length can be easily measured. Measuring boards are, however, bulky and cannot be introduced into cots. More recently a neonatal measuring instrument has been designed (Fig. 7.3). Where such aids are not available measurements can be made against a firm ruler of suitable length or with a tape measure.

Head circumference is generally measured with a tape measure (Fig. 7.4). Moulding of the head during delivery will affect the head circumference and it is more appropriate for this measurement to be taken on the third day. The maximum circumference of the head in the occipito-frontal plane should be measured. With any tape or instrument used precautions must be taken to prevent the possibility of transfer of organisms from one infant to another (Chap. 13).

The percentile distributions for weight, crown–heel length and head circumference for male and female term infants are given in Table 7.1. The 10th percentile includes the 10 per cent of infants who are smaller than this measurement. The 90th percentile includes 90 per cent of infants measured and only 10 per cent of infants will be larger than this. It will be noted that the figures are all given in the metric system. The equipment used should record in this system.

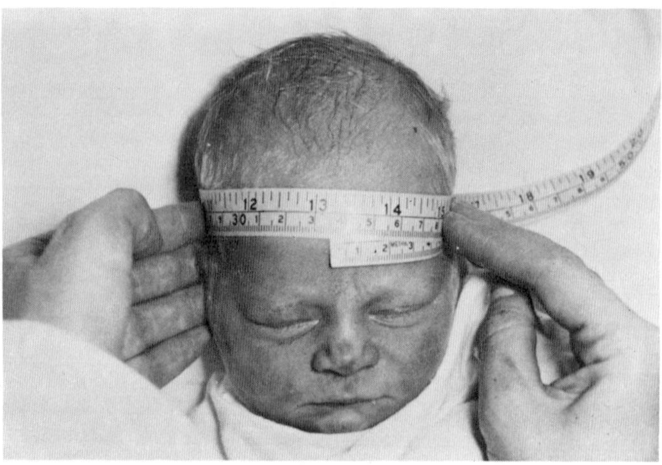

Figure 7.4 Measurement of occipito-frontal circumference.

Attempts at taking measurements in other systems and calculating the metric equivalent from conversion tables are most unsatisfactory and liable to lead to serious errors.

Table 7.1 Distribution by percentiles of weight, length and head circumference of term infants. (Based on figures from the Harvard School of Public Health.)

	Percentiles					
	Males			Females		
	10th	50th	90th	10th	50th	90th
Weight (g)	2860	3400	4130	2810	3360	3900
Length (cm)	48.1	50.6	53.3	47.8	50.2	51.9
Head circumference (cm)	33.5	35.3	37.0	33.4	34.7	36.0

Recognition of discrepancy. It is useful to have the basic measurements discussed above available at the time of the first detailed examination. This does not preclude their being taken separately as the disturbance caused may upset the infant and make physical examination more difficult. Whenever they are taken it is essential that the midwife or doctor making the measurements should be trained in the use of equipment involved and be capable of recognizing discrepant results so that these can be checked before they are recorded. The overall assessment of the infant under examination will include both a visual estimation of size and reference to the measurements taken. Should these appear to be discrepant the identity of the infant and the name on the documents must be compared to make sure that they coincide. More detailed inspection should follow to compare the relative size of the head, trunk and limbs and to check for any evidence of asymmetry.

POSTURE

Posture and movement should be observed. The healthy newborn infant when lying in the supine position will generally show partial flexion of the arms and legs (Fig. 7.5) and the head is commonly turned a little to one side. Even without a napkin to hold them apart the hip joints are partially abducted. If turned into the prone position the flexion of the limbs becomes more marked so that the buttocks are raised and the knees take much of the weight of the lower body. The head is turned to one side (Fig. 7.6).

Movement is most evident in the face and limbs. Asymmetry, unusual movements or lack of movement should be noted. The response to stimuli will be considered later under Neurological Examination, but at this stage any evidence of irritability or undue apathy should be looked for.

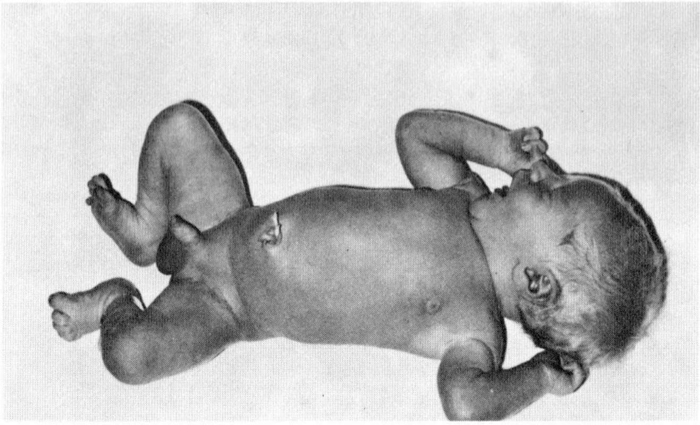

Figure 7.5 Posture of term infant in supine position.

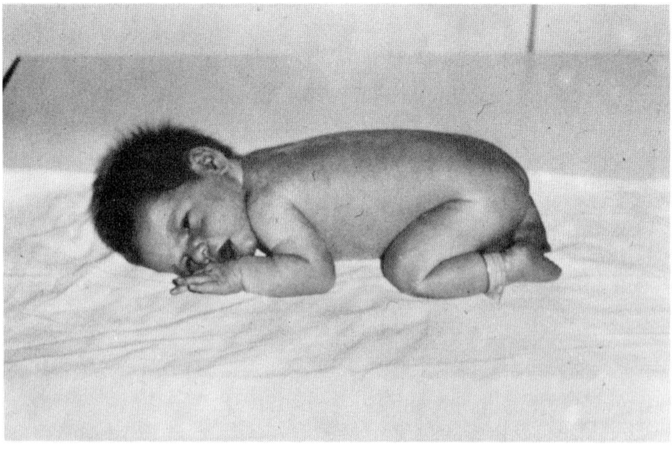

Figure 7.6 Posture of term infant in prone position.

SKIN

Inspection of the whole infant should continue with observation of skin colour with particular reference to pallor, cyanosis, haemorrhage, jaundice, rashes or birthmarks.

Vernix caseosa. At birth the skin is covered with vernix caseosa (Fig. 7.7). This is a greasy substance which is secreted by the fetal sebaceous glands and which disappears in the course of a few days if not removed by bathing.

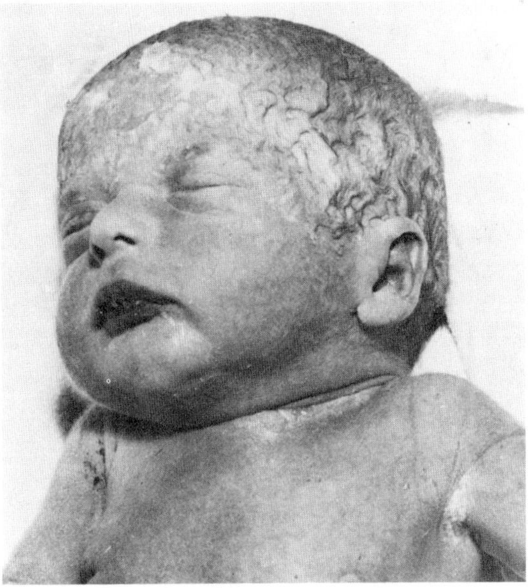

Figure 7.7 Vernix caseosa.

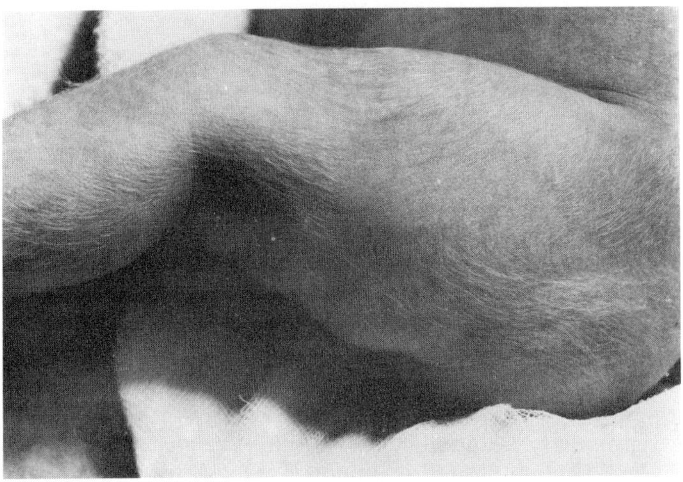

Figure 7.8 Lanugo.

Lanugo. Fine, scarcely perceptible hair known as lanugo (Fig. 7.8) can frequently be detected, being most obvious in dark-haired babies (Fig. 7.9).

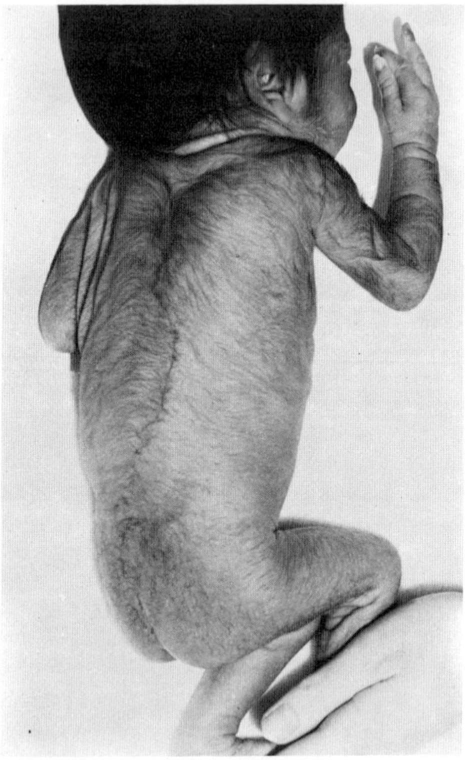

Figure 7.9 The plentiful dark hair often present at birth in babies of Eastern races.

Peeling. Some degree of exfoliation of the skin may take place a few days after birth. Peeling is usually most marked on the hands and feet. The skin of light-for-dates infants is often dry and scaly (Chap. 9).

Hair. Much of the hair of the scalp present at birth may fall out during the first few weeks of life. The exact colour of the hair in the early weeks of life rarely persists into later childhood.

Colour. Skin colour changes quite rapidly with changes in blood flow through the skin capillaries, vasoconstriction causing pallor, vasodilatation redness and slowing of the circulation peripheral cyanosis. The changes are not always uniform.

Harlequin. A striking clinical picture occasionally results with one half of the body, e.g. the right side red and the left white. This is called the 'harlequin sign' and is not of significance.

Cyanosis. A blotchy discoloration of the skin is generally an indication of poor peripheral circulation and the cause should be looked for. If cyanosis is present its distribution should be noted and in particular whether it is uniformly distributed or present only in the periphery. The distribution and character of haemorrhage, e.g. petechiae or ecchymoses, should be recorded for comparison with the findings at later examinations. Skin abrasions or incisions must be noted.

Stork marks. Many babies show 'stork marks', or naevi flammei, which are temporary areas of redness over the root of the nose, the upper eyelids or the nape of the neck. They disappear gradually but may reappear when the baby is hot, as after a hot bath, or following crying.

Milia. Small white opalescent spots on the nose and surrounding structures are called milia (Fig. 7.10). They are blocked sebaceous glands which clear spontaneously. No treatment is required and it is important to distinguish milia from skin pustules.

Birthmarks. Small birthmarks which are mainly haemangiomata

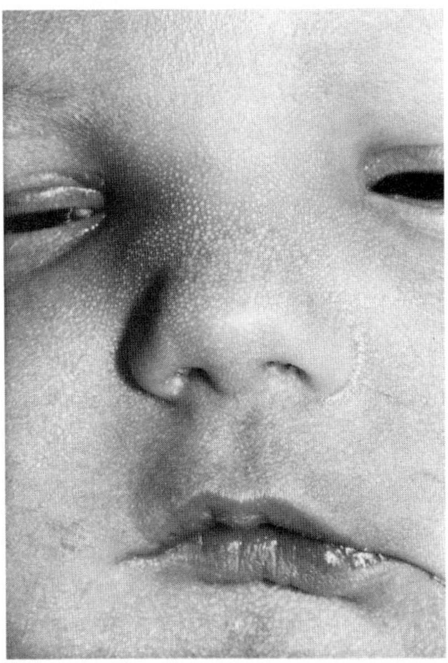

Figure 7.10 Milia.

often disappear within a few years without treatment although they may increase in size before regressing. This applies particularly to the cavernous type (Chap. 11).

Blue patches are areas of a deep bluish pigmentation over the buttocks and back seen in dark-skinned races (Fig. 7.11).

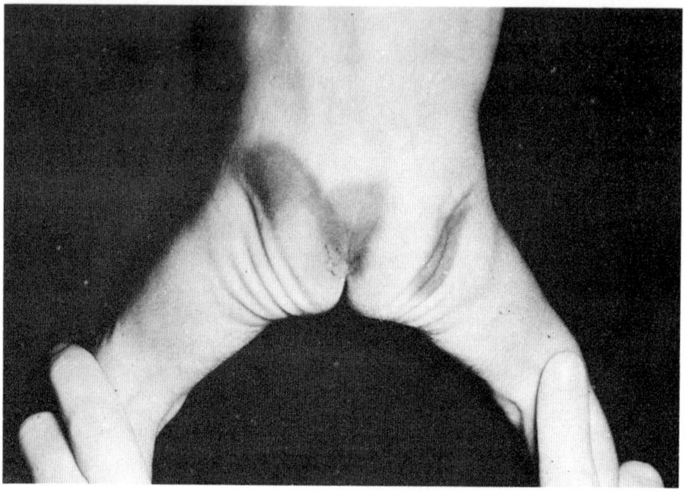

Figure 7.11 Blue patches.

RASHES

The skin of the newborn is readily irritated by a wide range of physical and chemical agents. As a result rashes are common but are frequently transient and it is not always easy to identify the specific cause although midwives are often convinced that they know the offending agent. Transient erythema often occurs over pressure points particularly where there has been any friction.

Urticaria neonatorum (sometimes inappropriately called erythema toxicum) is a common rash seen in the first week of life (Fig. 7.12). It resembles papular urticaria and consists of blotchy red areas with a raised central papule which is pale and which can be felt by the finger. This condition is not infective and requires no treatment. It must not be confused with staphylococcal skin pustules (Chap. 13).

Buttocks. The buttocks are a frequent site of erythema which generally occurs because of close contact with a moist stool on the napkin. In severe cases ulceration of the skin may occur. Such lesions are less frequently seen in breast-fed infants and may occur on change to cow's milk feeding. The erythema and ulceration is most

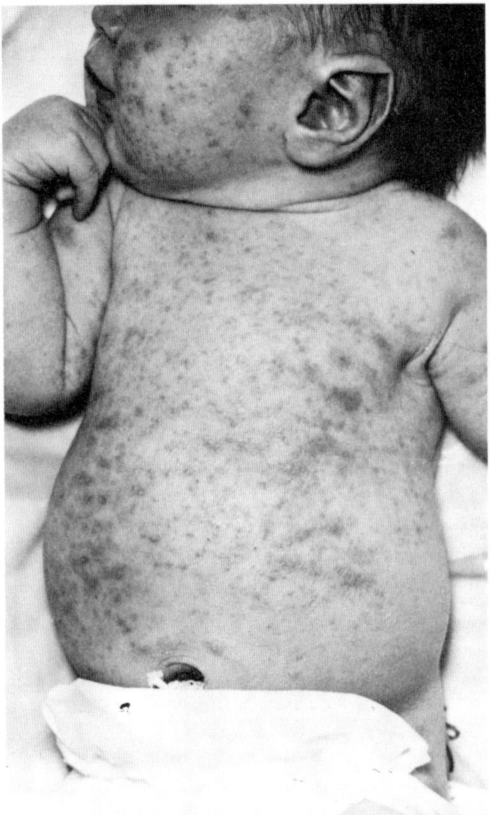

Figure 7.12 Urticaria neonatorum.

marked over the prominence of the buttocks and is absent in the immediate perianal area as opposed to monilial skin infection which spreads outwards from the anus. Treatment of simple erythema is by avoidance of contact with stool by nursing baby prone with the buttocks exposed to the air.

Sacrococcygeal dimple. Another common finding in this area is a sacrococcygeal dimple which is a small sinus, the bottom of which can be seen by everting the skin (Fig. 7.13). No treatment other than local hygiene is required. This simple condition has to be distinguished from the deeper forms of pilonidal sinus lying further up the sacrum. As these may communicate with the theca careful examination is called for.

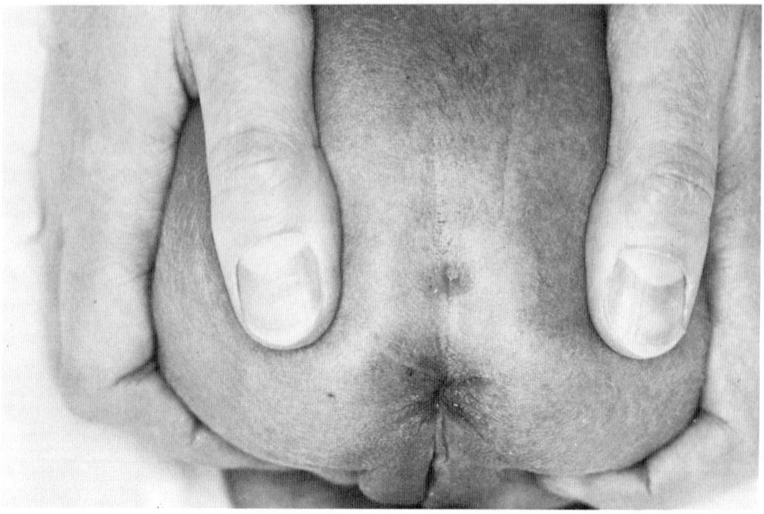

7.13 Sacrococcygeal dimple.

DETAILED EXAMINATION

Following the general inspection of the whole infant a more detailed examination is undertaken. It is generally more convenient to start at the head and work systematically down the body.

The Head

Head size and shape are assessed by both inspection and palpation. It was earlier noted that measurement of occipito-frontal circumference is more meaningful if deferred until the third day by which time much of the moulding often present at birth will have subsided.

Caput. Bruising and oedema of the scalp over the presenting part of the skull will remain evident for two or three days after birth. The skin should be inspected for any laceration which could be a potential source of entry of infection.

Moulding. The shape of the head may have been considerably distorted by moulding during delivery. Moulding can occur because of the pliability of the sutures and the relative softness of the cranial bones particularly in preterm infants. The resultant shape depends on the degree of flexion of the head during delivery. In a vertex presentation the head is lengthened in the mento-vertex axis (Fig. 7.14) whereas in a brow presentation the fronto-occipital axis is lengthened (Fig. 7.15). Overriding of the edges of the cranial bones

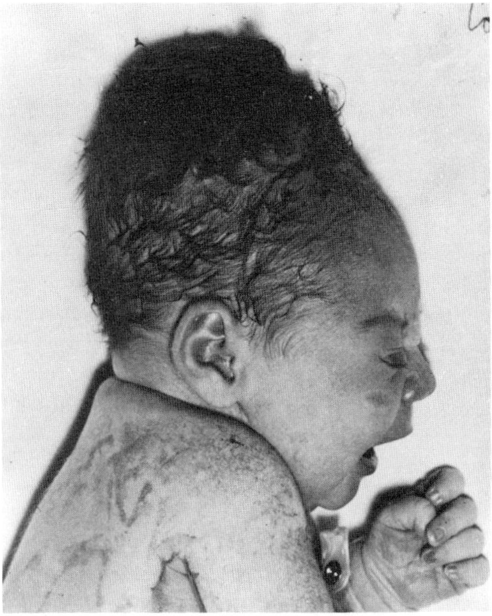

Figure 7.14 Head moulding in vertex delivery.

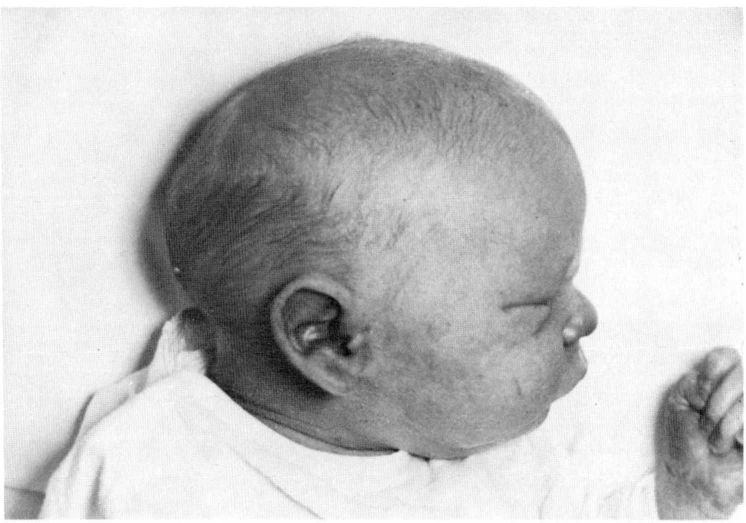

Figure 7.15 Head moulding in breech delivery.

may occur at the suture lines to make such moulding possible. Such changes in shape naturally call for a change in shape of the underlying blood vessels some of which may rupture. In the absence of signs of cerebral dysfunction or of rising intracranial pressure even marked degrees of moulding are, however, not of consequence. The shape of the skull returns to normal within a few days.

Fontanelles are wider areas of fibrous tissue occurring where two or more sutures join. The anterior and posterior fontanelles lie at either end of the saggital suture. The coronal sutures join the anterior fontanelle and the posterior fontanelle is joined by the lambdoidal sutures.

Plagiocephaly. Asymmetrical development of the skull produces the condition called plagiocephaly (Fig. 7.16). This commonly corrects itself to some extent but investigation is required if the condition appears to be progressive as unilateral craniosynostosis may be present.

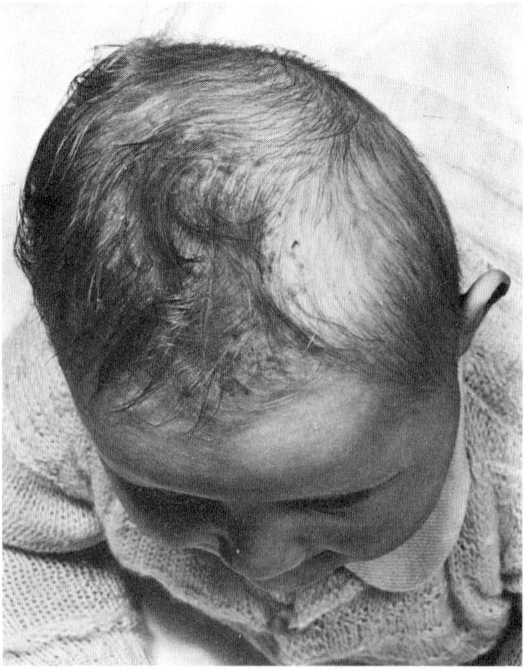

Figure 7.16 Plagiocephaly.

Craniotabes. Small areas of the parietal bones near the suture lines may be unusually soft and can be felt to click in and out on pressure. When localized this condition is harmless and is called craniotabes.

Cephalhaematoma, which is a collection of altered blood below the periosteum of one of the cranial vault bones, is rarely present in the first day of life (Chap. 12).

EARS

Before examining the facial features it is advisable to inspect the ears both for the general pattern of their development and for their position.

Accessory auricles. Small accessory auricles (Fig. 7.17) may be found on the line between the angle of the mouth and the ear. They

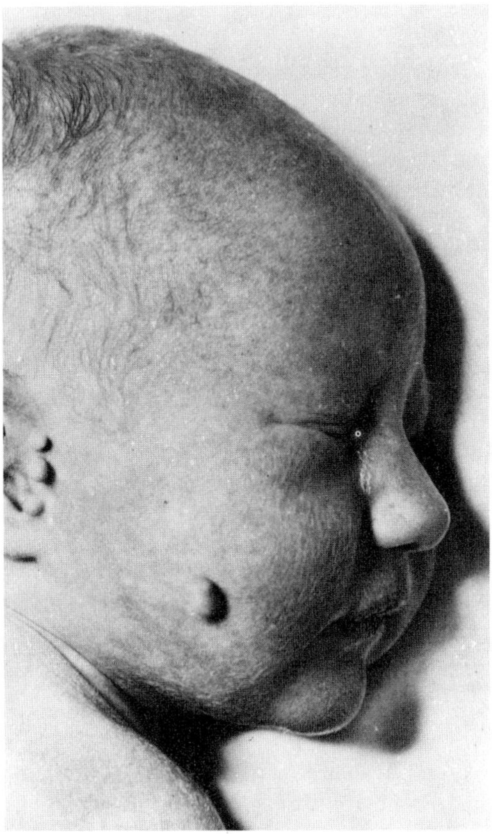

Figure 7.17 Accessory auricles.

commonly lie immediately anterior to the ear. If they have a sufficiently narrow peduncle they can be treated by ligation of the base so that the arterial blood supply is occluded.

FACE

The variations in facial features with different racial and familial backgrounds make it advisable to see the parents and siblings before deciding whether an infant's facies is abnormal. Some characteristics of abnormal facies are considered in Chapter 11.

The facial expression can be a useful guide to an infant's general state of health and should therefore be observed. Experience soon teaches the examiner to differentiate between the normal pattern, that of the over-reactive irritable infant and that of the seriously ill infant.

EYES

The eyes are difficult to examine but with patience can be seen in most infants. Future eye colour cannot be stated at birth as all infants have a greyish-blue iris. Eye movements are not fully coordinated and therefore momentary squinting is likely to occur. Tears are rarely seen and a discharge from the eyes generally indicates some degree of conjunctival irritation or blockage of the nasolacrimal duct. Small subconjunctival haemorrhages disappear without treatment. Vision at birth is present but limited. Ophthalmoscopic examination in the newborn is difficult and requires an expert skilled not only in the technique but also in the interpretation of findings. Cataracts are difficult to identify at birth unless well formed.

Epicanthus, a fold of skin over the inner canthus of the palpebral fissure, is common in young infants and generally disappears as the infant grows older. The length of the palpebral fissure varies but is abnormal if it does not allow the eyelids to part sufficiently for the dilated pupil to be uncovered completely.

Hypertelorism. The distance between the inner edge of each eyeball is normally the equivalent of the diameter of the eyeball. This can also be stated as the distance between the centre of each pupil being twice the diameter of the eyeball. Wider separation is called hypertelorism.

NOSE

Determination of the patency of both nasal airways should be part of the routine examination of the newborn. This can be done by ensuring that the mouth is closed and then occluding each side of the nostril in turn. Slight indrawing of the chest wall may result as the nasal passages are narrow but gross distress and indrawing indicate a blocked airway.

MOUTH

Examination of the mouth begins with an assessment of mandibular development with particular reference to underdevelopment or gross asymmetry.

'*Sucking blisters*' (Fig. 7.18) on the lips can be accepted as normal and occur particularly in babies fed at the breast.

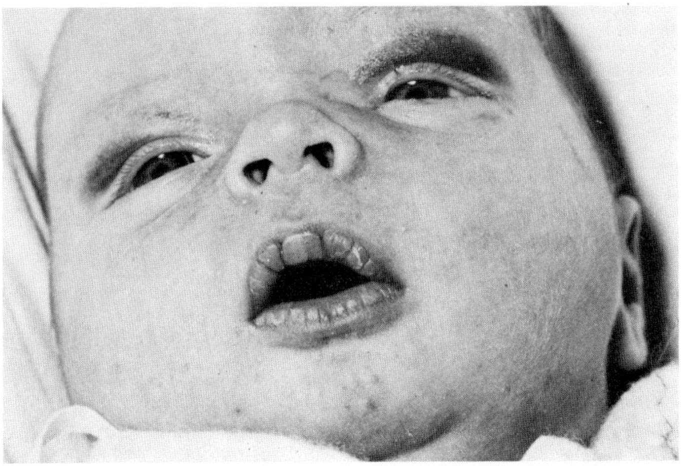

Figure 7.18 Sucking blisters.

Tongue. The size and position of the tongue are of considerable significance as glossoptosis (Chap. 11) is a potential cause of airway obstruction. The frenulum is attached near the tip of the tongue and rarely interferes with normal tongue movement at this stage of life. As described in Chapter 8 movement of the tongue pressing the nipple or teat against the roof of the mouth is essential in feeding and the ability to do this should be checked.

Palate. At the same time the hard and soft palate should be inspected. Small greyish white areas on either side of the midline posteriorly on the hard palate are called *Epstein's pearls* and are a normal finding. The soft palate should be capable of closing off the nasopharynx.

Teeth. Occasionally one or more teeth, generally lower incisors, are present at birth (Fig. 7.19). They are often loose and either fall out or are readily removed if they are causing damage to mother's nipples.

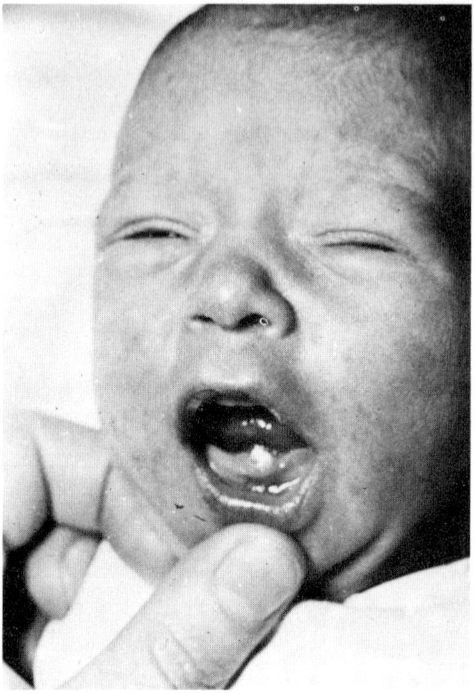

Figure 7.19 Tooth at birth.

NECK

The neck of the newborn is short and therefore difficult to examine. The range of movement is greater than in adult life and infant's heads can be turned to look directly over either shoulder. Soft tissue swellings or abnormal range of movement should be noted.

The Chest

Following examination of the head and neck attention most naturally passes to the chest, beginning with a general assessment of shape, size, symmetry and movement.

Nipples. The position of the nipples, their form and contour and the presence of accessory nipples should be checked.

Breast. Breast engorgement may occur in both male and female infants. It reaches a maximum between the third and fifth days and regresses spontaneously although the breasts may remain enlarged for several weeks. Secretion of colostrum occasionally occurs. Provided that infection is avoided the condition is harmless and requires no treatment.

The ribs are held more nearly horizontal in the newborn increasing the antero-posterior diameter of the chest and limiting movement of the thoracic cage. As the diaphragm therefore becomes a more important factor in respiratory movement inspection of the chest must take this into account. Some indrawing of the lower ribs which are softer than in later childhood is likely to occur on inspiration. The descent of the diaphragm displaces the abdominal contents and pushes the abdominal wall forward.

Respiratory movement can most easily be seen and counted in the upper central abdomen below the xiphisternum. The rate varies considerably with activity but is of the order of 40 cycles per minute at rest. Rates above 60 per minute should be considered abnormal.

The cardiac apex beat is generally difficult to localize by palpation. If not felt within the nipple line on the left side it should be felt for on both sides of the chest. The heart rate averages about 125 per minute on the first day of life with an acceptable as normal range from 70 to 180 per minute.

Percussion is of value only if carried out with a very light tap. With light percussion the area of cardiac dullness can be recognized. Absence of this dullness is of significance indicating emphysema or displacement of the heart.

Auscultation of the breath sounds is helpful in giving information about the volume of air entry in each part of the lung. The site of maximum intensity of the heart sounds aids localization of the position of the heart. Murmurs do not of themselves indicate cardiac abnormality unless they persist or are accompanied by other evidence of abnormality. No murmur may be heard in an infant with a major cardiac defect.

The Abdomen

Before turning baby over to examine the back of his thorax it is generally convenient to continue with the examination of the abdomen. Inspection is most important to observe the degree of prominence of the abdomen, comparing particularly the upper and lower segments.

Distension. Upper abdominal distension is common after feeds. Absence of lower abdominal distension, marked peristalsis or gross distension without peristalsis are abnormal and indicate the need for immediate investigation (Chap. 11).

THE CORD

Inspection of the cord including the number of vessels which it contains should have been made at the initial examination in the labour ward but should be repeated. At the same time the efficiency of the clamp, elastic band or ligature is checked. Shrinkage of the cord with drying occurs rapidly after birth as the umbilical arteries close depriving the tissue of a blood supply. Separation of the cord generally takes place between the fifth and tenth days. The longer interval is found where the cord has been kept moist and when excessive bacterial colonization has occurred. Exposure of the cord and local application of antispetics prevents delay in separation (Chap. 6). A discharge from the cord stump after separation warrants further investigation.

Granuloma. A collection of granulomatous tissue at the site of separation has to be distinguished from an umbilical polyp which is persistence of part of the mesenteric duct which requires surgical removal. A cord granuloma can be treated by local application of a copper sulphate crystal or silver nitrate stick.

Hernia. Umbilical hernia may be present at birth but more commonly develops within the first month particularly in low birth-weight infants. Spontaneous remission is common by 1 year of life.

Palpation. Palpation of the abdomen in the newborn requires patience and a delicate touch. By waiting for the abdominal wall to relax and wrapping the fingers around the abdominal contour more is gained than by irritating the baby with prodding finger tips. Examination is generally simplest during a feed but care must be taken not to cause vomiting.

The liver is normally palpable in the epigastrium and the edge can be felt round to the right costal margin in the midaxillary line on inspiration. The left lobe of the liver is sometimes mistaken for the spleen.

The spleen. The spleen when enlarged, presents more laterally than in older children and its tip points to the left rather than the right loin. Palpation of the spleen must bear this in mind. Ability to palpate the tip of the spleen on deep inspiration is not always an indication of abnormality but should be considered along with other findings.

Kidneys. During the first day or two before the bowel is fully distended both kidneys may be palpable readily and experience is required to decide whether they are enlarged. After the third day only the lower pole of the kidneys is palpable unless they are enlarged or the abdomen is unusually soft.

The bladder is an abdominal organ in infancy and is easily palpable or outlined by percussion when full. It should not be palpable after the baby has passed urine.

Femoral pulse. Examination of the groins should include palpation of the femoral arteries and comparison of the timing of the pulse stroke with that felt in the radial artery at the wrist.

The site, consistency and mobility of any swelling must be noted.

Genitalia

The external genitalia will already have been examined at birth when the sex was decided. Further more detailed inspection and palpation is now necessary. Identification of the urethral opening is important in both sexes. In males both gonads should be palpable and capable of being brought into the scrotum.

Hydrocele of the tunica vaginalis is common generally with small collections of fluid (Fig. 7.20). These disappear within a few days.

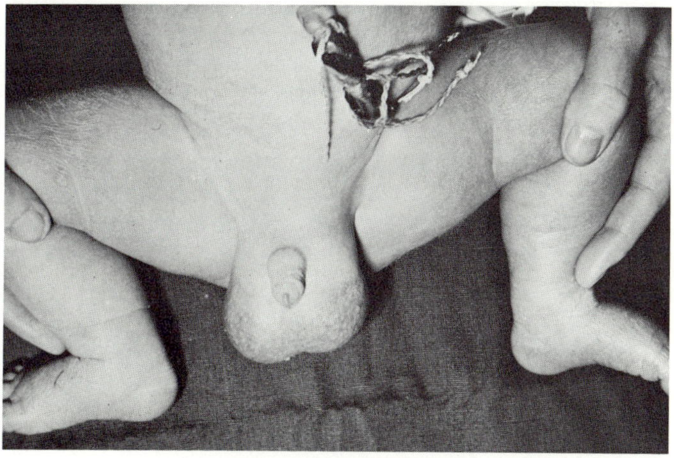

Figure 7.20 Hydrocele.

Larger collections of fluid particularly around the cord should lead to examination for inguinal hernia (Chap. 11).

Penis. There is considerable variation in the size of the penis and scrotum and in the anterior attachment of the skin web between penis and scrotum. The foreskin is adherent and should not be retracted. Urine should pass in a free stream without ballooning of the prepuce.

Labia. The female genitalia show considerable differences from the form found later in childhood, the clitoris and labia minora being more prominent. A thick white vaginal discharge may be evident shortly after birth. Small skin tags are not significant and generally disappear spontaneously. Bleeding as a result of oestrogen withdrawal is not abnormal unless the blood loss is excessive.

The Limbs

Following examination of the anterior part of the trunk, the limbs should be examined paying attention to the relative lengths of upper and lower segments and comparing the two sides.

Digits. The fingers and toes must be counted and separated to examine for webbing. Digits should be felt for the number of phalanges and the nails should be inspected.

Palms. Examination of the palm of the hand gives information about the shape and form of the creases but prints are necessary before the ridge pattern can be seen accurately.

HIP JOINTS

Assessment of the range of movement at each joint should conclude with examination for the stability of the hip joints. With the infant lying supine the pelvis is stabilized by the left hand while the right hand holds the left femur between the thumb and forefinger with the end of the finger lying over the greater trochanter (Fig. 7.21). With the femur held vertically pressure is applied downward

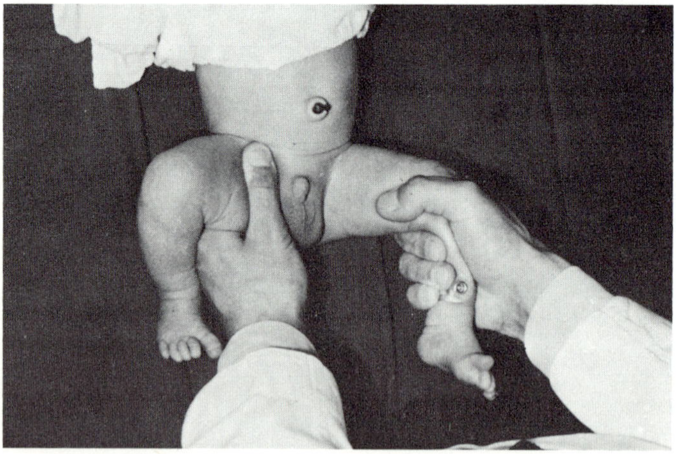

Figure 7.21 Examination for congenital dislocation of the hip.

and outward and then the femur is lifted forward and pressed inward. If the joint is unstable the head of the femur will be felt to ride forward and inward as it re-enters the acetabulum. This movement may be accompanied by a low-pitched clonk. High-pitched clicks without the sensation of the head of the femur leaving or re-entering the acetabulum are not significant. After the left hip has been examined the position of the hands should be reversed and the right hip examined.

Unstable hips. The presence of instability of the hip joint on the first day of life does not necessarily indicate liability to subsequent dislocation of the joint. Many unstable joints, particularly following breech delivery, become stable within a few days. The demonstration of instability of either or both hips is an indication for re-examination after an interval of about four days. If there is still evidence of instability long-term follow-up is indicated.

Dislocated hips. At the original examination a hip may be found to be lying in the dislocated position without pressure being applied. Such a situation is always abnormal. In true dislocation abduction at the affected hip joint is limited and difficulty in abducting either hip to 80° should always raise suspicion of congenital dislocation. The management of the dislocatable and the dislocated hip is discussed in Chapter 11.

The Back

The infant should now be turned into the prone position and careful inspection and palpation be made of the back including the buttocks and natal cleft. By running a finger down the spines of the vertebral bodies abnormalities of the vertebral column can often be detected more readily than by visual inspection. Examination of the thorax is completed by auscultation of the lungs from behind.

Posture

Having completed the anatomical examination attention is paid to those aspects of the infant's posture and movements which can be used as an assessment of his behaviour and motor function. A detailed description of the techniques required for the full neurological assessment of the newborn will be found in more specialized publications. Every routine examination should, however, include a less detailed neurological examination of the following type.

Muscle Tone

After observation of the infant's posture in the supine and prone position noting particularly the degree of activity, the pattern of movement and any obvious asymmetry, muscle tone is assessed by passive manipulation of the limbs. Greater resistance is normally found to extension as opposed to flexion. In the mature baby when the arms are extended and then released they return to their flexed position. Similar movements take place when the leg is extended in the supine position.

Other specific responses are elicited when the appropriate stimulus is applied. The response may be suppressed if the infant is drowsy or has been disturbed and is crying. Skill and patience are required in carrying out these tests and in interpreting the results.

REFLEXES

The grasp reflex in both hands and feet is elicited by pressing a finger lightly against the palm or sole (Fig. 7.22). The tightness of the grasp is often sufficient to allow immediate progress to testing for the traction response but it is generally safer to do this by holding the infant's wrist and pulling him slowly to the sitting position. The infant flexes his elbows as if trying to assist the movement and there may be an attempt to hold the head in line with the trunk as it is raised.

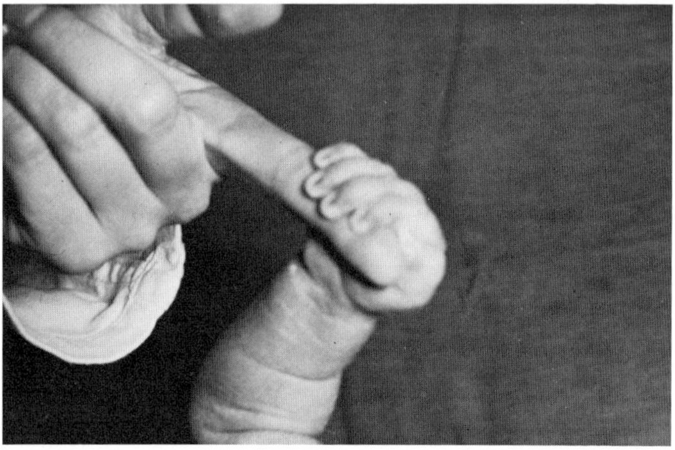

Figure 7.22 The grasp reflex.

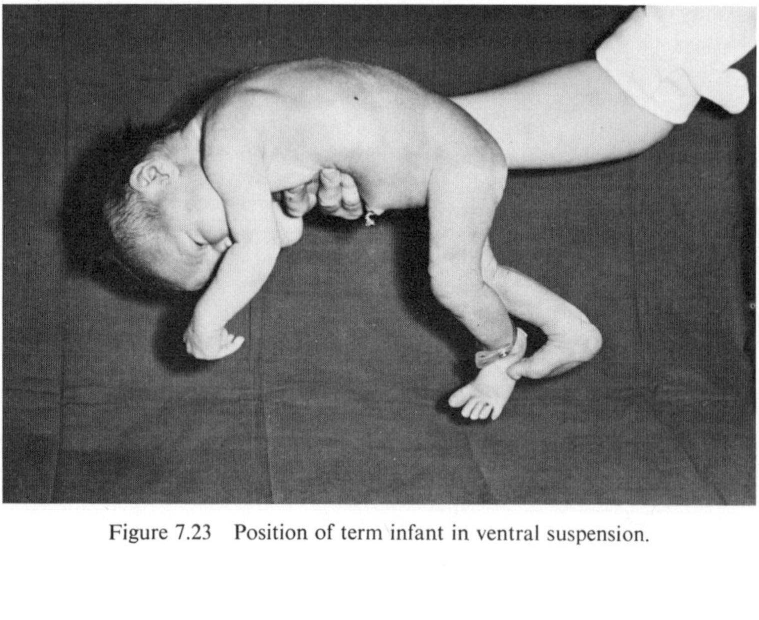

Figure 7.23 Position of term infant in ventral suspension.

The crossed extension response is elicited by extending one leg and tickling the sole. A positive response is a movement of extension possibly with adduction of the other leg.

Stepping movement. When held erect with the feet on a firm surface a full-term infant attempts to straighten the trunk and make stepping movements with his legs.

Ventral suspension. Before laying the baby down the position adopted when held in ventral suspension should be examined (Fig. 7.23). The spine and limbs are normally flexed but there may be momentary extension of the neck.

Moro reflex. As the infant is returned to its cot in the supine position the Moro response can be elicited by a sudden movement such as allowing the head to fall back unsupported for a short distance. The normal reaction is a sudden extension and abduction of the limbs followed by a slower adduction and flexion to the resting position.

The rooting response is tested by touching the infant's cheek, the normal reaction of an alert hungry baby being to turn eagerly to the side stimulated in the hope of finding a nipple or teat.

Tonic neck reflex. Passive rotation of the head to one side is used to test the tonic neck reflex in which the limbs on the side to which the head is turned extend. This reflex is not always easy to elicit but may be observed to occur spontaneously when the infant turns the head to one side (Fig. 7.24).

Eye movements. If eye movements are visible when the head is rotated a movement of the eyes in the opposite direction may be seen. This is sometimes called the doll's eye phenomenon.

Glabellar reflex. A tap over the root of the nose produces a screwing up of the eyes, the glabellar reflex.

The responsiveness of an individual infant to the tests indicated depends on a large number of factors including the degree of alertness, of hunger, of contentment or frustration. Interpretation of results must bear such factors in mind and the significance of absence of the expected response be tested by repeat stimulation under more favourable circumstances.

OTHER OBSERVATIONS

Further important information about an infant can be gained by noting his ability to maintain a constant temperature, by assessing the speed with which he returns to a normal resting state after being disturbed and by watching his vigour while feeding. At the same time reports on urine ouput, number and nature of stools, vomiting, undue crying should be available.

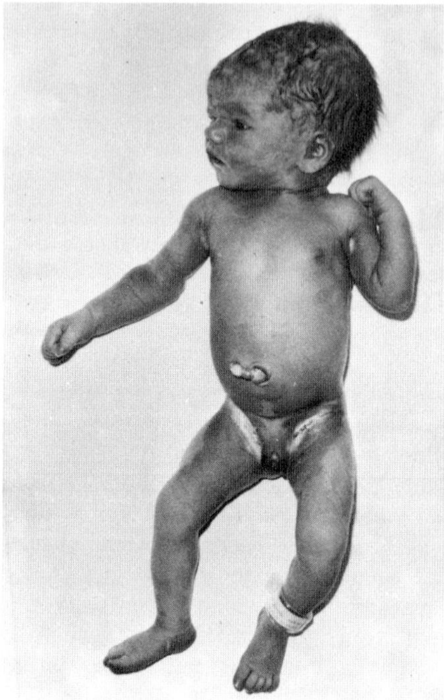

Figure 7.24 Tonic neck reflex: right arm and leg are extended as head turns to right.

SECOND EXAMINATION

Some of these features will be of more value at the second examination when charts of progress will be available. If the second examination takes place on the sixth day or later other special examinations such as collection of capillary blood for the Guthrie test for phenylalaninaemia and other metabolic disorders will be appropriate.

8
Feeding

In order to maintain after birth a rate of growth approaching that achieved by the fetus before birth the newborn infant must be adequately fed. Any method of feeding which provides the basis for normal growth and health and which keeps the infant and mother happy is acceptable.

CHANGING FASHION

Infant feeding is the subject of so many dogmatic statements that it has become a highly emotive affair to many mothers, fathers, midwives and doctors who each have their own favourite recipe. A review of practice in different countries and at varying periods of time forces one to the conclusion that fashions in feeding can be as changeable as the length of skirts. The sociologist and psychologist can, no doubt, produce good reasons to explain the changing pattern of fashion. In the individual situation, however, mother's choice of feed is often based on meagre information as to the options available and the relative advantage of one method over another.

PRIORITIES

In the world situation, although infant mortality remains high and malnutrition is a major problem in underdeveloped countries, our chief problem is a population explosion. Even under adverse conditions, therefore, infant nutrition does not present an insuperable problem. The human race existed for thousands of years without an understanding of nutritional requirements. We must not allow the wealth of scientific information now available about dietary requirements to obscure the relatively simple needs of an infant for food.

MEASURING SUCCESS

Most mothers find infant feeding, whether by breast or bottle, uncomplicated, enjoyable and successful. If she sees that her child is thriving and contented mother too will be happy and will not be interested in theoretical calculations as to what her baby 'should' be having.

The infant's well-being in the short and long term is the most important measure of success in infant feeding. It is essential that readers accept this basic premise before we embark upon an examination of some of the anatomical, physiological, biochemical and psychosocial aspects of the feeding of infants. Knowledge of these subjects is not essential to a mother feeding her infant but is necessary for those to whom she may turn for advice and reassurance.

CHANGING REQUIREMENTS

Infant feeding is a progressive affair involving different requirements and different diets as the infant grows and develops. As this book is concerned with the care of the newly born infant attention will be focused on the establishment of feeding and its continuation during the first month of life. For a further discussion of both early and later feeding the reader is referred to one or other of the excellent books listed at the end of this chapter.

As we are dealing with the early days of feeding when problems of delivery may be as important as the content of the food delivered we feel that it is appropriate to begin with a consideration of the sucking, swallowing and digestive mechanisms of a newborn infant. These mechanisms are the same for both breast- and bottle-fed infants.

Sucking

The healthy newborn infant is capable of performing the complicated manoeuvre of taking milk from his mother's nipple or from a bottle teat from the time of birth. In order to simplify matters further description will be limited to the baby feeding from his mother's breast. Similar considerations apply to the bottle-fed infant.

The infant draws the nipple well into his mouth so that the areola of the nipple lies at the level of his gums (Fig. 8.1). This is termed fixing on the breast. By closing the gums and by a rolling movement of the tongue milk is then squeezed from the milk ducts which are compressed against the infant's palate. Milk enters the pharynx and passes by co-ordinated muscular action into the oesophagus and stomach. The gums and tongue are relaxed while the milk ducts refill and a further cycle commences.

During each cycle the mouth is sealed anteriorly by the closure of the lips and the nasopharynx is closed off by the soft palate. Between sucks the mouth is closed posteriorly by apposition of the tongue and soft palate and the infant can breathe.

FEEDING DIFFICULTY

Nasal obstruction. If the nose is completely or partly obstructed nasal breathing may be impossible or difficult and the infant has to stop feeding in order to breathe through his mouth. Nasal airway obstruction is a common cause of feeding difficulty.

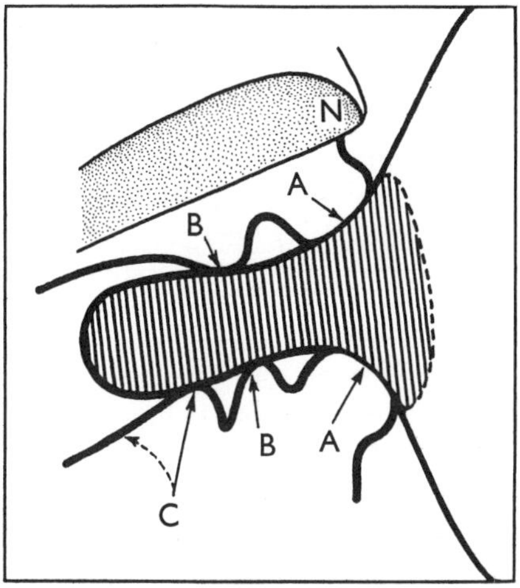

Figure 8.1 Fixing on the breast: A, lips applied well back on the areola; B, Gum margins pressing over the sinuses; C, Rolling movement of the tongue squeezing the nipple against the hard palate; N, Anterior nares clear of breast allowing air entry.

Muscular inco-ordination. Normal sucking and swallowing requires a co-ordination of several movements. This co-ordination may be lacking in immature infants and in those with brain damage.

Cleft palate. Infants with structural abnormalities such as hare lip or cleft palate have difficulty in sealing the lips round the nipple or in producing the stripping movement required to remove milk. Special feeding arrangements may be required.

Immaturity. In immature infants the milk may have to be delivered directly into the stomach by a nasogastric tube or very occasionally through a gastrostomy. Extremely small or very ill infants may not even tolerate gastric feeds and their needs have to be supplied by intravenous feeding. This subject will be considered briefly later in this chapter.

Swallowing

The fetus swallows small volumes of liquor amnii from about the fifth month. The stomach is relatively small at birth but capable of considerable expansion in the first week or two after birth. As soon as the infant cries after birth air enters the stomach and passes on through the small intestine reaching the colon by three hours. At each sucking movement air as well as milk is swallowed, the smaller the volume of milk the greater is the volume of air likely to be swallowed and vice versa. Particularly during crying considerable quantities of air may be swallowed. Most of the swallowed air is eructated but some may pass through the intestines to be discharged at the anus as flatus.

The Stomach

The gastric contents are normally passed on to the intestine via the pylorus but gastric emptying may take place in the reverse direction in the form of vomiting which is readily induced in young infants. Little digestive activity takes place in the stomach during the first few weeks of life and curdling of milk protein is the chief chemical activity present. Whereas the whey portion of curdled milk leaves the stomach within an hour or so casein curds may remain for several hours and are deposited on the surface of residue from earlier feeds as an outer layer. The layered curd is then broken down in the pyloric antrum before passage through the pylorus.

Digestion

The small intestine is the principal site of digestion and absorption. In the newborn infant the processes involved are virtually identical with those occurring in the adult but some differences relating chiefly to the maturity of the enzyme systems involved have implications as far as feeding at this age is concerned. Only small amounts of amylase, the starch-splitting enzyme are, available in the first two or three months of life and introduction of starch in the first month or two is therefore not justifiable. Lactase, the enzyme which splits milk sugar, lactose, into its components glucose and galactose, is not present in maximal quantity until term. Preterm infants may therefore have difficulty in dealing with large quantities of lactose. The fat-splitting enzyme, lipase, is also present in limited quantity during the first two or three months of life and dietary overload with fat may occur.

Stools

Mothers are frequently concerned about the appearance or smell of their infant's stool.

MECONIUM

Meconium, which is passed during the first one to three days after birth is a dark green sticky paste consisting of swallowed amniotic fluid, desquamated cells and digestive juices. It is odourless.

CHANGING STOOL

As food residues reach the lower bowel a mixture of meconium and stool called a 'changing', or 'transitional', stool is passed. By the third or fourth day the infant is passing stools composed of dietary residue, digestive juices and desquamated cells.

MILK STOOLS

In the breast-fed baby the stool is yellow and has a slightly sour smell. The stool of the baby fed on cow's milk is often paler at first and has a more definite faecal smell. Defaecation is involuntary and may occur several times a day or, particularly in the breast-fed baby, only once every second day.

NUTRITIONAL REQUIREMENTS

The nutritional requirements of an infant have to be considered under various headings including the total amounts of fluid, calories, protein, fat, carbohydrate, minerals and vitamins necessary for normal health and growth. In addition the frequency of feeding and the content of each individual feed is of importance. By using a feed which contains the necessary constituents in the correct proportions the infant, by taking an appropriate volume, is supplied with all the necessary nutritional requirements. If in addition the food is palatable and satisfying to the infant, presented at a suitable temperature and available at short notice the ideal situation is achieved.

Human Milk

Such, in essence, is the situation when an infant feeds from his mother's breast. In the case of the breast-fed infant volume of feed is the only assessment of adequacy of feed whereas in a bottle-fed infant it is also necessary to know the composition of the feed in order to check its nutritional efficiency. With one or two minor exceptions human breast milk can be accepted as a suitable parameter against which to measure any alternative preparation with regard to its nutritional value.

COLOSTRUM

Human breast milk varies slightly in its constitution with stages of lactation and even during an individual feed. During the first two or three days after birth the maternal breast secretes colostrum, which increases progressively in volume and alters in composition until by the third or fourth day milk is being produced together with colostrum which declines in volume thereafter. Colostrum is a translucent fluid with a high protein content but less sugar and fat than milk. The large globulin fraction includes immunoglobulins, some of which may be absorbed by the infant. Since the human infant obtains most of his immunoglobulins transplacentally the contribution of immunoglobulins from colostrum is probably not significant.

CONSTITUTION OF BREAST MILK

As milk flow increases the protein content falls slowly until it reaches a stable level of about 2 per cent at the end of the first week of life and thereafter there is a slow fall to levels of about 1 per cent at one year. At the same time there is a rise in the content of lactose. Fat content is variable both within an individual feed and at different times of the day. Any figures given for the content of human milk have therefore to be averages and these are shown in Table 8.1. The calorie content is of the order of 67 Cal. per 100 ml.

Table 8.1 Average constitution of human and cow's milk

Constituent	Human milk (per 100 ml)	Cow's milk (per 100 ml)
Protein	1.25 g	3.50 g
Casein	0.50 g	3.00 g
Lactalbumin	0.75 g	0.50 g
Lactose	7.50 g	4.50 g
Fat	3.50 g	4.00 g
Minerals	0.20 g	0.70 g
Water	88.00 g	88.00 g
Calories	67	67

With the basic information given above and a knowledge of the volume of breast milk taken by healthy infants who are growing normally an indication of an infant's nutritional requirements can be made.

Volume

By the end of the first week of life an average daily intake would be 150 ml per kg of body weight but this may rise to 190 ml per kg by the end of the first month. Thereafter there is a fall to 150 ml per kg by the fourth month. Intake is highest at the period of maximum growth.

AVERAGE REQUIREMENTS

Taking an average fluid requirement of 150 ml per kg per day and using breast milk as a guide the figures shown in Table 8.2 give the average intake for a healthy infant growing normally and can be accepted as the nutritional requirements of such an infant. Not all infants require the same dietary intake for health and growth and it is important to realize that there is a range of normality, some infants requiring more, some less than the average. The infant's progress remains the best short-term measure of the adequacy of his diet.

Table 8.2 Average daily intake of an infant fed on 150 ml/kg of human milk

	Daily intake (g/kg body weight)
Protein	2.00
Carbohydrate	11.00
Fat	5.25
Calories	100

Information with regard to vitamin requirements has to take into account maximum as well as minimum levels. Minerals cannot be considered in isolation from one another or from other constituents of the diet. Recommended daily intakes of selected vitamins and minerals are shown in Table 8.3. Human breast milk may not contain sufficient iron or vitamin D for the requirement of a rapidly growing infant and in this respect breast milk cannot be accepted as the parameter by which to assess requirements. In order to achieve the amounts described in Table 8.3, infants fed on human and cow's milk will both require dietary supplements after the first month of life.

Table 8.3 Average daily requirement in infancy

Vitamin A	1500 iu
Vitamin C	15 mg
Vitamin D	400 iu
Calcium	600 mg
Iron	6 mg

LONG-TERM EFFECTS

Long-term effects of variations in diet cannot be assessed rapidly and may only become evident as the infant passes through childhood into adult life. Such long-term effects may be due to changes in the mineral or vitamin content of the diet and in some instances to the precise nature of the protein, fat and carbohydrate. Changes may be noted in bone structure, in dental enamel, in the tendency to obesity or hypertension. Infant feeding may have some relation to subsequent character and behaviour. As such problems may be related to factors other than diet in infancy it is not always easy to give recommendations as to optimal requirements.

PHYSIOLOGY OF LACTATION

Having accepted human breast milk as a suitably balanced diet attention will now be paid to the physiology of lactation and to the establishment of lactation.

The Breast

The change in contour of the breast at puberty is due to deposition of fat. At the same time there is development of the areola and nipple with some increase in the duct system. Further development of the duct system occurs in early pregnancy and the alveolar system which consists of secretory cells, differentiates in the middle trimester. Colostrum is present in the breast from the sixteenth week of pregnancy. No milk is produced, however, until after delivery.

THE LACTATING BREAST

The lactating breast (Fig. 8.2) has 18 to 20 segments each consisting of large numbers of secretory alveoli which are drained by small ducts which join others to form a large duct in each segment which eventually leads to a separate opening in the nipple. The walls of the duct contain smooth muscle which can propel milk towards

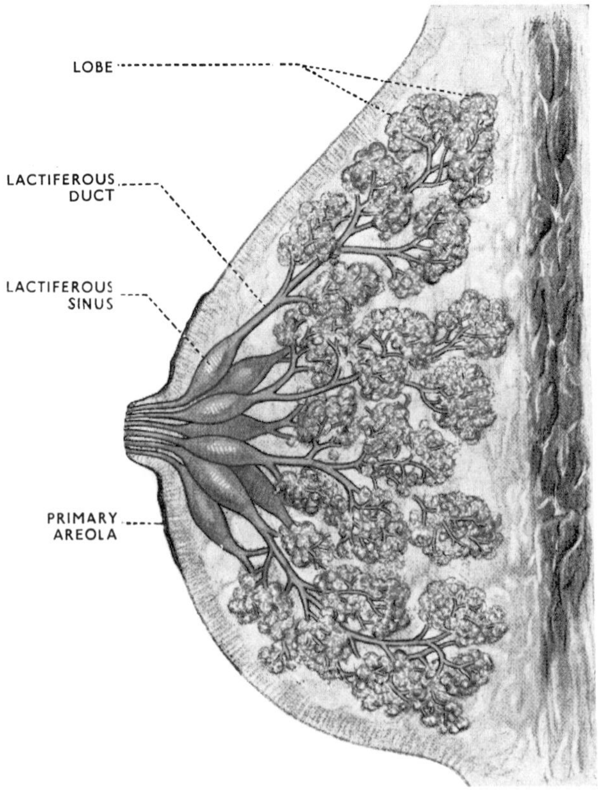

Figure 8.2 The lactating breast.

the nipple. Proximal to the nipple the lactiferous sinus, a distensible segment of the main duct, acts as a small temporary reservoir for milk. When the infant fixes at the breast and draws the nipple well into his mouth the sinuses lie under the areola between the infant's gums. Pressure by the gums helps to eject milk.

CONTROL OF LACTATION

The growth and development of the breast and the production of milk are controlled by hormones the most important of which are oestrogens and prolactin. After delivery the level of oestrogens falls and this fall together with the higher levels of prolactin said to be produced during labour are probably the factors responsible for the initiation of lactation. Once the breast has begun to secrete milk suckling appears to be the strongest stimulant to further milk production. In the early postpartum period lactation used to be inhibited by oestrogens administered to the mother. This practice is no longer acceptable because of the risk of venous thrombosis.

Draught reflex. Milk secretion takes place in the alveoli continuously but muscle sphincters at the nipple prevent leakage between feeds. A variety of stimuli, principally placing the infant to the breast, produces a reflex propulsion of milk from the alveoli and relaxation of the nipple sphincters. This is called the draught reflex (milk flow or milk ejection reflex) and is often recognized by the mother as a prickly sensation in the breast. Once the draught reflex has been initiated milk may continue to flow from both breasts even when the infant is not sucking. Ideally the draught reflex is initiated shortly after the infant fixes on the breast and fortunately most mothers and infants achieve this without difficulty. If the mother is not relaxed at the beginning of a feed the draught reflex may be delayed and the infant is likely to become frustrated.

Relaxation. The successful establishment of breast feeding depends to a considerable extent on the mother's ability to relax before and during a feed. She can be greatly helped in this by the attitude of those around her and by being in a pleasant, comfortable situation. If antenatal instruction has prepared her well and if her attendants are confident and sympathetic a mother is much more likely to be relaxed and to feed her baby at her breast without problems. The example of other mothers calmly and happily feeding their infants has a strong influence and it is often noted that the incidence of breast feeding in a lying-in ward rises as newcomers try to imitate the example of a mother and infant who are clearly enjoying breast feeding. Emotional factors have a big part to play in determining the success of feeding baby at the breast.

INSTRUCTION

Mothers do not know, without an example to follow, how to get their babies to fix at their breasts. Instruction is required. Even those mothers who have attended regularly at antenatal classes on breast feeding find it reassuring to have a sympathetic nurse to help them at the first few feeds. This is a situation requiring calm and patience and time must be allowed so that this can be achieved. The hustle and bustle of hospital life must take a large load of the responsibility for the present decline in breast feeding.

In a quiet, settled atmosphere mother must be shown how to arrange herself and her baby so that both can lie or sit at ease. Mother should hold her baby in the crook of her arm supporting baby's back and buttocks (Fig. 8.3). Baby's head is directed to-

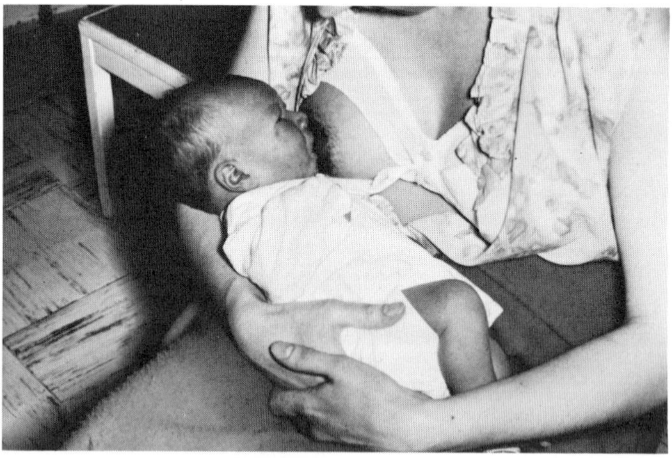

Figure 8.3 Comfortable position for breast feeding.

wards the nipple which should be allowed to touch baby's cheek. The rooting reflex is then stimulated and baby will hunt for the nipple. Mother may help by holding the breast between the fore and middle finger thus protruding the nipple and areola (Fig. 8.4) so that they pass well into baby's mouth. It is important to ensure that baby's nasal airway is not obstructed and that he can breathe freely.

FIRST FEED

The first feed should be offered in the first 12 hours after delivery at a convenient time with short periods of about two minutes at each breast. There appears to be more advantage than disadvantage in continuing feeds of short duration but at frequent intervals until the

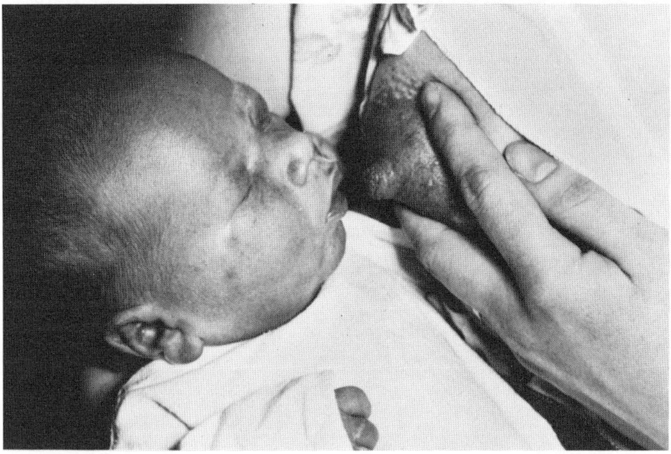

Figure 8.4 Guiding the nipple into baby's mouth.

milk comes in as this helps to establish a good draught reflex with free passage of colostrum and later of milk. The duration of early feeds has to be limited in order to protect mother's nipple, particularly where there is minimal pigmentation.

ENGORGEMENT

The onset of lactation on the third or fourth day after delivery is accompanied in some mothers, particularly primiparae, by a variable degree of engorgement of the breast. Accumulation of milk causes parts of the breast to become tense and tender and there may be oedema of the overlying skin. This is most likely to happen to mothers with small breasts and inelastic skin.

Manual expression. The milk may not flow when the infant feeds but may be removed by manual expression of the breast (Fig. 8.5). Hot bathing of the breast may make this easier. Mothers who have been taught the technique of manual expression in antenatal classes and who practise it as soon as they feel tension rising in the breast have little difficulty in overcoming engorgement and subsequently maintain a free flow of milk. Others find mechanical aids such as the Humolactor helpful.

If the breast is allowed to become severely engorged milk production may be permanently suppressed in the areas affected. The pain of severe engorgement and the poor subsequent lactation put some mothers off further attempts at breast feeding. It is essential, therefore, that this subject be discussed antenatally and that mothers are taught how to cope with the problem before it becomes severe.

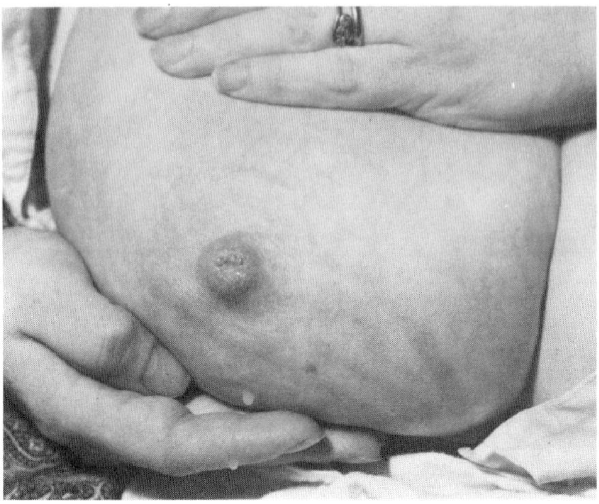

Figure 8.5 Manual expression of engorged breast.

Milk Flow

The flow of milk during a feed is not constant, being largest in the first minute during which up to 50 ml may be taken. Following this rapid flow there are further phases of flow at gradually lengthening intervals. During the intervals the infant may stop sucking temporarily and then induce a further flow by a rapid movement of his jaw and settle again to the slower regular sucking action. It is probable that the breast is not completely emptied at each feed. Prolonged overfilling appears to reduce the volume of milk secreted.

ALTERNATING THE BREASTS

If a mother feeds her baby on the right breast first she may be able to satisfy his needs and should put him to the left breast at the next feed. If the infant is not satisfied at the first breast he should then be placed at the other breast but it is unlikely that he will get as much milk from the second as from the first breast. This is because the draught reflex initiated by his sucking at the first breast occurs in both breasts but generally the nipple sphincters relax only in the breast at which he is feeding probably because of the warmth of his mouth. By the time he is placed at the second breast the draught reflex may be more difficult to initiate and less milk be expelled. The second breast will probably have a considerable volume of milk left at the end of the feed and should be used first at the next feed.

If the supply of milk appears to be diminishing it is important that the infant be put to both breasts at each feed. On the other hand if supply is too plentiful only one breast should be used at each feed.

DEMAND FEEDING

The importance of the draught reflex has been stressed because of its place in the establishment of breast feeding. As with other involuntary reflexes there is ample evidence that it can become conditioned to a variety of stimuli experienced by the mother. Among these, in addition to the stimulus of the infant being placed at the breast, are hearing her infant cry, knowing that it is the usual feed time and warmth applied to the nipple area. Should the reflex be initiated and suckling not start within a few minutes the infant may have difficulty in inducing the reflex again if put to the breast within the next hour. Until a satisfactory regime is established baby should be put to the breast when he appears hungry or if mother senses the draught reflex. This may result at first in frequent feeds at irregular intervals and is a strong indication for leaving infants beside their mothers so that feeding can take place on demand. Mothers must be reassured that the frequency of feeds diminishes over the first few days and that they should have no difficulty in establishing a routine which suits both infant and mother and allows suitable time for her other household duties when she returns home.

CONTINUATION OF LACTATION

The length of time during which lactation continued in women who in the past offered their services as wet nurses shows that milk secretion will continue for many years provided that the stimulus of an infant feeding from the breast continues. There is evidence that if in a period more than one infant was being fed milk production increased while the demand increased but decreased again if the wet nurse again fed only one infant.

The decline in popularity of breast feeding by mothers in this country has been associated with a reduction in the average length of time for which an infant is put to the breast. If an infant is given other foods or fluids he will take less from the breast and with decreasing demand the supply of milk diminishes and eventually ceases. For the comfort of the mother breast feeding should not be stopped suddenly. Once lactation is established oestrogens are much less effective as inhibitors of lactation than they are in the immediate postpartum period and, because of the danger of venous thrombosis, should not be used.

Choice of Feed

BEFORE BIRTH

It follows from what has been stated so far that the management of breast feeding starts with preparatory instruction to the mother when she attends the antenatal clinic. Even more useful may be talks and demonstrations to girls at school (Chap. 3). As the father's attitude can be very important in encouraging or dissuading his wife to breast feed, perhaps the boys should also be included.

PHYSICAL EFFECTS

Encouragement to breast feed can be overdone and harm may result from an overzealous exposition of its advantages which are marginal in any situation where there is a readily available alternative and where standards of hygiene are high. Breast-fed babies are less prone to infections, particularly of the gastrointestinal tract, and are less likely to develop tetany associated with raised levels of phosphate and lowered levels of calcium in the blood. On the other hand breast-fed infants are more liable to deficiency of vitamin K resulting in haemorrhagic disease and, in some families, are more likely to become jaundiced.

EMOTIONAL EFFECTS

Breast- and bottle-fed babies will both thrive if receiving a satisfactory intake. Mother and baby are in close contact with each other in either method. The mother who breast feeds her baby successfully has, however, a greater sense of achievement and this may help to establish a more satisfactory emotional relationship with her infant. Equally it must be recognized that the mother who is forced to breast feed may develop an antipathy not only to breast feeding but even to her infant. The establishment of a satisfactory feeding regime and a happy relationship between mother and infant is more important than theoretical considerations of the relative advantage of one feed over another. Breast feeding is not the ideal solution in every situation. It is unfortunate, however, that it is so infrequently given a trial.

CONTRAINDICATIONS TO BREAST FEEDING

In addition to the situation in which mother chooses not to put her baby to the breast there are a small number of circumstances in which mothers should be advised against breast feeding. These in general are conditions in which mother's health would be harmed to a greater extent than the infant's health would benefit from breast feeding.

Maternal illness. When breast feeding is well established a mother has an additional load on her metabolic activity of up to 1000 calories a day. Mothers with chronic respiratory, renal, or cardiac disease find this extra effort difficult to achieve. Several drugs taken by the mother may be excreted in her milk but the small concentrations occurring only rarely have any clinical effect on her infant and are seldom an indication for stopping breast feeding although there may be an indication for withdrawal of the drugs.

Low birth weight and congenital abnormalities occurring in the infant may make feeding from the breast difficult. If the problem is temporary mother can be encouraged to empty her breasts by manual expression and her milk can be given to her infant by bottle or tube until her infant is able to fix at the breast.

Faulty advice. The reasons given by many mothers for wishing to give up breast feeding after a short trial are often based on faulty advice given by those with no real interest in supporting mother's attempt to feed her baby herself. Very often the antenatal preparation has been inadequate and mother has not been helped enough to gain confidence in her ability to breast feed.

ALTERNATIVE FEEDS

Alternative methods of feeding when breast feeding is not chosen are readily available and, as they are widely advertised, better known by the mother. Two factors have to be considered, the type of milk and the method of delivery. These will be considered separately beginning with the milk. The milk of other mammals is not identical to human milk and whichever milk is chosen some modification is likely to be required to render it suitable for human infants.

COW'S MILK

Because cow's milk is readily available in one form or another in most parts of the world it is the commonest milk to be used. The average constitution of cow's milk when compared with human milk is shown in Table 8.1. The calorie content of the two milks is the same. Fat content varies in both but on average is similar. There is, however, a difference in the protein and carbohydrate components. Human milk has less total protein but more lactalbumin. Casein is present in higher concentration in cow's milk and this makes the total protein content of cow's milk greater. Milk sugar, lactose, is the carbohydrate in both milks and is present in human milk in a higher concentration. Cow's milk contains the same minerals as human milk but in greater quantities.

Modification

Unmodified cow's milk is not well tolerated in the newborn period, the infant having particular difficulty with the large curd formed by casein. Modifications of cow's milk are aimed at reducing the difficulties caused by its casein content. This can be done by a variety of methods including boiling, partial evaporation of water or complete drying. Further alteration is achieved by dilution and restoration of the original calorie value by addition of sugar.

EVAPORATED MILK

Partial evaporation of water from milk leaves a concentrated solution which can be stored in vacuum-packed tins for long periods. Once the tin is opened the evaporated milk is exposed to the same risk of infection and in the same way as is fresh milk and both have a limited duration of usefulness which can be extended by the use of refrigeration. Tinned evaporated milk was the original type of infant feed which could be stored and is still very popular in many parts of the world. Reconstitution to cow's milk is achieved by adding $1\frac{1}{2}$ parts of water to 1 part of evaporated milk.

POWDERED MILK

Reducing milk to the form of a dried powder diminishes its bulk very considerably and makes transport and storage more economical. Because of the presence of fat and a very small amount of moisture it is possible for dried milk to go rancid after very prolonged storage and expiry dates are indicated on packets. As this date is seldom approached in practice it is customary in this country to pack most dried milks in polythene bags within cardboard cartons thus reducing the cost to the consumer. The method employed in drying the milk has an effect on the technique used for reconstitution and some effect on its digestibility by the infant.

DRYING PROCESSES

Roller drying. The first process to be used was introduced at the beginning of this century and involved passage of a thin film of partially evaporated and preheated milk over hot rollers. As the water evaporates the milk leaves the rollers as a thin sheet which is subsequently broken up into a fine powder (Fig. 8.6).

Spray drying. More recently spray drying has become increasingly used. In this process the partially evaporated milk after heating is sprayed either from a nozzle or from a revolving disk into a large chamber in which there is a continuous current of hot air. The resulting dried powder has a finer consistency than that produced by the roller-drying process.

Further improvement is obtained by the 'instantizing' process in which by the addition of a wetting agent the powder becomes more readily soluble in water and can be reconstituted at room temperatures. Roller dried milks are less rapidly reconstituted and require hot water and careful mixing.

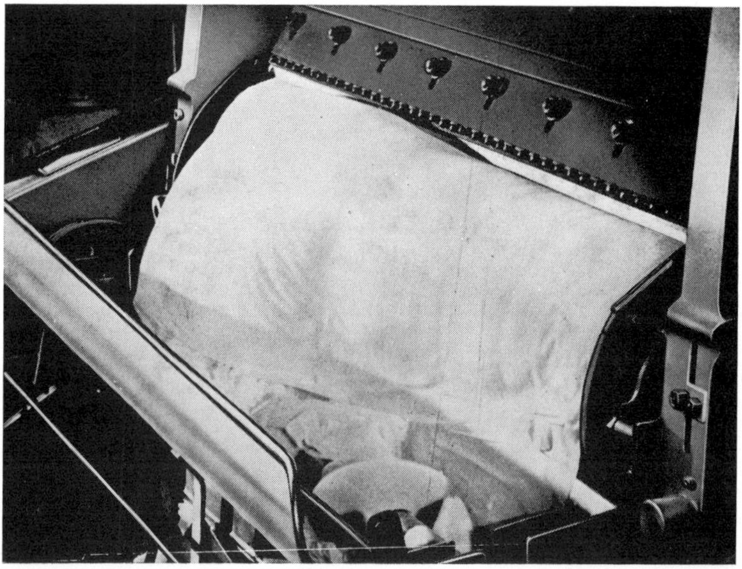

Figure 8.6 Roller drying of milk. (Photograph by courtesy of Cow and Gate Baby Foods.)

Dried Milk Preparations

Before the drying process takes place the manufacturers standardize the milk to a set fat or protein content and in most cases add vitamins and iron. Further alteration of the milk before drying can be carried out to produce milk powders with different fat or carbohydrate content. Fully skimmed milk will keep for very long periods as a dried powder and is used commercially, particularly in the catering industry. It is not, however, suitable as a standard infant feed. It may, however, be used as the basis of an infant feed which is completed by the addition of fats of vegetable origin, lactose, minerals and vitamins, to achieve a final composition which is closely similar to that of human milk. Such adaptations increase the cost of the milk. As most infants thrive on simpler and therefore cheaper modifications of milk the more synthetic milks have not received universal acceptance in this country in spite of their potential advantages. Other forms of humanized milks retain the butter fat but have a modified fat content. The standard dried milks are still offered in two basic forms: half cream, or no. 1; and full cream, or no. 2. Half-cream milks are modified by some firms by partial skimming and addition of carbohydrate. Other firms add extra skimmed milk powder and carbohydrate thus effectively reducing the fat content.

RECONSTITUTION

The final constitution of a dried-milk preparation fed to an infant depends upon the volume of water added to reconstitute the powder. Instructions are given by the makers. In general, where the milk has not been modified before drying, one scoop of the powder in 30 ml of water will reconstitute full-strength cow's milk.

Dilution. Most infants under one month have difficulty in digesting full-strength cow's milk and further modification by dilution is necessary. This is indicated in the manufacturer's directions.

Addition of sugar. As the dilution reduces the calorie content carbohydrate is added in the amount recommended if this has not already been done by the manufacturers. Cane sugar, lactose or maltose-dextrimaltose may be used.

The dilution of the milk is at its greatest in the first week or so and is progressively lessened as the total volume of feeds increases until the infant is fed undiluted reconstituted cow's milk after the first or second month according to his tolerance. Dilution of feeds is also advisable when using evaporated milks so that instead of using 1 part in $1\frac{1}{2}$ parts water it is usual to start feeds with 1 part evaporated milk and 2 parts water and to add sugar.

MINERALS

The mineral content of cow's milk which is proportionately higher than that of human milk causes difficulty to some infants.

Phosphate. In particular they may have difficulty in dealing with the higher levels of phosphate in cow's milk. This results in hyperphosphataemia and, as an indirect consequence, hypocalcaemia, which may be evident as twitching or convulsions (Chap. 16).

Calcium. Some manufacturers add calcium to dried milk powder to maintain a more satisfactory balance between the calcium and phosphate content.

Iron. It has already been mentioned that most manufacturers now add iron in the form of iron and ammonium citrate to milk before drying.

Concentration. It is important to appreciate that adding too small a volume of water to a powdered milk will increase the concentration of all the constituents beyond that in cow's milk. This may be particularly dangerous with minerals such as sodium. Severe brain damage and death have occurred after infants have been fed on concentrated feeds.

VITAMINS

All manufacturers are required to add vitamin D to milk feeds in specified amounts. Vitamin A is generally added with the vitamin D.

After the milk has been dried or evaporated vitamin C is added to some preparations. Other vitamins and minerals are added to the 'humanized' and 'synthetic' preparations. The vitamin and mineral content of dried or evaporated milks is stated on the container. Certain highly specialized feeds which are only required in the treatment of metabolic disorders may not have added vitamins or iron and supplements have to be provided. As these are not generally necessary in the first month of life no further details will be given here.

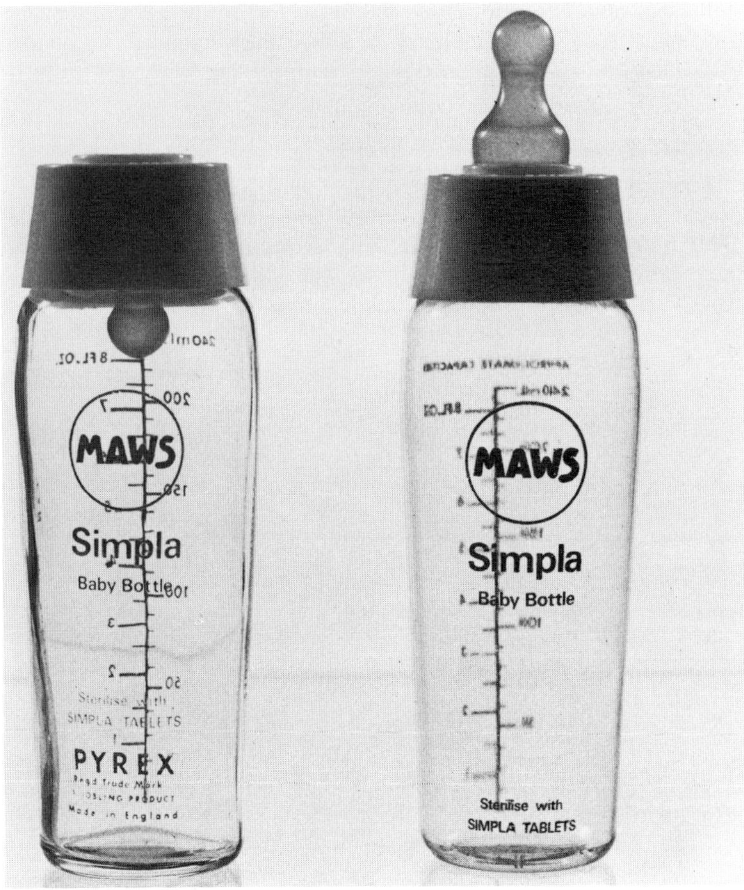

Figure 8.7 Maw's Simpla baby bottle. (Photograph by courtesy of Henleys Medical Supplies Ltd.)

Bottles and Teats

Feeding with cow's milk involves the use of a delivery system which will be accepted by the infant and which protects him from the danger of aspiration of food or of infection from a contaminated bottle or teat. Design of bottles and teats has improved greatly in recent years and the commonly used wide-necked bottles are easier to clean and sterilize than the narrow-necked bottles previously used. Screw-on caps with the teat held in the reverse position (Fig. 8.7) allow feeds to be carried around after preparation without fear of spillage or contamination. Reversal of the teat to the normal feeding position is readily accomplished without touching the bulb of the teat. Disposable plastic bottles or feeding bags have not proved popular in this country.

Prepared Feeds

Recently a number of firms have marketed a range of feeds prepared and sterilized in the factory and issued in a sealed bottle containing 120 ml of feed (Fig. 8.8). A separate sterile disposable teat is also supplied (Fig. 8.9). By the use of such prepared feeds the work carried out in hospital milk kitchens is obviated. The system is

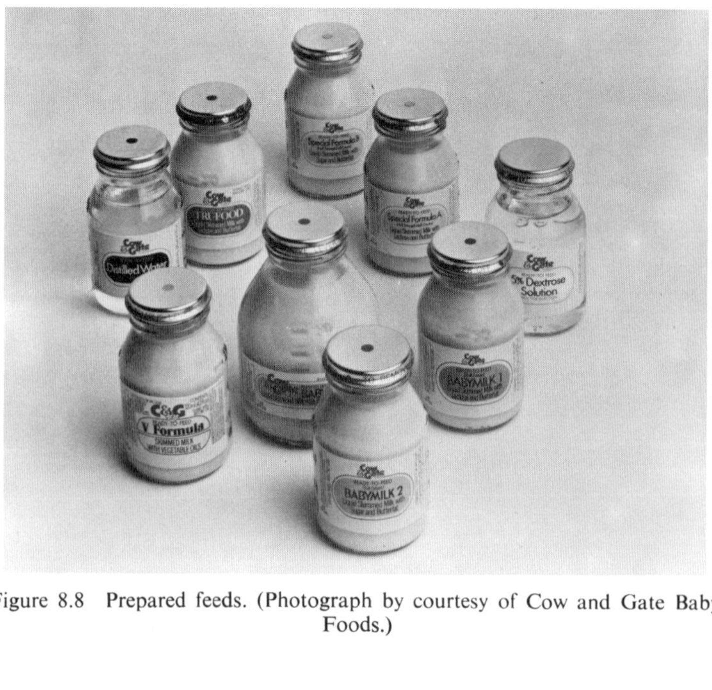

Figure 8.8 Prepared feeds. (Photograph by courtesy of Cow and Gate Baby Foods.)

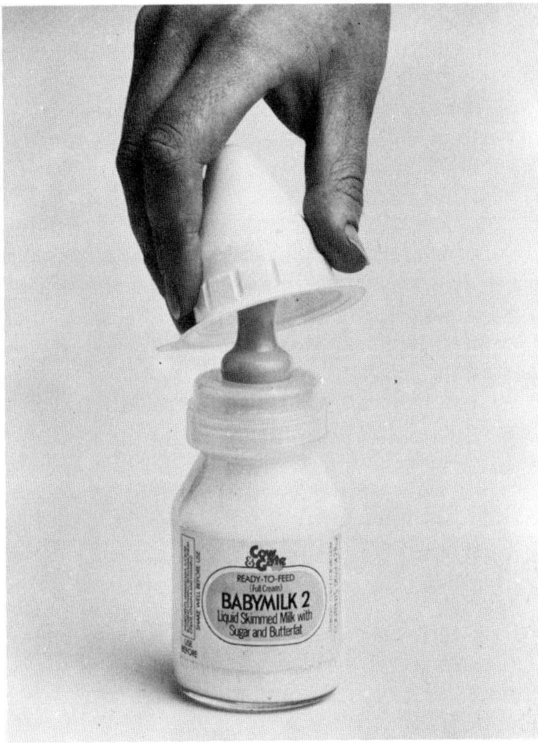

Figure 8.9 Sterile disposable teat attached to prepared feed bottle. (Photograph by courtesy of Cow and Gate Baby Foods.)

more costly per individual feed than feeds prepared in a milk kitchen but the cost can be reduced by resterilizing the teat and using it on more than one occasion. As the expense of providing or maintaining and staffing a milk kitchen is no longer necessary many hospital authorities find that this method of feeding justifies the expense involved. At present it is unlikely that prepared feeds will become available at a price to attract the mother to use them at home.

Sterilization

Even in hospitals using factory-prepared feeds it is essential that medical and nursing staff should be knowledgeable about sterilization of feeds, bottles and teats and that they should be able to instruct mothers in methods suitable for use at home.

Cleaning is a very important part of this process and must be done thoroughly beginning with cold water to remove protein before coagulation and then with hot water to remove the film of fat. Teats should be thoroughly rinsed and turned inside out to ensure that all particles of milk are removed.

Sterilization by complete immersion of bottles and teats in a solution of sodium hypochlorite (Milton) or sodium dichloroiso-cyanurate (Maw's Simpla) for a period of at least four hours is as effective as heat sterilization.

These methods are suitable for use at home and suitable containers are available commercially. Instructions for use are given by the manufacturers. It is important in any chemical method of sterilization to ensure that the bottle and teat are completely immersed and that all air has been expelled. Most mothers find that the convenience of chemical sterilization justifies the small extra cost involved. Sterilizing fluids such as sodium hypochlorite should be replaced every 24 hours. Manufacturers' instructions with regard to concentrations to be used must be observed. It is common practice to rinse bottles and teats after sterilization but this is not absolutely necessary provided that bottle and teat are emptied of sterilizing agent.

Preparation of Feed

WATER

In most areas tap water taken directly from the mains supply is virtually sterile and it is unnecessary to boil it before use. If water is obtained from a tank or if there is any doubt about its sterility it should be boiled before use for mixing feeds.

Mixing. Roller-dried milks have to be mixed in hot water whereas instantized spray-dried milks, such as Golden Ostermilk, can be mixed with water at room temperature as can evaporated milks. Hospitals preparing feeds in large numbers find a mechanical mixer useful when reconstituting roller-dried milks.

Bulk preparation of feeds so that the 24-hour requirements are prepared at one time is economical on staffing in hospital milk kitchens and may equally prove suitable to mother at home. Sterile feeds in sterile screw-top type bottles can be safely stored for up to 24 hours and refrigeration is not essential.

Temperature. If feeds are stored at room temperature there is no need to warm them further. Feeds stored in a refrigerator should be warmed to room temperature before being offered to a baby. There is a risk that in heating feeds mothers will bring them to temperatures which could harm baby's mouth. If heating is applied it is essential that the temperature of the milk be tested by shaking a drop on to the back of mother's hand to test whether it is unpleasantly hot.

Breast Milk Banks

Many maternity hospitals with special-care baby units encourage mothers who are lactating well to empty their breasts after they have fed their infants and to donate the surplus milk to a breast milk bank. Milk from several mothers may be pooled and is then sterilized by boiling in bottles which can subsequently be sealed so that a vacuum is created as the milk cools. Such sterile breast milk can then be stored in a refrigerator at a temperature below 5°C. Bacteriological sampling for sterility should be undertaken regularly. When the milk is required the bottle is heated and then shaken to disperse the fat before opening. After the bottle has been opened any milk left after 12 hours should be resterilized.

Feeding Technique

The technique of feeding a baby from the bottle is just as important as the technique of preparing the feed. As with the mother who breast feeds, relaxation is essential. This implies that mother has the feed prepared and ready to give before she settles in a comfortable position with her infant held securely but not tensely. The bottle must be held so that the teat is always full of milk and this must be checked frequently during a feed. As with the nipple it is important that the teat be allowed to pass well into baby's mouth so that he fixes on the teat in the same way that the breast-fed baby fixes on the nipple.

RATE OF FLOW

Although too fast a flow for baby's comfort may occur with a well-worn teat, particularly if the hole has been enlarged, trouble is more likely to arise from too small a hole with a flow rate lower than that hoped for by the baby. This is most likely to occur with a new teat which is still firm. The hole can most readily be widened by jabbing a red hot needle tip into the hole and then washing away the burned material. It is wise to hold the other end of the needle in forceps or pliers or to push it into a cork before heating. A satisfactory hole allows milk to emerge from the bottle when inverted at a fast flow of drops but not as a continuous stream.

TIME TAKEN

Most babies will finish their feed within 15 minutes. If they are taking longer than this the rate of milk flow may be too low and baby is expending more energy than is advisable. Slow feeding is often accompanied by swallowing of excess air which may cause baby discomfort.

The teat. The consistency and shape of the teat are also of importance. Most babies take the bulb-ended type of teat well. Some, particularly small infants, prefer a soft teat while more vigorous infants do better with a firmer teat.

BREAKING WIND

Breaking wind is a time-honoured custom which allows mother and infant a break during the feed. Positioning of the infant so that the air rises to the fundus of the stomach makes it less likely that milk will be brought up when wind is broken. The other manoeuvres commonly applied such as rubbing or patting the back seem to be aimed at giving mother something to do and therefore may serve some purpose. It is very important for midwives and mothers to appreciate that a good burp by the infant is an indication of faulty feeding technique allowing excess air swallowing rather than a source of pride to whoever is feeding the infant.

FREQUENCY OF FEEDS

As with breast feeding the frequency of feeds can in the first few days be left to the demands of the infant. In hospitals in which babies are kept separately from their mothers this is not easy to achieve and an artificially fixed time interval between feeds is imposed more for the benefit of hospital staff than for the babies' well-being. Small babies may not be able to take sufficient volume at each feed to obtain their total requirement in the five or six feeds available on a four-hourly regime. With a three-hourly regime up to eight feeds in a day can be given and the total volume for each feed thereby reduced. Each infant has to be considered on his own merits and some may start with six or seven feeds at three-hourly intervals and proceed to five feeds at four-hourly intervals as their capacity for taking an individual feed increases.

VOLUME

The volume of feed to be offered should be related to the average taken by babies of the particular age and weight concerned. Such average volumes must only be considered as a guide-line and the appetite and activity of individual babies must always be considered. A breast-fed baby does not take the same volume at each feed and there appears to be no reason to expect the bottle-fed baby to be any more regular in his habits.

Baby's choice. The increasing use of prepared feeds in bottles containing 120 ml makes it easier to allow infants to choose how much they wish to take at individual feeds. If a check is required on the amount taken this can easily be calculated by subtracting the volume of milk left from the initial total of 120 ml using the markings on the bottle. Table 8.4 shows the volumes of feed taken by a group of 40 term babies in one of our hospitals during the first five days of life. Feeding continued until the infant appeared satisfied. For each day of life the table shows the mean or average volume taken by all of the babies together with the maximum and minimum taken by one infant on that day. The babies were all thriving satisfactorily in spite of the large differences in the volume of feed taken.

Table 8.4 Daily intake of 40 term infants allowed to choose their own volume of feed. Day 1 refers to the first 24 hours after feeding commenced

	Daily intake (ml/kg)	
Day	Average	Range
1	63	30 to 103
2	89	50 to 130
3	115	77 to 153
4	127	80 to 170
5	136	90 to 183

Average requirements. It is important that mothers as well as midwives and doctors should be aware of such variations and that a rigid pattern should not be imposed on all infants. At the same time it is useful to have guide-lines so that the inexperienced mother can have some idea of what to expect her baby to take. As most mothers think of volumes of feed in relation to single feeds, the average daily intake of the infant expressed as ml per kg per 24 hours has to be divided by the number of feeds being given in the day to reach a measure of the individual feed. The figures shown in Table 8.4 can be taken as a guide for the first five days of life. By the seventh to tenth day of life term babies will generally be taking 150 ml per kg per 24 hours in five feeds. For a baby of 3.5 kg this will be 100 ml per feed. In recording feeds it is useful to keep a record of the total daily intake.

Low Birth-weight Infants

The feeding of low birth-weight infants requires special consideration and is considered in more detail in Chapters 9 and 10. Fluid and calorie requirements are higher than for mature infants but a longer period is required before the infant can accept the full volume which will often rise to 200 ml per kg body weight per day. Small infants may not be able to suck from the breast or bottle. Such infants are most safely fed by a nasogastric tube. In order to avoid over-distension of the stomach feeds may have to be given in small volumes more frequently, for instance every hour or every two hours. In the smallest infants even this may not be tolerated and feeds can be given by slow infusion into the stomach. A few very small or very ill infants may not tolerate this and intravenous feeding has to be used. When this involves total feeding by the intravenous route specialized knowledge is necessary, and this method should only be used by those fully conversant with the techniques and problems involved.

REASSESSMENT OF FEEDS

The feeding of infants requires periodic reassessment of the total feed given and the content of the feed. As the early very rapid rate of growth with its high energy requirement is followed by a slower rate of growth the need for food becomes relatively less great and mothers have to be taught this. Much of the overfeeding of infants later in the first year of life may stem from a reluctance to accept that the infant's requirements do not continue at the extremely high level of the newborn period. Such overfeeding may establish a pattern which persists into later childhood and adult life resulting in obesity.

As this book is confined to consideration of the care of the newly born the later feeding of infants will not be considered here.

EMOTIONAL RELATIONSHIP

One other aspect in which early feeding patterns may affect subsequent well-being is the emotional relationship which it establishes betweeen a mother and her baby. Feeding is a social occasion in which mother and baby establish a very close contact which should be enjoyed by both. The baby not only enjoys the satisfaction of his hunger being satisfied but also obviously welcomes a feeling of warmth and security by being cradled in his mother's arms, by being handled and spoken to. Mothers also feel pleasure in feeding, as does anyone who bottle-feeds an infant who is feeding well.

Tensions can, however, easily arise either because mother is not relaxed in the first place or because baby is not thought to be feeding well and mother becomes anxious and strained. Overanxiety by parents or attendants, frequent handling of the baby at every whimper, attempts to give feeds when they are not wanted all create an atmosphere of tension which distresses the infant as much as his attendants and which may persist into later life as a factor in preventing normal emotional development.

SATISFACTION

For a satisfactory relationship to be established mother and baby must be confident, relaxed and satisfied with the method of feeding and the type of feed being used. This brings us back to a phrase used at the beginning of this chapter—any method of feeding which provides the basis for normal growth and development and which keeps the infant and mother happy is acceptable.

FURTHER READING

British Medical Journal (1973). Fashions in infant feeding, ii, 727–728.

Catz, C. S. & Giacora, G. P. (1972). Drugs and breast milk. *Pediatric Clinics of North America*, **19**, 151–166.

Gunther, M. (1970). *Infant feeding*. London: Methuen.

Hanson, L. A. & Winberg, J. (1972). Breast milk and defence against infection in the newborn. *Archives of Disease in Childhood*, **47**, 845–848.

Her Majesty's Stationery Office (1970). Recommended intakes of nutrients for the United Kingdom. *Reports on Public Health and Medical Subjects*, no. 120. London: HMSO.

MacKeith, R. & Wood, C. (1971). *Infant Feeding and Feeding Difficulties*, 4th edn. London: Churchill.

Shukla, A., Forsyth, H. A., Anderson, C. M. & Marwah, S. M. (1972). Infantile overnutrition in the first year of life. A field study in Dudley, Worcestershire. *British Medical Journal*, iv, 507–515.

Scottish Home and Health Department (1970). *Principles of Infant Feeding*. Report of the Joint Subcommittee, Standing Nursery and Midwifery Advisory Committees. Edinburgh.

9

Low Birth-Weight Infants

Delivery at term, that is between the 37th and the end of the 41st weeks of pregnancy, increases the chances of an infant's survival whereas delivery before or after term increases the risk of perinatal death. Although the danger of early delivery has always been recognized no means of assessing the degree of risk of what was generally called prematurity was available until agreement was reached on the definition of prematurity.

Definitions

In earlier editions of this book, in accordance with an international agreement, the word premature was used to describe all babies weighing 2500 g or less at birth. This artificial weight barrier had the merit of simplicity when used as a definition for statistical purposes. It failed to take into account those babies who, although born at term and healthy, weigh less than 2500 g. The weight range of term babies varies in different parts of the world and birth weight is not in itself an adequate measure of maturity.

LOW BIRTH WEIGHT

The last statement does not, however, mean that we should abandon the weight of 2500 g as a line of division. The group of infants weighing 2500 g or less at birth are at a major disadvantage compared with the much larger group weighing over 2500 g. The dividing line, although not ideal, is acceptable provided that we designate those of 2500 g or less at birth as low birth-weight infants.

Significance. More than 50 per cent of stillbirths in the United Kingdom and almost 70 per cent of neonatal deaths are associated with low birth weight, although only 7 per cent of deliveries in the United Kingdom fall into this group. Of infants who die within four weeks of birth more than half are of low birth weight. The scale of the problem, which is the concern of the sociologist no less than the doctor and midwife, is evident in the fact that annually more than 5500 registered deaths in England and Wales are attributable to low birth weight or to conditions associated with low birth weight. More than 80 per cent of these deaths occur during the first week and more than 50 per cent during the first 24 hours of life. Together with the infant death rate, the neonatal and perinatal death rates are accepted as reliable indices of socioeconomic progress. The problem of low birth weight is the most important single challenge confronting those responsible for the care of the newly born.

PRETERM INFANTS

Menstrual age. The antenatal examinations of the mother used for assessing menstrual age have been discussed in Chapter 4. Term is defined as a menstrual age of 259 to 293 days (37 to 41 weeks). A preterm infant is one delivered before 259 days (37 weeks) as based on the menstrual age of the pregnancy (Table 9.1).

Table 9.1 Definition of menstrual age of the fetus

Preterm	Less than 259 days (37 weeks)
Term	259 to 293 days (37 to 41 weeks)
Post-term	294 days and over (42 weeks and over)

Postnatal examination. A method of assessing the infant's state of development at birth which allows an estimate to be made of the stage of pregnancy at which it was born is described later.

Weight. Most preterm infants are of low birth weight and weigh less than 2500 g at birth.

WEIGHT FOR GESTATIONAL AGE

Birth weight is not an acceptable measure of maturity because low birth weight may be caused either by preterm delivery or by slow fetal growth (Table 9.2). A further definition is therefore required taking into account menstrual age. Infants less than the 10th percentile of the weight distribution for their particular menstrual (gestational) age are termed light-for-dates and infants over the 90th percentile are termed heavy-for-dates.

Table 9.2 Outline of causes of low birth weight

Preterm delivery
Maternal ill-health
Complications of pregnancy
Fetal abnormality
Slow fetal growth
Malnutrition *in utero*
Poor placental function
Hypoplasia
Constitutional
Chromosome abnormality
Combination of 1 and 2

Light-for-dates. Table 9.3 shows a percentile distribution of weight at different gestational ages. It will be seen that some light-for-dates infants born at term will be 2500 g or less at birth. Infants who are below the 10th percentile for their gestational age at birth have often been noted at earlier stages of pregnancy to be small and their smallness is associated with failure of adequate growth through much of pregnancy. Possible reasons for this have already been discussed in Chapter 4. In general they can be classified as malnourished or hypoplastic.

Table 9.3 Weight percentiles for gestational age. (Reproduced with permission from Brown, R. J. K. & Valman, H. B. (1971) *Practical Neonatal Paediatrics*. Oxford: Blackwell.)

Completed week from L.M.P.	Percentiles of birth weight (g) 10th	50th	90th*
28	700	1140	
29	850	1280	
30	1000	1440	
31	1160	1640	
32	1330	1870	
33	1530	2110	
34	1740	2340	3100
35	1950	2550	3330
36	2160	2750	3520
37	2370	2950	3670
38	2570	3100	3780
39	2720	3240	3880
40	2820	3370	3970
41	2880	3450	4040
42	2910	3500	4100
43	2880	3510	4120
44	2850	3460	4140

* Cannot be reliably established below 34 weeks.

Usefulness of classification. Does this classification serve any useful purpose? The answer is very definitely yes as it is only by thorough assessment at birth that we can plan adequately that infant's future management and prevent those complications to which he is most exposed. In particular we must learn to recognize those infants who have failed to grow adequately *in utero* as they have problems of a different nature from those low birth-weight babies who are adequately nourished but who were delivered before term.

Postnatal Assessment of Maturity

As a check on the information available from antenatal examinations it is useful to have methods of assessment of maturity which are

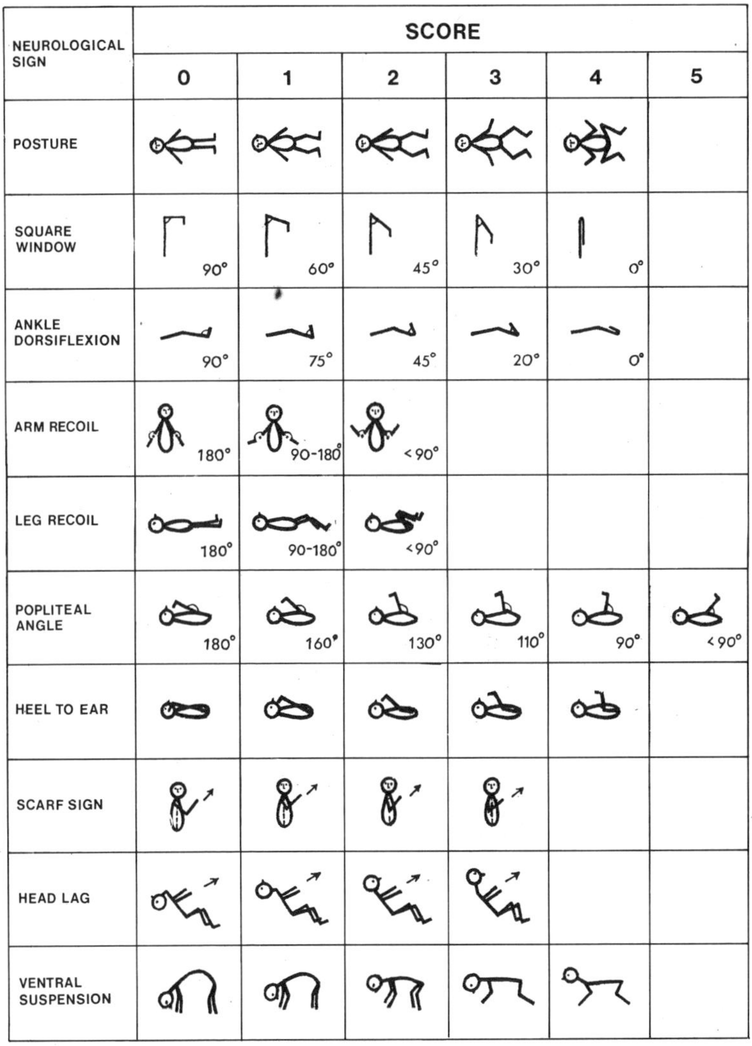

Figure 9.1 Scoring system for neurological signs.

(Figures 9.1 and 9.2 are reproduced by kind permission of the authors and C. V. Mosby Company from Dubowitz, L. M. S., Dubowitz, V., & Goldberg, C. (1970). Clinical assessment of gestational age in the newborn infant, *Journal of Pediatrics*, 77, 1–10.)

Table 9.4 Scoring system for external criteria

External sign	Score* 0	1	2	3	4
Oedema	Obvious oedema of hands and feet; pitting over tibia	No obvious oedema of hands and feet; pitting over tibia	No oedema		
Skin texture	Very thin gelatinous	Thin and smooth	Smooth; medium thickness. Rash or superficial peeling	Slight thickening. Superficial cracking and peeling especially of hands and feet	Thick and parchment-like: superficial or deep cracking
Skin colour	Dark red	Uniformly pink	Pale pink; variable over body	Pale: only pink over ears, lips, palms, or soles	
Skin opacity (trunk)	Numerous veins and venules clearly seen, especially over abdomen	Veins and tributaries seen	A few large vessels clearly seen over abdomen	A few large vessels seen indistinctly over abdomen	No blood vessels seen
Lanugo (over back)	No lanugo	Abundant; long and thick over whole back	Hair thinning especially over lower back	Small amount of lanugo and bald area	At least half of back devoid of lanugo
Plantar creases	No skin creases	Faint red marks over anterior half of	Definite red marks over > anterior $\frac{1}{2}$;	Indentations over > anterior $\frac{1}{3}$	Definite deep indentations over

		flat, diameter < 0.75 cm	diameter < 0.75 cm	meter > 0.75 cm
Breast size	No breast tissue palpable	Breast tissue on one or both sides, < 0.5 cm. diameter	Breast tissue both sides; one or both 0.5–1.0 cm	Breast tissue both sides; one or both > 1 cm
Ear form	Pinna flat and shapeless, little or no incurving of edge	Incurving of part of edge of pinna	Partial incurving whole of upper pinna	Well-defined in-curving whole of upper pinna
Ear firmness	Pinna soft, easily folded, no recoil	Pinna soft, easily folded, slow recoil	Cartilage to edge of pinna, but soft in places, ready recoil	Pinna firm, cartilage to edge; instant recoil
Genitals Male	Neither testis in scrotum	At least one testis high in scrotum	At least one testis right down	
Female (with hips half abducted)	Labia majora widely separated, labia minora protruding	Labia majora almost cover labia minora	Labia majora com-pletely cover labia minora	

* If score differs on two sides, take the mean.

From Dubowitz, M. S., Dubowitz, V. & Goldberg, C. (1970). Clinical assessment of gestational age in the newborn infant, *Journal of Pediatrics*, **77,** 1–10; adapted from Farr and associates (1966) *Developmental Medicine and Child Neurology*, **8,** 507.

based on examination of the infant at birth. Before we consider the particular problem facing preterm and light-for-dates babies we

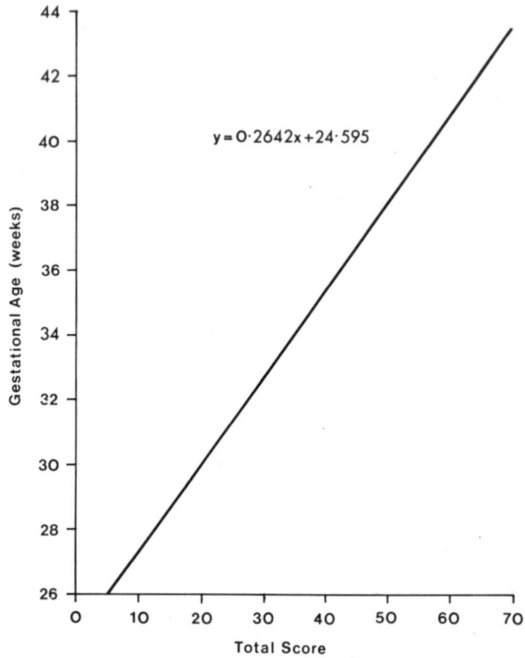

Figure 9.2 Graph for calculation of gestational age from total score.

shall therefore, consider methods of assessment of maturity after delivery.

The examination to be described is based on that described by Dubowitz, Dubowitz and Goldberg (1970). It can be carried out at any time during the first five days of life provided that there is no evidence of birth injury. The method is easily learned and with practice the examination can be completed in about 10 minutes.

The assessment is based on a series of external characteristics and a number of neurological signs based on posture and primitive reflexes. Each sign is given a score.

EXTERNAL CHARACTERISTICS

The external signs and the scoring system used are shown in Table 9.4. Some of these signs are less easy to score than others but in general little difficulty is found. As each sign is explained in the table no further comment will be made here.

NEUROLOGICAL SIGNS

The signs used and the scores given are demonstrated diagrammatically in Figure 9.1. The legend describes the techniques of assessment of the neurological criteria.

FINAL SCORE

The maximum score of 70 is equally divided between the external characteristics and the neurological signs. The score achieved by an infant is plotted on a graph (Fig. 9.2) which correlates the score with gestational age.

THE PRETERM INFANT

The significance of low birth weight has been discussed earlier in this chapter. Preterm delivery is a major cause of low birth weight and is associated with a greatly increased risk of mortality and morbidity. The degree of risk increases progressively the longer before term that an infant is born. Improved methods of management have increased the chance and quality of survival of small preterm infants but the risk of complications remains sufficiently high to justify every effort being taken to prevent preterm delivery.

Prevention of Preterm Delivery

Prevention of preterm delivery requires knowledge about the factors which predispose to the onset of labour before term. As

Table 9.5 Factors carrying a high risk of preterm delivery

MATERNAL
General
Age: below 20 years
Height: less than 155 cm
Poor socioeconomic status
Unmarried
Obstetric
Primiparity
Pre-eclamptic toxaemia
Antepartum haemorrhage
Chronic ill-health
Smoking
Previous history of preterm delivery
FETAL
Multiple pregnancy
Congenital abnormalities
Slow intrauterine growth

knowledge of the factors responsible for the onset of labour at term is incomplete it is not surprising that we are also ignorant about many of the reasons why women go into labour before term.

FACTORS PREDISPOSING TO PRETERM DELIVERY

Some factors are recognized as carrying a high risk of inducing premature labour and these are listed in Table 9.5.

PREVENTIVE MEASURES

Improvement in socioeconomic status. As will be seen some of the factors such as poor social circumstances, poor nutrition and small stature are not amenable to short-term medical treatment. They still constitute a considerable problem in the United Kingdom but are a major cause of preterm delivery in underdeveloped countries. Raising the general standard of living in a community lowers the incidence of preterm delivery and political or economic efforts to achieve this end are likely to produce a reduction in preterm delivery more readily than advances in medical knowledge.

Antenatal care. Regular and careful supervision during the antenatal period improves the chance of early recognition and treatment of complications of pregnancy which may lead to preterm delivery. Education of the mother in general health care and in the recognition of early warning signs of developing problems will all help to allow improved antenatal care. In many mothers 'at risk' pregnancy can be prolonged by such simple measures as bed rest for which hospital admission may be necessary.

Obstetric care. If a mother goes into labour before term every effort should be made to get her to a maternity unit with a special-care baby unit for delivery and care of her baby. Mothers must be told in the antenatal clinic of the action they should take should they suspect that labour is starting. The greatly increased risk of delivery of a small preterm infant at home must be stressed. The mother's uterus is the ideal transport incubator for bringing such an infant to hospital.

Delivery and Resuscitation

Midwifery, obstetric, anaesthetic and paediatric staff may be involved in the care of the infant at delivery. It is essential that all those likely to be involved should have been trained in resuscitative procedures and be aware of the need to maintain the infant's body heat. Resuscitative measures are discussed in Chapter 19. When the need for resuscitation is anticipated before delivery an experienced member of the paediatric team should be present in the delivery room. If an emergency arises in the absence of paediatric staff the individual on the spot who is best qualified should be responsible for the vital process of resuscitation.

WARMTH

Early cooling can be avoided by carrying out resuscitation under a suitably designed infant warmer of which a number of varying designs are commercially available.

Transfer to nursery. When the baby is transferred from the labour ward to another hospital, or even to another ward in the same hospital, there is always the danger of hypothermia and such

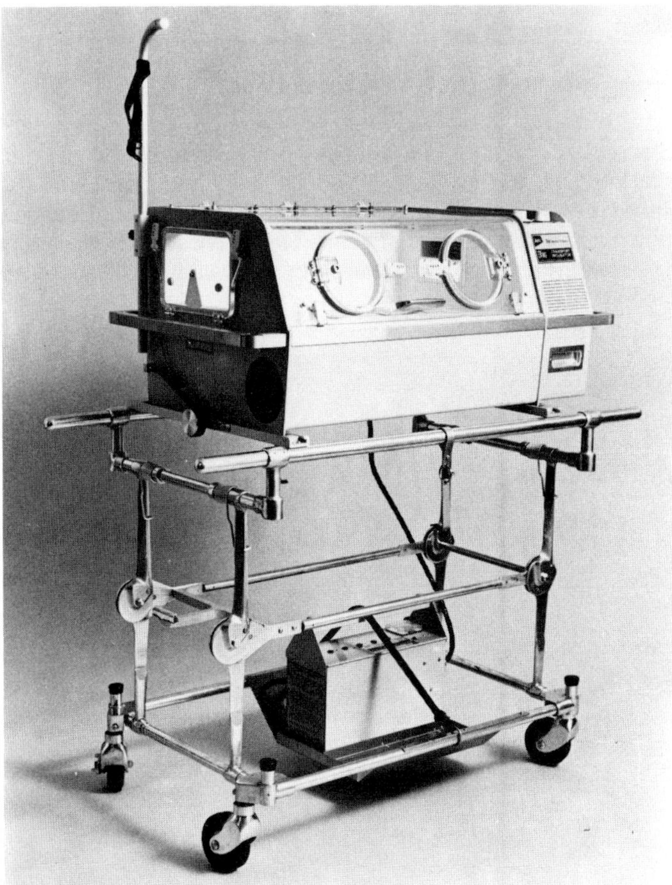

Figure 9.3 Ohio transport incubator. (Photograph by courtesy of P. K. Morgan Ltd.)

journeys should always take place in a portable incubator. A heated portable incubator, ready for immediate use, should be retained in the labour ward (Fig. 9.3). In the absence of a portable incubator the baby should be wrapped in a warm dry towel or a blanket or enclosed in an aluminium swaddler while being moved.

Indications for special care nursery. Not all low birth-weight infants require the facilities of a special-care baby unit. It is probable, however, that most infants of 2000 g or less will require extra attention and all infants of that weight should be admitted in the first place to special-care wards for observation. Any infant over 2000 g who is showing evidence of respiratory difficulty or who is not maintaining his temperature readily should also be in the special-care unit until fit for return to his mother.

General Characteristics of the Preterm Baby

APPEARANCE

The preterm infant's head and abdomen are large and his thorax small (Fig. 9.4). Hands and feet appear ungainly. The skin is soft, slightly velvet-like in texture and moderately elastic, and the colour pale or more usually a delicate pink. The forehead may be wrinkled, and frequently in the very small baby the veins of the head show

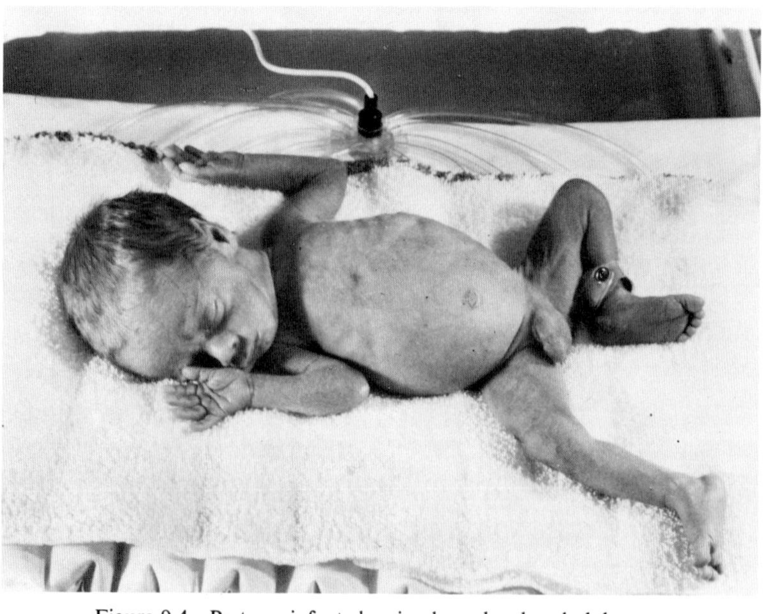

Figure 9.4 Preterm infant showing large head and abdomen.

prominently. In the female the labia minora are visible and not hidden by the labia majora as in the term infant. The testes have often not descended into the scrotum in the preterm male infant. The nails may not reach the tips of the digits, an observation which does not deserve the importance sometimes attached to it. A generalized lack of subcutaneous tissue results in prominence of the body skeleton.

ACTIVITY

The preterm baby is commonly described as being inactive and as sleeping throughout the day except when disturbed for feeding. In point of fact there are few preterm babies who are absolutely still even in sleep. If a preterm baby is observed in an incubator his breathing will be seen to be rhythmical but not wholly regular. His abdominal muscles are constantly moving. Every now and again a limb will flex and relax. At one time he may be seen lying on his back, his arms lazily outstretched and at another lying easily on his side, his lower limbs gently flexed at hips and knees. Occasionally a very small infant shows remarkable activity (it might almost be called agility) during the first day or two of life after which his behaviour resembles that of other larger preterm babies. In the course of time increasing bodily vigour affords unmistakable evidence of growing strength.

CHANGES AFTER BIRTH

Weight. Following birth there is a physiological loss of weight comparable with that of the full-term child. For a variable period extending over a number of days there is a progressive slight loss of subcutaneous tissue, usually evident in the face, trunk and limbs. Reversal of the trend is gradual.

Muscle tone. As tissue tone improves, muscle groups become more clearly defined. This is first evident in the calf muscles. The nasolabial and other skin folds become more prominent about the same time. Later, but only slowly, the musculature and related tissues increase in bulk, until eventually the face acquires a contour suggestive of rotund 'chubbiness'.

Respiration. For some time following birth, respiration is often irregularly erratic in rate, rythm and amplitude. A more constant pattern slowly evolves, but breathing remains essentially abdominal in character.

Changes in activity. In the course of time activity increases in vigour, and this is reflected in the increasing strength of the cry and in the growing determination with which nourishment is taken. As body tone increases, the infant periodically indulges in a slow, deliberate stretching of the entire body reminiscent of an adult awakening from a satisfying sleep. Yawning is characteristic and sneezing common. In a way difficult to describe, the delicate colour of the skin gives place to a 'bloom' indicative of increasing vitality.

Jaundice may mask this change, but is less likely to do so if the baby is disturbed before observations on the colour of the skin are made. As compared with that in the full-term infant, physiological jaundice is often both more pronounced and more prolonged (Chap. 14). Jaundice in the small preterm baby must always be kept under close observation and kernicterus prevented by early treatment (Chap. 14).

Nursing Care

The most significant factor in the survival of a low birth-weight infant is the standard of nursing care provided to meet his requirements. Advances in the understanding of physiological processes and the provision of complicated electronic equipment help to improve the service which the nurse provides but do not replace it. This aspect of the care of the preterm infant is so important that a separate chapter (Chap. 10) is devoted to it. In order to preserve some continuity of thought in this chapter a brief outline of the most important aspects of nursing care is presented.

STAFFING

The staffing requirements of special-care nurseries have already been considered in Chapter 2, where it was shown that a high nurse–patient ratio will be required. At all times nurses who have been trained in the care of preterm babies should be available. As the nursing staff are those most directly and most constantly involved in the observation of the infant and the management of his environment they must be constantly aware of the potential problems which may arise and know what action to institute if any abnormality is observed.

Temperature control. As the small infant's most important problems are temperature control and maintenance of adequate respiration nursing staff must bear in mind the possible effect on these factors of any nursing procedure they plan to carry out.

Oxygen. The dangers of some forms of management such as exposure of the infant to high concentrations of oxygen have to be remembered.

Infection. The particular risk to preterm infants of infection (Chap. 13) places a further responsibility on attendant nurses as spread of infection should be preventible by good nursing technique.

Feeding

IMPORTANCE

Feeding is essential for the further growth of all infants and is of particular importance to the preterm infant. This is because the very high intrauterine rate of growth and development can only be achieved after birth with a high intake of the factors essential for growth. Among other things these include fluid, calories and amino acids. Most preterm infants cannot accept their full requirements of all these factors immediately after birth and feeding has to be adjusted very carefully to make sure that the infant receives as much as he can tolerate of an appropriate food until he is able to take sufficient to re-establish a normal rate of growth.

Changed policy. Earlier and more liberal feeding of preterm infants is now a generally accepted policy. Previously the risks attached to early feeding, which included the possibility of aspiration after vomiting a feed, were considered too great to justify feeding before the third or fourth day. Now it is clear that the harm caused by delayed feeding, with the resultant metabolic acidosis, hypoglycaemia, jaundice and serious brain damage, is greater than the risks of early feeding, which, with a good standard of supervision, are relatively low.

EARLY FEEDING

The policy of early feeding has resulted in a fall in such problems as hypoglycaemia and jaundice, in improved growth and in improved later neurological development.

The first feed can be given at about 3 hours of age. Some adjustment may be necessary because of the infant's condition but it is essential to start some form of nutrition before 12 hours of age and preferably before 6 hours in all preterm infants including those who are ill.

METHOD

The most mature infants of over 35 weeks gestation who will weigh more than 2000 g will generally have little difficulty in feeding from the breast or from a bottle.

Infants of about 32 to 35 weeks gestation may be able to take some feeds by bottle particularly during the first day or two, but as they become quickly tired by bottle feeding they must be supervised very carefully and tube-fed whenever they become exhausted.

Tube feeding will be required at some stage for most infants of less than 35 weeks gestation and for some more mature infants. The risks of this method have been greatly reduced since the introduction of disposable feeding tubes which can be left in place for longer periods than untreated rubber tubes. Complications of tube feeding do still occur and must always be borne in mind. They include faulty passage of a tube into the trachea with a major risk of the infant's death, if a feed is given before the mistake has been recognized. Leaving a nasogastric tube in place for long periods leads to the risk of ulceration of the nose or pharynx and of perforation of the stomach. Repeated withdrawal of a tube increases the risk of aspiration. Most of these dangers can be reduced by good nursing technique. The nursing aspects of tube feeding are dealt with in Chapter 10.

Frequency. As discussed in Chapter 8 the frequency of feeding will depend upon the volume of feed which the infant can tolerate at an individual feed. This volume of tolerance will increase progressively but as the infant's total volume requirements may not be reached for two to three weeks after birth small and frequent feeds are likely to be required by most preterm infants. For the smallest, of the order of 1000 g, a continuous intragastric infusion is required. Others will require half-hourly, hourly, two-hourly or three-hourly feeds according to the volume which they can tolerate. The interval between feeds is progressively increased as the volume tolerated per feed increases. Most mothers find it difficult to give more than six feeds a day when their baby returns home, and the feeding regime should be arranged to bring the total number of feeds down to this number by the time of baby's discharge.

Volumes. Guide-lines only can be given as to the total volume of feed to be given in the 24 hours. Much will depend upon the infant's capacity to tolerate these volumes and this capacity may vary from day to day with changes in the infant's condition. Preterm infants have a greater fluid and calorie requirement than term infants. Total 24 hour volumes on the first day should be of the order of 30 to 50 ml per kg rising by 10 to 20 ml per kg per day as tolerated with the aim of achieving a total volume of 150 ml per kg per day by the end of the second week, and increasing up to 200 ml per kg per day by the end of the third week of life, if this is indicated and tolerated.

As an example an infant of 32 weeks gestation weighing 1300 g at birth could be offered eight feeds of 6 ml in the first 24 hours. If these are accepted three-hourly feeding could be continued, giving eight feeds in the day and increasing the volume to 8 ml on the second day, 10 ml on the third day, and increasing by 1 or 2 ml per feed per day, aiming at 20 ml feeds by the 10th day and 25 ml by the 15th day and 30 ml by the 20th day.

If this volume of feeding caused vomiting or distress on the second or third day the volume per feed would be reduced and the frequency increased so that on the third day instead of eight feeds of 10 ml at three-hourly intervals, 12 feeds of 7 ml would be given at two-hourly intervals.

MILK

Composition. Giving an infant a suitable volume of feed is only an indication of satisfactory nutrition if the feed is of a satisfactory composition. As stated in Chapter 8 human breast milk can be accepted as having a model content for the feeding of human infants. No completely satisfactory substitute has been marketed but many preterm infants can thrive satisfactorily on a modification of cow's milk.

Breast milk. Experience has shown that for the smallest infants human breast milk is a safer feed in that it is less likely to lead to digestive and other complications. Wherever possible infants below 1500 g should be started on feeds of expressed breast milk (Chap. 8).

Modified cow's milk. Opinions range widely as to the optimal formula for modification of cow's milk feeds for preterm infants. The policy of using so-called half-cream preparations is difficult to justify as it implies giving a feed with more than 10 per cent carbohydrate. This is liable to overload the disaccharide-splitting capacity and result in loose stools and possible metabolic acidosis. The mineral content of most full-cream preparations may cause problems. Further modification of milk as in S.M.A. overcomes some of these difficulties. Two new modified milk preparations were introduced in the U.K. in 1973. These are Cow and Gate V Formula and Ostermilk New Ready to Feed Milk Food. A period of assessment is advisable before any recommendations are made about their suitability for routine use with preterm infants.

Calories. Satisfactory weight gain is generally achieved and maintained on a daily intake of 110 to 130 Cal per kg. Human breast milk has 67 Cal per 100 ml and it is advisable to maintain the same calorie content in artificial feeds.

Protein. Human breast milk contains approximately 1.5 g protein per 100 ml. A preterm infant requires a minimum protein intake of 2 g per kg per day and cannot tolerate more than 6 g per kg per day. A preterm infant fed on breast milk must therefore take 150 ml per kg per day before his minimum protein requirements are satisfied.

The advocates of giving higher protein intakes than can be achieved with breast milk feeding alone have yet to prove the long-term advantage of such feeds. As the proportion of casein to lactalbumin is higher in unmodified cow's milk and as infants find greater difficulty in utilizing casein the higher protein content of cow's milk (3.5 g per 100 ml) is not readily used by the infant.

Minerals. The mineral content of breast milk (0.2 per cent) is lower than that of cow's milk (0.7 per cent). Increasing the solute load of a feed adds problems to the feeding of small preterm infants. This factor must be remembered when calculating the concentration of milk to be given.

Choice of milk. In spite of its lower protein content we are happy to accept human breast milk as the ideal preparation for feeding preterm infants. Of the modifications of cow's milk which have been fully assessed S.M.A. appears to have most advantages for the very smallest infants but larger infants thrive satisfactorily on preparations used for feeding term infants.

INTRAVENOUS FEEDING

The ability of infants to tolerate gastric feeds may be so limited that they cannot be given an adequate intake by this method. This is most likely to occur in infants who have respiratory or other problems. In such circumstances fluid must be given intravenously. For short periods simple solutions such as dextrose and saline may suffice, but they cannot provide sufficient calories for growth and there is no protein being given. Much has yet to be learned about the intravenous feeding of small preterm infants with amino acid and lipid preparations and this subject will not be discussed here.

Since the more extensive use of feeding by constant infusion of breast milk into the stomach the need for intravenous feeding of very small but healthy infants has been greatly reduced.

RECORDING OF FEEDS

As the progress of preterm infants is so dependent on a sufficient intake of fluid, calories and protein it is essential that a very careful record should be made of what each infant is receiving.

A feed chart should be kept for each infant showing the time, the type of feed, the volume given, the method by which it was given and how the infant reacted. In addition the total volume of feed given in each 24-hour period should be calculated and recorded. It is very useful to have this total volume recorded on the daily record so that the weight pattern can be checked against the volume of intake.

As most nurseries will be using a standard feed it is essential that the composition of that feed—its calorie, protein and mineral content—should be known to those in charge of feeding so that a check on these factors can be kept.

SUPPLEMENTS

As explained in Chapter 8 the vitamin and iron content of both human and cow's milk is not generally sufficient to supply the requirements of the preterm infant during its most rapid period of growth. Vitamin supplements should be given from 1 month of age and continued during the first year of life. Multivitamin preparations such as Abidec (Parke Davis) 0.6 ml per day together with the vitamins A and D added to artificial milks is generally sufficient to cover the preterm infant's requirements of up to 800 iu vitamin D and 50 mg vitamin C daily.

Supplements of iron should be added during the second month of life and continued until baby is fully weaned. This is to prevent the late anaemia of prematurity (Chap. 17).

Complications of Preterm Delivery

The complications associated with preterm delivery are really a reflection of the structural and functional immaturity of the individual organs of the baby as compared with their counterparts in an infant who has gone to term. The cerebral centres share in this immaturity of development and theoretically it can be argued that cerebral immaturity contributes in varying degree to most of the handicaps experienced by the preterm baby. Although the implications of immature development of cerebral centres are not fully understood, knowledge concerning other factors giving rise to handicap are more precise.

The principal handicaps in question relate to temperature control, respiratory, renal and alimentary function. Additional to these are the immature infant's liability to haemorrhage, anaemia, jaundice, infection and hypoglycaemia.

HYPOTHERMIA

Central temperature. Throughout this chapter reference is frequently made to the need to prevent loss of heat from preterm babies so that body temperature can be maintained. The most significant body temperature is that which applies to the internal organs and which is referred to as central, or core, temperature. Skin, or superficial, temperature is dependent on a number of factors which may change rapidly. Central, or core, temperature changes more slowly and, particularly in small preterm infants, is affected by skin temperature. In a satisfactory environment (Table 9.6) central

Table 9.6 Suggested incubator temperatures

Weight of infant	Temperature of incubator
1 kg	35°C
2 kg	34°C
3 kg	33°C

temperature will remain stable within a small range of normal and skin temperature will not differ by more than 0.5°C from central temperature. An environment which satisfies these conditions is called a neutral thermal environment and is the environment which we should aim at creating for all low birth-weight infants. The precise conditions required for a neutral thermal environment may be slightly different for each infant and therefore the situation has to be assessed separately for each baby.

Heat loss. The means by which infants produce and lose heat have already been discussed in Chapter 5. Preterm infants are able to produce heat by metabolic activity including the burning of brown fat. Unless they are in a suitable environment, however, their ability to produce heat is readily overburdened by the ease with which they lose heat. Heat loss takes place from the skin by radiation, convection and conduction, by evaporation of moisture from the lungs and airways, and the urine and faeces. The relatively larger surface area increases skin loss and the lack of subcutaneous fat means that the deeper tissues are less well insulated from the effect of fall in skin temperature. Hypoxia is accompanied by reduced metabolic activity and a fall in body temperature.

Neonatal cold injury. Loss of heat greater than that which can be replaced by the infant leads to hypothermia. Initially this is evident as lowering of skin temperature and later as a fall in central temperature. If the fall in skin temperature can be corrected rapidly the fall in central temperature can be prevented. Severe hypothermia with progressive fall in central temperature is a serious complication and may be irreversible. Before the dangers of hypothermia were fully appreciated infants developed what was called neonatal cold injury in which the subcutaneous tissues particularly of the cheeks, buttocks and limbs became increasingly firm until movement was prevented (Fig. 9.5). Such infants often had very low blood sugars, bowel movement ceased, and internal haemorrhages occurred. Death was common. Treatment in the later stages was seldom successful and the only useful line of management is prevention of heat loss and the recognition of early stages of fall in skin temperature.

The significance with regard to nursing techniques and medical procedures is discussed in Chapters 10 and 19.

RESPIRATORY DISTRESS

Embarrassment of respiratory function may manifest itself in rapid shallow respirations, attacks of cyanosis, increased subcostal recession, movement of the alae nasi, or periods of apnoea. The underlying problem may be in the respiratory system but is not necessarily so. As the diaphragm is the main muscle involved and the thoracic

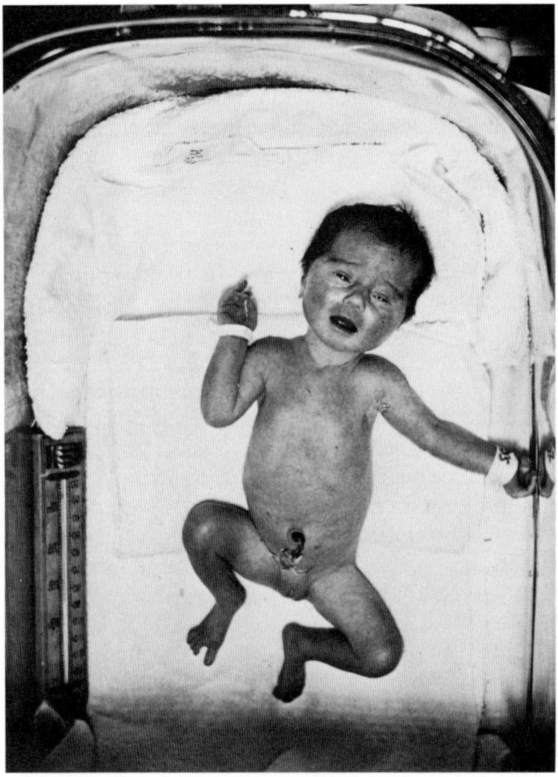

Figure 9.5 Neonatal cold injury with sclerema (hardening) of subcutaneous tissues.

cage is soft any obstruction to the airway will produce marked subcostal, intercostal and suprasternal indrawing. The diminished cough reflex creates difficulty in clearing mucus or other matter blocking the trachea or bronchus. Extra muscular effort is required and the infant may become exhausted. Inefficient oxygen exchange may occur in the alveoli because of inadequacy of the pulmonary vascular circulation. Any depression of central nervous function reduces muscle activity including respiration. This in turn may be due to a wide variety of conditions including hypoxia and haemorrhage.

Respiratory distress syndrome (Chap. 15) is a major cause of death in immature infants. The disorder is related to immaturity of the lungs, being rare in term infants, and occurring with increasing frequency and severity at decreasing gestational ages. Other factors which probably predispose to respiratory distress syndrome are intrauterine hypoxia and antepartum haemorrhage. Other possible factors are maternal diabetes and caesarean section. Though the aetiology of the condition is not fully understood, it seems clear that absence from the lungs of surfactant (Chap. 15) plays an important part. There is also increased pulmonary vascular resistance and reduced pulmonary blood flow, leading to right-to-left shunting of blood, arterial hypoxaemia, and cyanosis.

Apnoeic attacks commonly complicate respiratory distress syndrome. They also occur in the most immature babies especially those below about 32 to 33 weeks gestation. In severe apnoeic attacks the baby becomes cyanosed and the heart slows, possibly followed by cardiac arrest. Apnoeic attacks may be a sign of infection, intracranial haemorrhage or hypoglycaemia, but frequently there is no obvious cause. Increasing the oxygen concentration of inspired air may diminish the frequency of apnoeic attacks. Artificial ventilation is indicated for prolonged apnoea.

Hypoglycaemia, which is common in light-for-dates babies, may also occur in preterm babies during the first 72 hours of life, but may develop in any baby under stress as, for example, in the respiratory distress syndrome, congestive cardiac failure, following exchange blood transfusion and in association with cerebral birth trauma. Hypoglycaemia may also be found in babies of diabetic mothers and also in infants heavier than the 90th percentile. As mentioned previously, early feeding of preterm babies has been adopted to overcome the problem of hypoglycaemia.

RENAL DYSFUNCTION

The kidney plays an essential part in the maintenance of the body's water and mineral content. Adaptation to the external environment exposes it to new problems and these are particularly difficult for the preterm infant (Chap. 5). The capacity for preterm infants to concentrate and dilute their urine and to modify their mineral salt excretion is somewhat limited but by no means absent. There is therefore a narrower range of tolerance of water and mineral load. This is a complicated subject in which advances in knowledge continue to be made and no attempt will be made here to discuss the imbalance which appears to be present between glomerular and tubular function.

Dietary load. The important lesson to be learned is that great care has to be taken in assessing the fluid and electrolyte state of preterm infants. Evidence of oedema or dehydration indicates that the range of the kidney's tolerance has been exceeded. By a better understanding of an infant's requirements for fluid and minerals and by arranging management accordingly it should be possible to avoid these signs of failure to respect the considerable but limited ability of the preterm infant's kidney to deal with the load presented to it.

DIGESTIVE PROBLEMS

In the matter of alimentary function the preterm infant is subject to both mechanical and secretory handicaps. Immature development of the muscular layer of the alimentary tract makes for ineffective neuromuscular control, which may account for regurgitation of feeds, passage of loose stools and possibly functional intestinal obstruction. The physical effort involved in sucking may prove too exhausting. Extreme frailty may be associated with inability to swallow. In either event tube feeding is necessary. The ability of a preterm infant to digest and absorb food within a few hours of birth is evident from the success achieved with early feeding using human breast milk.

Limit of tolerance. It is clear, however, that there is a limit of tolerance which applies both as to the volume given at one feed and the amount of the individual constituents of the diet. Much attention has been paid in the past to the fat and protein content of the preterm infant's feed. It is now also recognized that until the enzyme systems of the small intestine are fully developed there is a limit to the infant's tolerance for carbohydrates such as lactose. Some of the disorders previously attributed to fat intolerance may have been due to lactose overload.

Functional intestinal obstruction produces the signs of an intestinal obstruction without an organic obstruction to the bowel being demonstrable. The abdomen becomes distended (Fig. 9.6) and bile-stained fluid is aspirated from the stomach or is vomited. There is

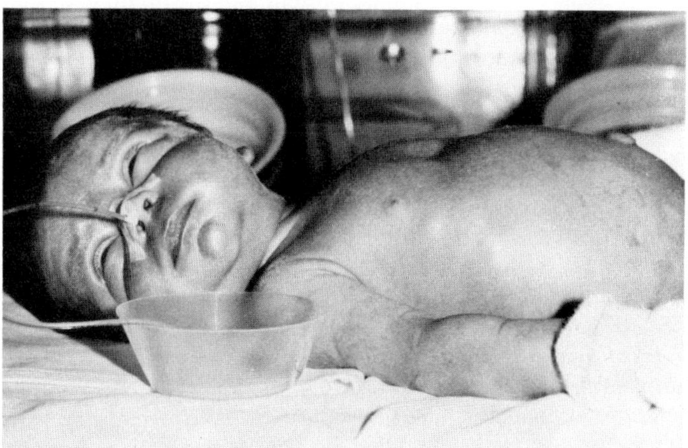

Figure 9.6 Abdominal distension due to functional intestinal obstruction.

delay in the passage of meconium. The condition often clears spontaneously within 24 hours to 48 hours, sometimes after the passage of a mucus plug (Fig. 9.7). A gastrografin enema given under careful supervision will help to exclude Hirschsprung's disease or

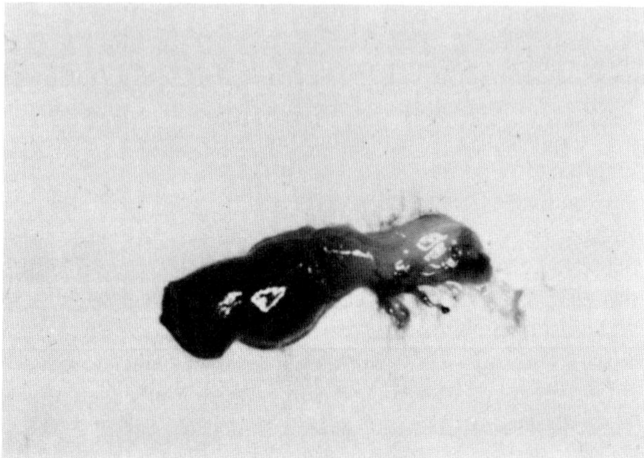

Figure 9.7 Mucus plug passed by baby shown in Figure 9.6 with relief of functional obstruction.

other organic abnormality and frequently hastens the passage of meconium and the return of normal bowel function.

Necrotizing enterocolitis is also associated with signs of intestinal obstruction but is a much more serious condition with a considerable mortality. Signs of obstruction are present and the infant is seriously ill. Radiological examination may show gas to be present in the intestinal wall. Haemorrhagic necrosis of the bowel wall may lead to perforation. Treatment is by gastric aspiration, intravenous fluids and systemic antibiotics. Laparotomy will be indicated if signs of perforation develop.

HAEMORRHAGE

The various factors responsible for bleeding will be fully discussed in Chapter 17. Sufficient here to say that two factors in particular favour bleeding—pronounced fragility and abnormal permeability of the capillaries together with slowness of the blood to clot.

Cerebral haemorrhage. The second commonest cause of death in preterm infants is haemorrhage into the lateral cerebral ventricles. Intraventricular haemorrhage may complicate the respiratory distress syndrome, or occur in the first few days of life in a preterm baby who has previously done well. The commonest clinical signs are apnoeic attacks, convulsions, or unexplained deterioration. There is no effective treatment, and mortality is high. In those who survive a ventricular haemorrhage a not infrequent complication is obstructive hydrocephalus signalled by a rapid increase in head size, vomiting and possibly convulsions.

INFECTION

The susceptibility of the preterm baby to infection is far greater even than that of the term infant. Infection has already been touched on earlier in this chapter and is discussed at length in Chapter 13.

Gram-negative infection. In most neonatal units in the United Kingdom Gram-negative organisms have displaced the staphylococci as the commonest pathogens. *Pseudomonas aeruginosa*—which flourishes in wet apparatus such as incubators, resuscitation equipment, and ventilators—is a particularly serious hazard to the immature baby. Since the signs of Gram-negative infection in the newborn are often non-specific, such infections should be suspected whenever a preterm baby becomes ill or has apnoeic attacks without any other obvious cause. In these circumstances it is wise to obtain cultures of blood, cerebrospinal fluid, and urine, and of nose, throat, and umbilical swabs; and, without waiting for the results of the cultures, to start treatment with systemic antibiotics.

JAUNDICE

Functional immaturity of the liver with defective conjugation of bilirubin accounts for the high levels of unconjugated bilirubin in the preterm baby. There is an increasing risk of kernicterus, causing death or permanent brain damage with the possible eventual development of microcephaly, deafness, athetoid cerebral palsy and mental handicap, if the serum bilirubin level rises above 15 mg per 100 ml. Kernicterus is more likely to occur if the baby is hypoxic or acidotic. In seriously ill babies kernicterus may occur at lower serum bilirubin levels. Exchange blood transfusion should be carried out if the serum bilirubin approaches a dangerous level.

Prevention. Clinical experience has taught that babies are less likely to develop a high serum bilirubin level if they are given adequate fluid and calories soon after birth. Phototherapy and the giving of phenobarbitone both reduce the level of serum bilirubin, but there is still considerable debate as to their place in routine treatment of hyperbilirubinaemia. The blue light emitted by the phototherapy unit converts the bilirubin in the baby's skin into, among other products, water-soluble pyrroles which are then excreted. Phenobarbitone induces the formation of the conjugating enzyme, glucuronyl transferase, in the liver (Chap. 14).

Prognosis of Preterm Delivery

In general terms the prospects of survival are directly related to birth weight, except in so far as a small infant born near term is more likely to live than an infant of greater weight but of shorter gestation period.

SHORT-TERM PROGNOSIS

Although a fetus born after the 28th week of pregnancy is considered to be viable, the prospects of an infant born before the 30th week are poor. As a pointer to short-term prognosis it should be recalled that of deaths due to low birth weight, 50 per cent occur during the first 24 hours, 80 per cent occur during the first week and 100 per cent occur during the first six weeks of life. Put another way, the prospects of survival become progressively brighter as the baby successfully survives the first 24 hours, the first week and finally the first four to six weeks of life.

LONG-TERM PROGNOSIS

Past studies have shown a considerable incidence of cerebral palsy, mental retardation, fits, learning difficulties and behaviour problems in preterm babies. The incidence of neurological disorder, especially spastic diplegia, was particularly associated with preterm delivery. Prognosis has been directly related to birth weight. More recent studies suggest that even among those of less than 1500 g birth weight a higher proportion than in previous years are now surviving without obvious cerebral damage. It would appear that modern neonatal care which pays particular attention to warmth and correct feeding, and practises energetic and early treatment of hypoxia, hypoglycaemia and hyperbilirubinaemia, has greatly improved the outlook for preterm babies. Low birth-weight babies are among those 'at risk' and should be seen regularly in the follow-up clinic for developmental examinations including assessment of hearing and vision, so that any neurodevelopmental deficits can be detected and treated as soon as possible.

Follow-up. It is now reasonable to be optimistic about the prognosis for all except the very smallest preterm babies and those who have definite or prolonged neurological disturbances in the neonatal period. The importance of the long-term follow-up of preterm babies is discussed in Chapter 21.

THE LIGHT-FOR-DATES BABY

Much that has been written about the preterm baby applies to the light-for-dates baby. Only points of difference will be emphasized.

Causes of Slow Intrauterine Growth

Causes of slow intrauterine growth are shown in Table 9.7. It will be noted that there is a close similarity between this table and Table 9.5 which showed factors carrying a high risk of preterm onset of labour.

Table 9.7 Causes of intrauterine growth failure

MATERNAL
- General
  - Poor socioeconomic conditions
    - Malnutrition
    - Unmarried
  - Height: less than 155 cm
  - Living at high altitudes
  - Racial and constitutional
  - History of previous light-for-dates infants
- Obstetric
  - Complications of pregnancy
  - Poor placental function
  - Smoking
  - Poor antenatal care
  - Parity first or third onwards

FETAL
- Multiple pregnancy
- Congenital abnormalities
- Chromosomal abnormality

General Characteristics of the Light-for-Dates Baby

A number of clinical features are associated with the light-for-dates baby. Table 9.8 shows the contrasting features of preterm and light-for-dates infants.

SIZE

Usually undersized, the baby may be small both in terms of length and weight and not infrequently weight is disproportionately below average. The head appears large even for a newly born infant. There is an absence of subcutaneous fat giving rise to folds of apparently redundant skin in the axillae, the groins, the neck and over the abdomen (Fig. 9.8)

APPEARANCE

The skin is dry, coarse and inelastic, and shows signs of cracking or desquamation—features which, while they may occur in any situation, are most pronounced over the abdomen and on the dorsa of the feet and hands (Fig. 9.9, 9.10). In the severe case the face is wizened and the expression strangely old, although alert. Variations in

Table 9.8 Contrasting features of preterm and light-for-dates babies

Feature	Preterm	Light-for-Dates
Definition	Born before 37 weeks gestation	Birth weight below 10th percentile for gestational age
Vernix	Present in variable amounts	Little or absent
Skin	Red and transparent	Dry, folds of lax skin
Subcutaneous tissue	Sparse	Sparse
Skull	Bones soft and mobile	Bones hard with minimal mobility
Facies	Doll-like	Mature
Abdomen	Large	Scaphoid
Cord	Thick and fleshy	Thin, flabby and stained
Cry	Feeble	Mature
Muscle tone	Hypotonic, frog-like position	Variable. Usually active
Complications	Hypothermia Respiratory distress syndrome Infection Cerebral haemorrhage	Hypoglycaemia Hypocalcaemia Hypothermia

the clinical picture have been related to the duration of detrimental influences.

Other occasional findings include a scaphoid abdomen, and (in babies with a preceding history of fetal distress) green or yellow discoloration of the umbilical cord and nails. Should signs of persistent respiratory distress develop within a few hours of birth the possibility of massive meconium aspiration must be considered.

Feeding

The light-for-dates baby will usually be able to suck and swallow satisfactorily. Early and adequate feeding is especially important in

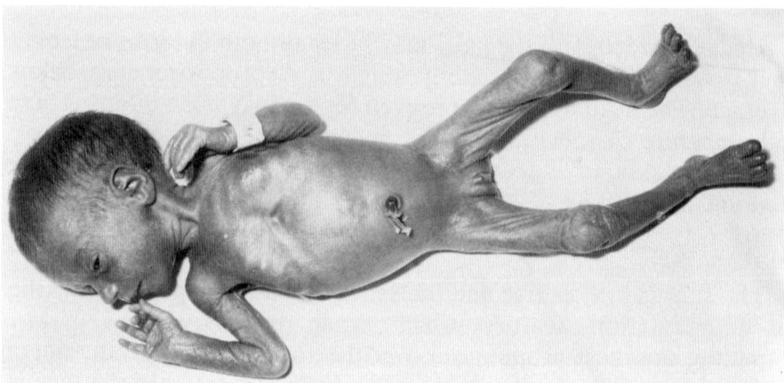

Figure 9.8 Light-for-dates infant showing lack of subcutaneous fat and dry skin.

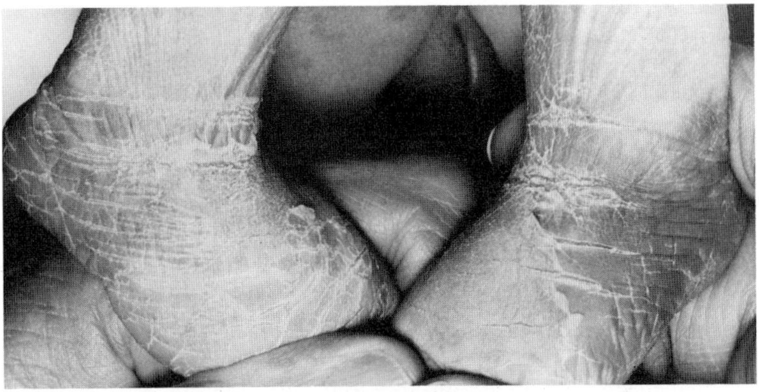

Figure 9.9 Dry skin over dorsum of feet.

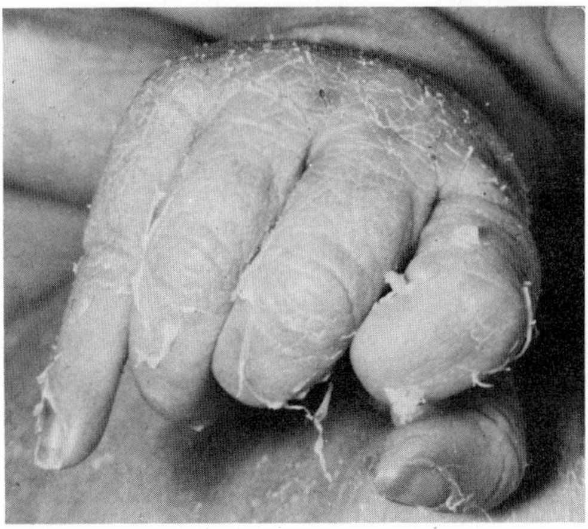

Figure 9.10 Dry scaly skin over fingers of light-for-dates baby.

the light-for-dates baby to correct metabolic acidosis, prevent hypoglycaemia and lessen the degree of physiological jaundice. Milk is an entirely satisfactory food and produces adequate growth for the first four or five months of life. The introduction of mixed feeding before the third month is therefore both unnecessary and undesirable.

Complications Associated with the Light-for-dates Baby

HYPOGLYCAEMIA

The light-for-dates baby is particularly subject to hypoglycaemia during the first 48 hours of life as a direct consequence of insufficient stores of energy-producing glycogen. Other important factors which contribute to the hypoglycaemia are the high consumption of glucose by the relatively large brain and disordered insulin secretion.

Asymptomatic. Blood-glucose levels are considerably lower in the first weeks of life than later, but in the light-for-dates baby particularly they may reach dangerously low levels, usually on the second and third days of life. Although hypoglycaemia is defined as a true blood-glucose level below 20 mg per 100 ml many babies have a lower blood-glucose level without ever exhibiting any abnormal signs or symptoms and probably do not develop any long-term neurological damage.

Symptomatic. On the other hand hypoglycaemia accompanied by unresponsiveness, periods of lethargy, failure to suck, apnoeic and cyanotic attacks and fits is associated with a considerable risk of permanent brain damage and intellectual retardation. Such symptomatic hypoglycaemia should not only be actively treated but also prevented and detected before symptoms occur.

Diagnosis. Dextrostix may be used as a screening test for hypoglycaemia, low readings being checked in the laboratory on a whole blood sample for true blood-glucose levels. Such screening tests should be carried out at 12 to 24 hours and another at 36 to 48 hours. In the presence of abnormal symptoms measurements of blood glucose should be made every four hours during the danger period.

Treatment. Hypoxia and chilling predispose to hypoglycaemia in the light-for-dates baby so resuscitation must be prompt and carried out in a warm environment. Early feeding of light-for-dates babies will prevent the development of hypoglycaemia in most cases. Ideally the feeds should be of breast milk starting with 60 ml per kg in the first 24 hours and increasing up to 150 ml per kg by the fourth day. If the mother is unable to meet the baby's demand and milk from a human breast is unobtainable then complementary feeds should be given. Additional benefits of early feeding include rapid correction of metabolic acidosis and the lessening of physiological jaundice.

Symptomatic hypoglycaemia should be a very rare occurrence so long as the instructions on prevention and early detection have been followed. When it does occur an immediate intravenous injection of glucose (1 g per kg body weight) should be given followed by an infusion of 10 per cent glucose at a rate of 75 ml per kg per day. The management of the baby with asymptomatic hypoglycaemia is controversial. There is not universal agreement about the necessity to treat asymptomatic hypoglycaemia.

HYPOTHERMIA

As the light-for-dates baby is poorly endowed with fat he chills readily. Chilling is more likely to occur in the presence of hypoxia, more especially if the birth weight is less than 2 kg. It follows that an essential part of nursing care is to maintain the body heat of light-for-dates babies.

OTHER PROBLEMS

Infection, functional intestinal obstruction, enterocolitis affect the light-for-dates baby in the same way as the preterm baby.

Hypothermia and hypoglycaemia may be further complicated by pulmonary haemorrhage. Better temperature control and correction of hypoglycaemia have reduced the incidence of this complication.

Congenital malformations and intrauterine viral infections are frequently the cause of intrauterine growth failure so the light-for-dates baby should be carefully examined for evidence of hidden malformations or intrauterine infections.

Prognosis

Early delivery of the malnourished fetus and the greater care employed to prevent the deleterious effects of hypoglycaemia have reduced the incidence of neurological handicap, including cerebral palsy, mental retardation, fits and learning difficulties, in the light-for-dates baby. Although modern neonatal care has considerably reduced the risk of permanent brain damage and intellectual retardation the light-for-dates baby usually remains small throughout life and can be identified by his short stature, triangular face, short upper arms and small, pointed chin.

Health Services for the Low Birth-Weight Infant

Not only the treatment of the ill low birth-weight baby but also the care of the healthy low birth-weight baby is very demanding in terms of medical and nursing staff, skill and equipment. The staffing of special-care and of intensive therapy nurseries has already been discussed in Chapters 2 and 6. Not all maternity departments will be able to achieve these levels of staffing and will not therefore be able to provide the high standards of care required by the very low birth-weight infant. In each area and district policy decisions with regard to services for low birth-weight infants will be required so that mothers going into labour before term can be delivered in a hospital where suitable facilities are available for the care of her infant.

Our prime objective must be the prevention of preterm delivery. Where preventive efforts are not successful the best service available must be provided for the infant in order to diminish the many hazards associated with preterm delivery.

FURTHER READING

ALDEN, E. R., MANDELKORN, T., WOODRUM, D. E., WENNBERG, C. P., PARKS, C. R. & HODSON, W. A. (1972). Morbidity and mortality of infants weighing less than 1000 g in an intensive care nursery. *Pediatrics*, **50**, 40–49.

CROSSE, V. M. (1972). *The Preterm Baby and Other Babies with Low Birth Weight.* 7th edn. Edinburgh: Churchill Livingstone.

DUBOWITZ, L. M. S., DUBOWITZ, V. & GOLDBERG, C. (1970). Clinical assessment of gestational age in the newborn infant. *Journal of Pediatrics*, 77, 1–10.

EXPERT GROUP ON SPECIAL CARE FOR BABIES (1971). *Reports on Public Health and Medical Subjects*, no. 127. London: HMSO.

LANCET (1971). Development and very low birth weight, i, 534.

LUBCHENCO, L. O. (1972). Long-term follow-up of studies of prematurely born infants: 1. Relationships of handicaps to nursery routines, *Journal of Pediatrics*, **80**, 501–508, 2. Influence of birth weight and gestational age on sequelae, *Journal of Pediatrics*, **80**, 509–512.

RAWLINGS, G., REYNOLDS, E. O. R., STEWART, A. & STRANG. L. B. (1971). Changing prognosis for infants of very low birth weight. *Lancet*, i, 516–519.

ROBINSON, R. (1971a). Problems of the newborn: the preterm baby. *British Medical Journal*, iv, 416–419.

ROBINSON, R. (1971b). Problems of the newborn: the small-for-dates baby. *British Medical Journal*, iv, 480–482.

10

Nursing Care of Low Birth-Weight Infants

Special Care Nurseries

In spite of advances in medical science and the provision of sophisticated equipment the survival of the low birth-weight baby still depends on the skill and attention of those providing his nursing care. Further training is required for those who undertake this highly specialized form of nursing, and a high staff to patient ratio is necessary to provide the intensive care called for in the successful rearing of low birth-weight infants. Nursing care can be made easier by the provision of suitable equipment housed in accommodation designed for the purpose. As discussed in Chapter 2 the maternity departments of district hospitals should each have a special care nursery designed or adapted for its specific function. A more limited number of regional intensive therapy nurseries are or will become available to deal with infants requiring highly specialized treatment.

Staffing. It will therefore be necessary for a considerable number of nurses or midwives to receive special training in the care of the newborn. The training of staff and the number of staff required have already been discussed in Chapter 2.

Design. Policy decisions about the design of nurseries may seem remote from the day-to-day nursing and medical care of the newborn. It is essential, however, that nurseries be designed and constructed with nursing procedures in mind. This involves the overall plan which should allow separation of dirty and clean traffic. The infants requiring most intensive care should be nearest to the nursing station and clearly visible. Adequate space must be allowed without causing unnecessary movement. Floors, walls, windows and surfaces must be easily cleaned. Facilities for the washing and drying of hands must be available in every room. It is a major advantage to have piped air, oxygen and suction available.

Temperature. The temperature of each nursery should be controllable within the range 25° to 30°C. As adequate ventilation is also essential an air-conditioning system is generally necessary to provide a satisfactory degree of control of the environment. Extra humidity is most readily provided within incubators. In a well-designed nursery it is possible to provide accommodation at different temperatures to suit the requirement of individual infants. The smallest babies even although in incubators should be in rooms kept at 30°C. This temperature should also be maintained in any room where procedures involving the undressing of infants are undertaken. Larger infants can be nursed in cots at a room temperature of 25°C. Before discharge home the infants should be nursed in cooler rooms with a temperature within the range of 20° to 25°C so that they become accustomed to a temperature which can be achieved in most homes with extra heating.

Mother and baby relationships. Much has already been said on this subject in Chapter 6, and in the case of the low birth-weight baby there may be a real danger of this relationship being damaged by the separation of the mother from her baby in a special care nursery. It was the practice in the past to allow the parents to see their babies only through a glass viewing panel. In recent years most paediatricians have encouraged the parents to come into the special care nursery, to handle their babies and to take part as far as possible in their care (Fig. 10.1).

A great deal of thought must be given to this problem in order to promote contact as much as possible. There are cases on record where a mother has rejected her baby after a prolonged stay in hospital in isolation from his mother.

All special care nurseries should have a mother and baby unit where the mother can be readmitted prior to the discharge of her baby. In this unit she is taught how to care for her baby under supervision. The atmosphere of this unit must be relaxed and as homely as possible.

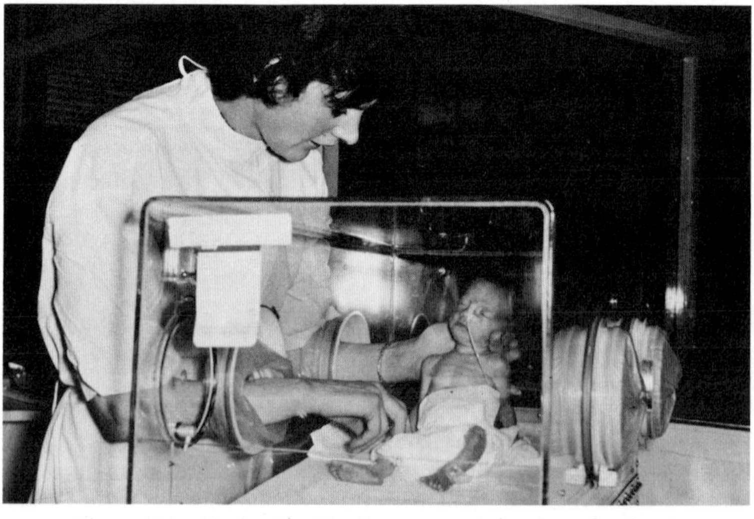

Figure 10.1 Mother handling her preterm infant in an incubator.

Equipment

Much of the nursing care of low birth-weight infants involves the use of special equipment such as incubators, monitors, infusion pumps and other intricate apparatus. The nursing staff must be trained in the use of such equipment. Instruction must include a description of the function of the machine and the limitations of its action, the correct method of usage, the responsibility of the nurse and the doctor with regard to the initial settings and subsequent changes and the action to be taken if the machine appears to be faulty. All doctors and nurses should be aware of the emergency electricity supply available should the main source fail. Similarly if all power should fail written instructions should be available as to the actions to be taken. There should always be at least one fully trained nurse on duty who is conversant with all the equipment available, where it is kept and how it should be connected to electricity, oxygen or air supply. Where the possibility exists that special equipment will be required this should be thoroughly checked in good time so that it is known to be in working order before it is required. The nursing staff should also be trained in the methods to be used in sterilizing special equipment and in precautions to be taken to avoid contamination of equipment.

Incubators

It is interesting at this juncture to take a look into the past at the development of the incubator and the early methods of provision of warmth which is so essential to a low birth-weight baby's survival. There are some reports in early writings of special attempts to preserve warmth in small babies; a Swiss monk of the 10th century reports on a premature baby being wrapped in animal fat to keep him warm. There is also a report of a baby who survived to become later a famous historian, being born in 1577 and at birth no bigger than the palm of his father's hand. He was noted to be perfectly formed, so his father gave instructions to keep him in an oven, and he was reared in this way!

The forerunner of the modern incubator was first used in Bordeaux in 1857. It was a double-lined cradle with a water jacket into which hot water was poured to maintain the correct temperature. A similar apparatus was used in Moscow in 1878. The first closed incubator was introduced by Farmer in 1881. It was a closed wooden box with air holes in the lid. A lower compartment contained water heated by gas, spirit or oil, with the water kept circulating. Modifications were made, the most important being an alarm bell which rang when the temperature rose too high. A thermostatic device which maintained a constant temperature was incorporated in the incubator which was in use at the City of London Lying-in Hospital in 1884. The use of incubators was very popular in France, and various charitable centres were opened for the care of low birth-weight babies which the public could visit on payment of a fee to see the babies in their incubators, as in fact more than one baby might share the same incubator. The practice of administering oxygen to premature babies was increased after the Second World War and produced many new designs of incubators to provide warmth and the administration of oxygen at the same time.

MODERN INCUBATORS

Various designs of incubators are now available and some are very expensive items of equipment. They are not indispensable but they are of great value in nursing care. The baby is nursed in an environment with regulation of temperature and humidity. The oxygen concentration can be monitored. Observation of the baby is much more satisfactory as he can be nursed without clothing. The respiratory pattern can be carefully studied and any change of colour noted immediately.

Servocontrol. Incubators provided with a temperature servocontrol mechanism are now widely used (Fig. 10.2). The infant's temperature is measured by a thermocouple attached to the skin. The temperature is read on a calibrated dial which gives a constant reading. At the same time the result is fed into a servocontrol mechanism which controls the heater of the incubator. The mechanism can be set to maintain the infant's skin temperature within a narrow range, the midpoint of which can be altered to suit the infant's requirements. Incubators without a servocontrol mechanism can be set to maintain a constant air temperature at a predetermined level.

Humidity. Control of humidity is much less precise but in most incubators there is a certain degree of control of the moisture content of the circulating air. In modern incubators the heated air is circulated by a fan, but in older models no fan was provided and convection circuits were relied upon to maintain a circulation of air.

Access. Incubators cannot be kept permanently closed and access is required for a number of nursing and medical procedures. Suitable access ports are provided. It must not be forgotten that frequent use of such ports affects the efficiency of the incubator.

Heat loss can be minimized by keeping the rooms in which incubators are used at a temperature of 30°C. This also reduces the heat loss from the incubator surfaces and prevents misting of the inner surface of the hood. Incubators with double-skinned perspex canopies have been constructed with the object of reducing radiant

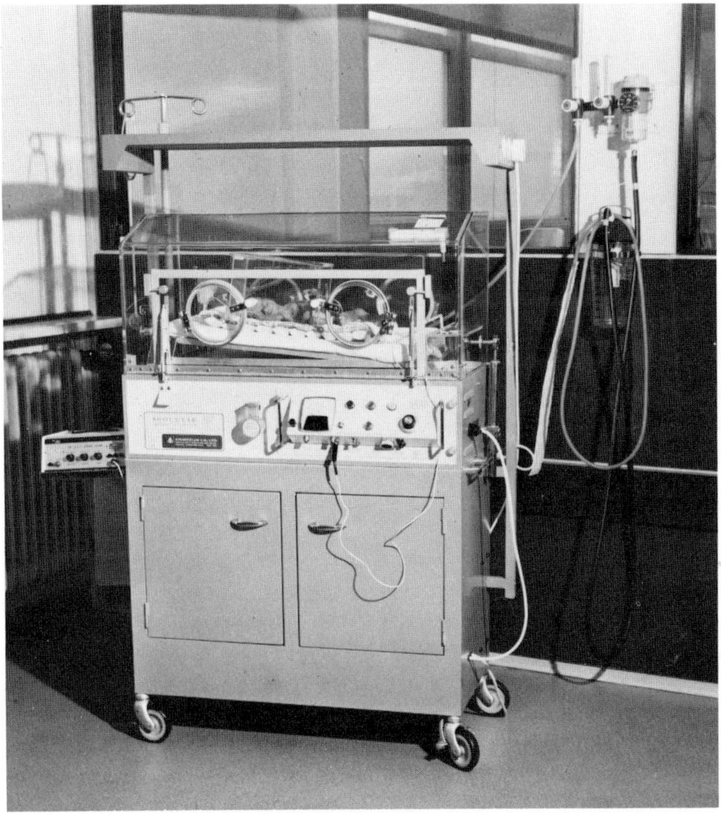

Figure 10.2 Isolette incubator with servocontrol for temperature regulation.

heat loss. For a variety of reasons they have not as yet proved to be better than the present single thickness models. Other methods of reducing heat loss such as the use of a perspex radiation shield and clothing the infant in an aluminium swaddler are discussed in Chapter 19.

Cots

In nurseries heated to 30°C many low birth-weight babies can be nursed in open cots as described in Chapter 6. Extra heat can be provided by overhead infrared heaters if necessary. Special covers are available for some cots so that oxygen can be given if required (Fig. 10.3)

Formerly many low birth-weight infants were successfully cared

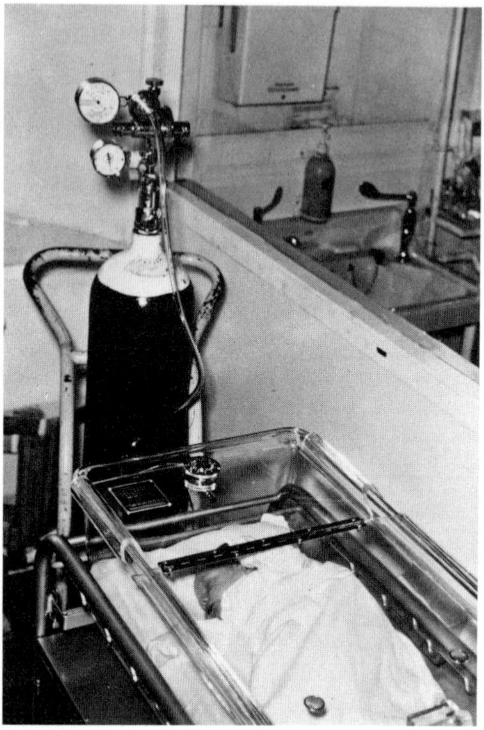

Figure 10.3 Cot covering to allow treatment with oxygen.

for in Sorrento cots with extra heat supplied by hot water bottles inserted into pockets in the canvas lining.

Other Equipment

MONITORS

The simplest forms of monitoring equipment which should be available in all special care nurseries are continuous temperature recorders, apnoea monitors and oxygen analysers. Highly complex and therefore expensive sets of monitoring equipment are available commercially. Such apparatus can give a continuous recording of the ECG, heart rate, respiratory rate and blood pressure. The high cost of such monitors will probably limit their use to regional intensive therapy nurseries.

Apnoea monitors are available in a number of forms, all of which produce an audible alarm after the infant has ceased to breathe for a preset period. They are relatively cheap and a most useful aid to nursing observation (Fig. 10.4).

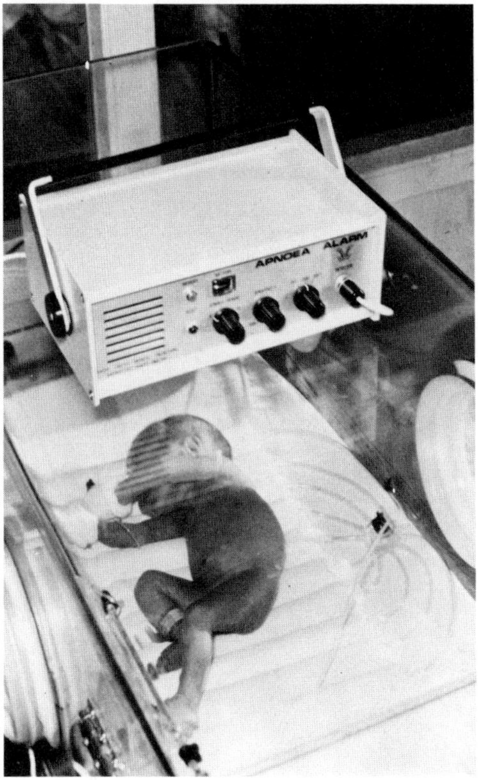

Figure 10.4 Apnoea alarm.

INFUSION PUMPS

High precision roller pumps are available which will deliver fluids at rates down to 1.0 ml per hour. These have made intragastric or intravenous feeding of very low birth-weight infants much easier and more successful. Servocontrolled drop counters can be used for the same purpose (Fig. 10.5).

RESPIRATORS

Simple respirators which are essentially mechanical means of providing intermittent positive pressure of limited total pressure are easy to operate and relatively cheap (Fig. 10.6). Although they are not sufficient for dealing with complicated respiratory problems they are suitable for maintaining respiration in the infant with recurrent temporary apnoea and are widely used in special care nurseries. The

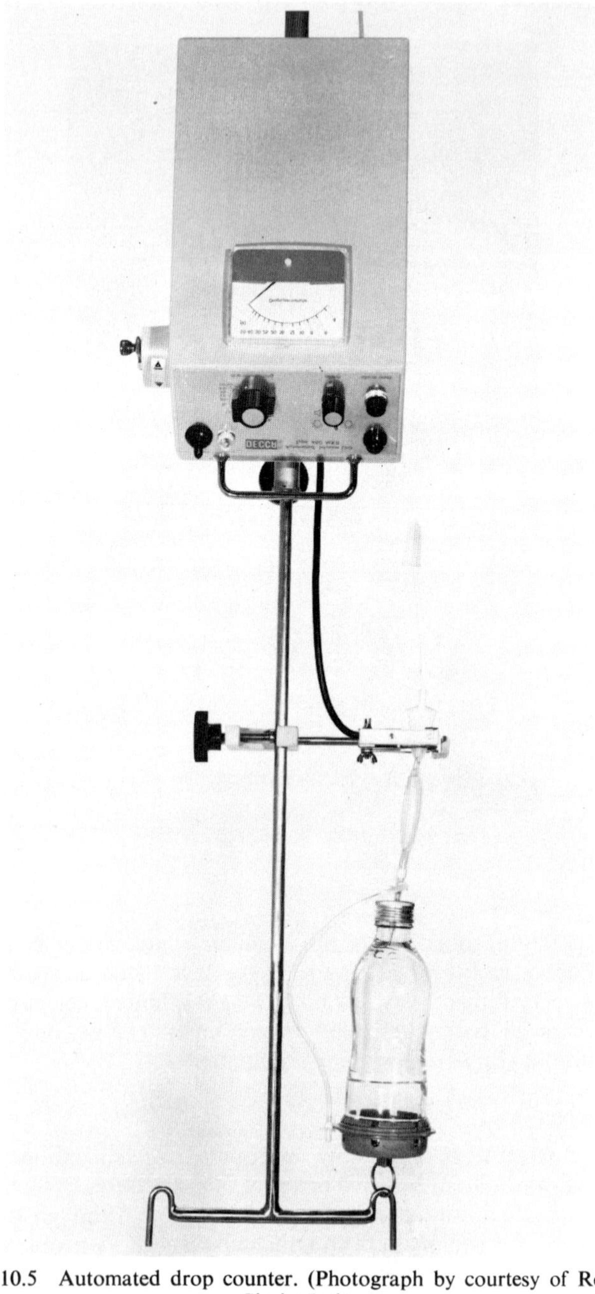

Figure 10.5 Automated drop counter. (Photograph by courtesy of Reid and Sigrist Ltd.)

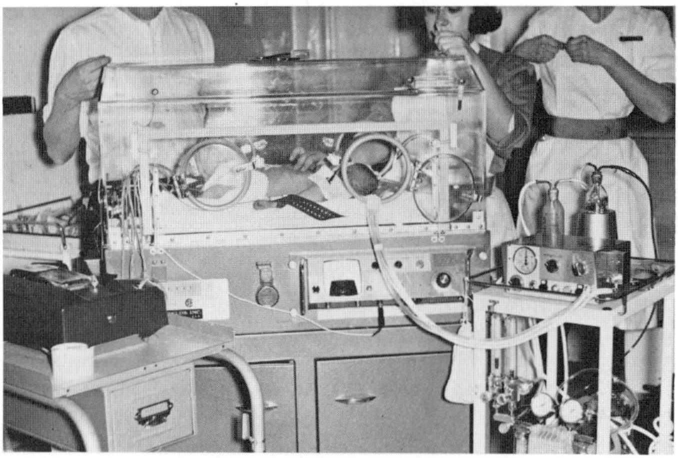

Figure 10.6 Loosco infant ventilator.

more highly sophisticated respirators are better reserved for intensive therapy nurseries.

ORGANIZATION OF NURSERIES

The successful running of special care nurseries requires the introduction of an agreed plan of policy with regard to almost all aspects of nursing and medical care. Such policies must be kept constantly under review and the effect of changes in policy assessed for both their short-term and long-term effects. It follows that a careful record must be kept of the date of introduction of any particular policy and it is useful to note the reason why previous policy was changed. A book stating current policy with regard to standard procedures for such items as reception and immediate care, prevention of infection, maintenance of respiration, maintenance of body temperature, feeding, skin and toilet care, nursing care in special circumstances, preparation for discharge, death of an infant, should be easily available for all staff to consult. It can most conveniently be in the form of a loose-leaf folder which can readily be altered. Space should be left for suggestions as to improvement in procedure.

It is important that parents be allowed to record their impressions as they can often make most useful suggestions.

Some of the items listed in the preceding paragraph are worthy of more detailed discussion.

Prevention of Infection

This subject is discussed in greater detail in Chapter 13.

Isolation facilities. Facilities should be available within or nearby any special care nursery for the separate nursing in isolation of any infants considered likely to have a clinical infection (Chap. 13). Nurses working in the isolation section should not have duties within the general special care nursery.

STAFF

Medical, nursing and ancillary staff entering the nursery should be free from infection. Earlier in this chapter the importance of parents entering the unit was discussed. Parents too must be carefully briefed on the prevention of infection. No one with a cold, sore throat, skin infection or diarrhoea should be allowed into the unit. It is the practice in many hospitals to screen all staff by taking nose, throat and rectal swabs before commencing duty in the unit and at intervals subsequently.

Clothing. Although some special care units expect all staff entering the unit to change into special clothing, as for entering an operating theatre, other units have not found this necessary or practicable. Medical staff must have their individual gowns or coats which should be changed daily. Nursing staff who are handling infants should use an individual gown for each infant, the gown being kept by the infant's cot or incubator with the outer side folded inward.

Provided that those staff with respiratory tract infections are excluded from nurseries there is insufficient evidence in their favour to justify the continued use of face masks for routine medical and nursing procedures.

Hand-washing is the most important basic procedure in the prevention of cross infection and must be carried out with meticulous care. Wash basins must be provided in each nursery with elbow taps together with a supply of paper towels to be used once only and discarded. All buckets or receptacles for soiled linen or paper should have foot-operated pedals. The hands and the forearms should be thoroughly washed with a liquid soap containing an antiseptic such as 3 per cent hexachlorophane (pHisoHex) or a povidone iodine scrub (Betadine) under running water.

Hand-washing must be carried out before any procedure in the unit and prior to handling each baby.

Domestic cleanliness. Domestic staff must be allocated to the special care nursery only and have no other duties outside that area. A cool short-sleeved uniform should be provided and gowns worn when entering the actual nursery areas. In-service education of domestic staff on the importance of their work being carried out with meticulous care is essential. Modern suction cleaning equipment for floors has greatly reduced the danger of flying dust. All surfaces, furniture and equipment must be damp-dusted with a disposable cleaning cloth wrung out in a solution of hexachlorophane. Walls and ceilings must be washed down frequently. Hand basins and water taps may harbour *Pseudomonas aeruginosa*, which can cause serious infections in the newborn, and require thorough cleaning.

It is excellent practice if possible to empty one cubicle or area in the special care nursery in rotation and thoroughly air and clean both it and the furniture. This procedure could be carried out so that the whole nursery (depending on its size) could be thoroughly cleaned every three to four weeks.

Soiled linen must be handled as little as possible by nursing staff and should be collected in a disposable bag and removed from the nursery area immediately. It should never be allowed to lie on the floor. There is now a wide range of disposable items on the market such as napkins, sheets and baby gowns, all of which are rapidly improving and in the future may completely replace the washable linen.

Cots, bassinets and mattresses should be thoroughly cleaned with an antiseptic solution when a baby has been discharged home. Canvas linings can be autoclaved.

Incubators can be a source of infection if not thoroughly cleaned. The makers give detailed instructions regarding dismantling of various parts for cleaning. These should be studied carefully and adequate time allowed to carry out the recommended procedures. *Pseudomonas aeruginosa* may contaminate water tanks. Milton 1 in 80 or a 1 per cent solution of acetic acid should be put into the tank for 1 hour. In some incubators the reservoirs and water taps can be detached and autoclaved.

Incubator sleeves may be a source of infection. They should be changed frequently and sterilized if not disposable. Care must be taken to use one set of sleeves for 'clean' procedures—such as feeding—and the other set of sleeves for 'dirty' procedures—such as changing napkins. Filters on the air inlet must be changed regularly and all tubing autoclaved. When cleaning is finished swabs are taken from the inside of the incubator and water tank for bacteriological examination, and the incubator should not be put into use until the reports prove that there is no infection present.

Equipment for suction and resuscitation must be dismantled and carefully sterilized either by autoclaving or immersion in an antiseptic solution depending on the type of material used.

Feeds. Special precautions against the risk of infection have to be taken where feeds are being prepared. This has already been discussed in Chapter 8.

IMMEDIATE CARE

As stated earlier at least one incubator fully prepared and warmed should always be available for the reception of infants from the delivery rooms or elsewhere. On admission to the special care nursery the infant's name should be checked against the name on the records provided and information about the pregnancy and delivery recorded. Meanwhile the infant's immediate requirements are being assessed and a decision made as to whether incubator nursing is required. This decision will depend upon the infant's maturity, weight, temperature and general condition.

The following observations are made:

Temperature, recording both skin and rectal temperature
Colour, noting pallor, cyanosis or jaundice
Respiration with particular reference to rate, depth and periodicity
Heart rate
Activity—observing movements and strength of cry
Time of passage of urine
Time of passage of meconium
Umbilical cord is checked for control of bleeding
Abnormal signs such as convulsions are reported
The incubator temperature is recorded
The oxygen content is measured and recorded.

Respiratory pattern. Any infant who shows any evidence of respiratory distress, whether this be excessive chest movement, indrawing, grunting, cyanosis or apnoea, should be reported immediately. In cases of apnoea or severe sudden distress suction should be applied to the pharynx and if this does not cause improvement IPPR should be administered by face mask and bag until tracheal intubation can be carried out. The time of apnoea must be carefully noted. Infants having episodes of apnoea should be nursed on an apnoea monitor. This gives an audible warning if the infant stops breathing for a set period such as 10 seconds. A Silverman score sheet (see Table 15.1) should be kept for all infants showing any evidence of respiratory distress. Respiratory distress syndrome is discussed in Chapter 15. Should the infant's Silverman score be 6 or more it is probable that arterial blood-gas samples will be taken and the appropriate equipment should be in readiness (Chap. 19).

MAINTENANCE OF BODY TEMPERATURE

This is one of the greatest problems in nursing low birth-weight babies, who lose heat readily and have limited powers of heat production (Chap. 5). Each baby must have his own low-reading thermometer giving readings down to 25°C. Every care must be taken during nursing procedures to prevent heat loss by avoiding unnecessary exposure and preventing excessive air movements.

FEEDING

The type of feeds and amounts given have already been dealt with in Chapters 8 and 9. The method of feeding is important as low birth-weight babies may have poor sucking and swallowing reflexes. The cardiac sphincter is poorly developed and regurgitation of food occurs readily. The cough reflex is feeble and inhalation of the feed may occur. Large feeds must be avoided and the baby handled after feeding as little as possible.

The lower the gestational age the weaker the powers of digestion and abdominal distension may occur following feeds and give rise to cyanotic attacks. The method of feeding employed depends on the baby's condition and gestational age.

Breast feeding. Most babies who weigh 2000 g and over and who are in good general condition will cope well with breast feeding. Breast feeding must be carefully supervised and care must be taken not to allow the baby to become exhausted by prolonged attempts to feed. It is a wise plan to allow a set time at the breast. If necessary following test weighing a complementary feed with mothers' own expressed breast milk may be given by bottle or tube. Enthusiasm and encouragement go a long way in achieving successful breast feeding.

Bottle feeding. It is essential to ensure that the teat is soft and has a hole large enough to permit a steady flow of drops when the bottle is inverted. The feed may be warmed or it may be given at room temperature.

If the baby is being fed in his incubator or cot the head of the incubator or cot must be raised and the baby turned on his right side. Care must be taken to ensure that the teat is always filled with milk to ensure that air is not being sucked in by the baby. A finger under the chin assists the baby to suck and if the baby is being fed out of his cot he should be held with the spine and head well supported. In the middle and at the end of the feed the baby is supported in a sitting position with the spine extended and 'winded'. Following the feed the baby is left lying on his right side and the incubator tray or cot left tilted for 20 to 30 minutes. The prone position is favoured by many following feeds as it has been shown that the stomach empties more quickly in this position. Careful attention to detail is essential during bottle feeding of a low birth-weight baby.

Intragastric tube feeding. In babies of low gestational age and those whose general condition is poor tube feeding is used to ensure an adequate intake and to prevent exhaustion. This method of feeding must only be carried out by nurses who have had experience in nursing low birth-weight babies. If carried out with meticulous care it is a safe and most suitable method of feeding. The baby receives the feed with no physical effort and minimal handling.

The technique most widely practised is to use a sterile disposable infant feeding catheter which is left *in situ* and only requires to be changed every 5 to 7 days. Sterile disposable infant feeding sets are readily available.

The head of the cot is raised. Before the catheter is removed from its sterile wrapping, it is measured against the baby holding the tip at the xiphisternum and extending it upwards to the lobe of the ear and then forward to the bridge of the baby's nose, and the catheter is marked at this site.

After washing her hands, the midwife passes the catheter gently along the floor of the nostril and down into the oesophagus until the mark previously made is at the baby's nostrils. The mouth is inspected to ensure that the catheter has gone down into the oesophagus. The catheter is fixed to baby's skin with a narrow strip of an adhesive tape. A small amount of gastric juice is aspirated and tested with litmus paper. If the reaction is acid, the tube can be assumed to be in the stomach. The barrel of the syringe is then attached to the tube and a feed is poured in and the rate of flow regulated by raising or lowering the syringe. When the whole feed has been run into the catheter, 1 ml of sterile water is injected to clear the catheter and a small spigot may be inserted to seal the open end.

The baby must be very carefully observed throughout the feed for any colour change or apnoea, and following the feed for any regurgitation which so easily could be inhaled.

The baby's cot is left with the head tipped up for 20 to 30 minutes following feeds and the baby left on his right side. All aseptic precautions must be carefully observed with the equipment used and during the administration of a feed.

The amount of feed actually taken must be recorded on the baby's chart. Vitamins and iron preparations may be added to the feeds (Chap. 8).

GENERAL HANDLING AND DAILY CARE

The nursing care of low birth-weight babies demands the highest standard possible. The ultimate survival of the baby depends largely upon the standard of nursing care, constant observation and the keeping of accurate detailed records.

Minimal handling is essential especially in the babies of lower gestational age. Cleansing, changing, and weighing of the baby must be carried out prior to feeding to avoid the possibility of regurgitation. All procedures must be carried out in the cot or incubator and each baby must have his own equipment for his exclusive use.

Toilet. The skin may be cleaned using pHisoHex in water on a cotton wool swab. The skin folds (axillae, groins, neck and behind the ears) must be given special attention as abrasion of the skin surfaces by particles of debris may very easily occur. The napkin area also requires very careful cleansing. This treatment can be carried out daily until the baby reaches 2000 g, when he may be given a bath every second or third day gradually increasing to a daily bath.

The eyes should be gently cleansed once daily with swabs wrung out in warm sterile water. Separate swabs are used for each eye.

The mouth must be inspected at each feeding time. The tiny feeble baby may hold milk particles in the mouth and is prone to thrush infection which must be recognized and treated as soon as possible.

The cord is treated as already described in Chapter 6, but to the baby being nursed in an incubator there is an additional risk from infection with *Escherichia coli* and *Pseudomonas aeruginosa*.

Weighing. Frequency of weighing varies with the policy of units. The smallest babies can be weighed on a special scale inside the incubator. For larger babies the scales should be brought to the cot and the baby weighed lying on a sheet of disposable tissue which is changed between each baby. The baby may be weighed wrapped in his own cot blanket and then the blanket is weighed and the weight deducted. The weight usually falls (or remains stationary) during the first seven to ten days of life.

Thereafter the weight should slowly rise and the birth weight may be regained in two or three weeks. The babies of low gestational age will be slower to regain their birth weights.

NURSING CARE IN SPECIAL CIRCUMSTANCES

Oxygen therapy. Blindness in premature babies due to retrolental fibroplasia has been proved to be caused by the administration of excessive concentrations of oxygen. This condition has been most frequently seen in babies of low gestational age.

Oxygen may have to be given in high concentration but this should be used for as short a period of time as possible. There are various oxygen analysers available for measuring the oxygen content in an incubator. The concentration should be monitored regularly while the baby is receiving additional oxygen. Oxygen concentration should normally be kept below 30 per cent. A more accurate method of controlling oxygen therapy is by monitoring the level of the infant's arterial oxygen tension. A cannula is introduced into the umbilical artery with strict aseptic precautions. Samples of blood are withdrawn into a heparinized syringe and analysed (Chap. 19).

During phototherapy. Recent work has shown the value of phototherapy in reducing hyperbilirubinaemia (Chap. 14). The baby is nursed naked under the phototherapy unit. The eyes must be covered to prevent the light from damaging the retina and the body temperature carefully recorded. The length of treatment is governed by the infant's serum bilirubin level.

PREPARATION FOR DISCHARGE

Nursing staff in special care nurseries tend to become very attached to infants under their care. They must remember that they are acting on behalf of the infant's mother and that part of their duty is to teach mother to gain confidence in her ability to look after her baby at first in hospital then at home. Preparation for discharge of a low birth-weight infant who may need to remain in a special care nursery for two or three months must begin well before the baby is expected to be ready for discharge. Mother will already have been encouraged to handle her baby from the beginning. She now has to be shown how to take over the regular nursing management including feeding. Through contact with the health visitor and family doctor the suitability of the home is checked particularly with regard to heating.

FOLLOW-UP CARE

Most maternity units will arrange for follow-up attendances of low birth-weight infants during their first year or two of life. It is only when assessing the progress of infants who have been cared for in special care nurseries that the success or failure of the policies of management can be assessed. Through 'at risk' registers kept by local authorities the long-term prognosis for such infants is checked by reference to reports on their school health and education.

FURTHER READING

CROSSE, V. M. (1972). *The Preterm Baby and Other Babies with Low Birth Weight*. Edinburgh: Churchill Livingstone.

EXPERT GROUP ON SPECIAL CARE FOR BABIES (1971). *Report on Public Health and Medical Subjects*, no. 127. London: HMSO.

MYLES, M. F. (1971). *A Textbook for Midwives*, 7th edn. Edinburgh: Churchill Livingstone.

11

Congenital Abnormalities

In describing the development of the normal fetus in Chapter 4 mention was made of hereditary and environmental factors which might interfere with development of the fetus, and the value of genetic counselling was discussed. In this chapter attention will be concentrated on abnormalities of development which allow fetal life to progress until the age of potential viability and which are evident as abnormalities of form or function detectable at birth.

FETAL DEATH

It must be remembered, however, that the most seriously malformed products of gestation cause fetal death at an early stage of pregnancy and are generally unrecognized when they are aborted. The surviving abnormal fetuses are the smaller group whom we recognize at birth whether live- or stillborn as congenital abnormalities. This group is now of greater relative importance as a cause of perinatal mortality and morbidity as birth trauma, infection and other causes of perinatal death come under control.

Incidence

Recognition. Assessment of the incidence of congenital abnormalities is simplest when confined to major well-recognized abnormalities such as anencephaly or spina bifida which are clearly visible at birth. A firm diagnosis of cardiac, renal or cerebral abnormality is seldom possible at birth and it may be weeks or years before an abnormality is confirmed. With less serious forms of abnormality in which function may not be affected, as in the case of birthmarks, embarrassment may be the principal handicap. Opinions differ as to whether such conditions should be classified as abnormalities.

Range. Variations in frequency of examination, in interpretation of signs and in the period of follow-up as well as the skill of the physician concerned account for much of the range of incidence quoted in different surveys. Where the incidence of specifically defined abnormalities is studied and these errors are excluded considerable differences in incidence are still found in different parts of the world and in different parts of one country. Such studies of the epidemiology of congenital abnormalities can provide evidence as to aetiological factors.

THE BRITISH PERINATAL MORTALITY SURVEY (1958)

The British Perinatal Mortality Survey (1958) showed an incidence of malformation of 17.5 per 1000 total births. Almost half of these were stillborn or died in the neonatal period. They were almost equally divided between stillbirths and first-week deaths. Thus in this survey 4 or 5 of every 1000 liveborn infants died shortly after birth because of congenital abnormality and another 9 survived with a significant abnormality.

Multiple abnormalities. The majority of those who died had multiple abnormalities whereas most of those who survived were thought to have single abnormalities. In other surveys where more detailed examination has been carried out while the infants were in nurseries or where a longer term follow-up has been arranged the incidence of abnormality discovered in survivors has been much higher.

Perinatal deaths. In the British Perinatal Mortality Survey quoted above malformations accounted for 16 per cent of perinatal deaths. Although there is no evidence that the absolute incidence of congenital abnormality has changed since 1958 a recent survey of perinatal deaths in Edinburgh shows that 25 per cent are now due to this cause as deaths from other causes have declined. Congenital abnormalities are therefore a major cause of perinatal death and result in serious handicap to many surviving infants.

Causative Factors

Prevention is clearly the most acceptable form of management. This requires prior knowledge of the causative factors involved. These are many and frequently interaction between two or more such factors appears to be necessary. Table 11.1 lists some of the principal situations known to be associated with increased risk of congenital abnormality.

GENETIC

Inherited factors. The part played by inherited factors such as abnormal genes in the causation of congenital abnormality recognizable at birth is relatively small. Many inherited genetic disorders are of a metabolic nature and only become evident later in infancy or require special investigation for their detection at birth. Some inherited skeletal abnormalities such as achondroplasia can be recognized at birth or even in prenatal life by X-ray examination of the fetus.

Mutations. Chromosomal abnormalities, the majority of which are mutants, are an uncommon cause of congenital abnormality. The majority of infants with a chromosomal abnormality show no physical abnormality at birth. The autosomal trisomies are, however, associated with recognizable abnormality the commonest of which is Down's syndrome.

ENVIRONMENTAL

Of the adverse environmental factors liable to cause abnormality of the fetus most are only harmful during the period of organogenesis during the first trimester of pregnancy. Knowledge about the part played by viral infections is slowly increasing. A number of studies have now been carried out on the part played by drugs. More recently interest has focused on chemicals present in water and in foodstuffs. Epidemics of potato blight are said to be followed about two years later by an increased incidence of spina bifida and hydrocephalus. Oligohydramnios results in excessive pressure of the uterine wall on the growing fetus and may result in abnormalities of the limbs such as talipes (Fig. 11.1). More localized pressure changes from amniotic bands can cause local constriction around a limb which occasionally results in intrauterine amputation (Fig. 11.2, 11.3).

Unknown. As shown above a variety of causes of congenital abnormality are known but in the majority of cases no cause can be recognized.

Prevention

Of the causes listed in Table 11.1 some are capable of control by doctors and midwives with the co-operation of the mother.

Rubella immunization. Education with regard to the risk from rubella and the benefit of protective immunization could lead to

Table 11.1 Causes of congenital abnormality

GENETIC
Inherited
Mutations
ENVIRONMENTAL IN UTERO
Viral Infections
Rubella
Mumps
Herpes simplex
X-rays
Chemicals
(?Blighted potatoes)
Drugs
Mechanical
Pressure effects
Constricting bands
UNKNOWN

(a) 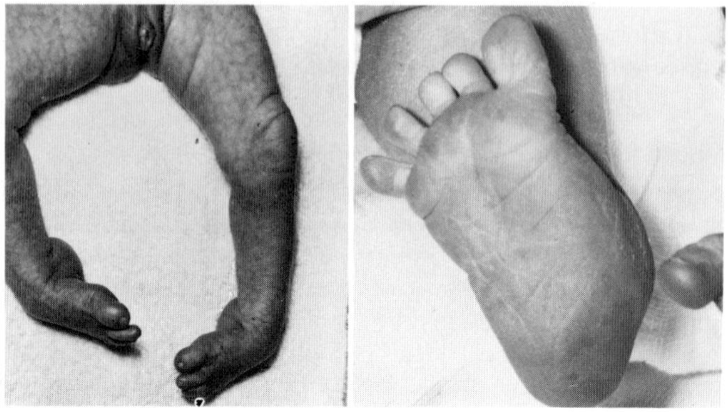 (b)

Figure 11.1 Talipes: (a) talipes equino-varus; (b) talipes calcaneo-valgus.

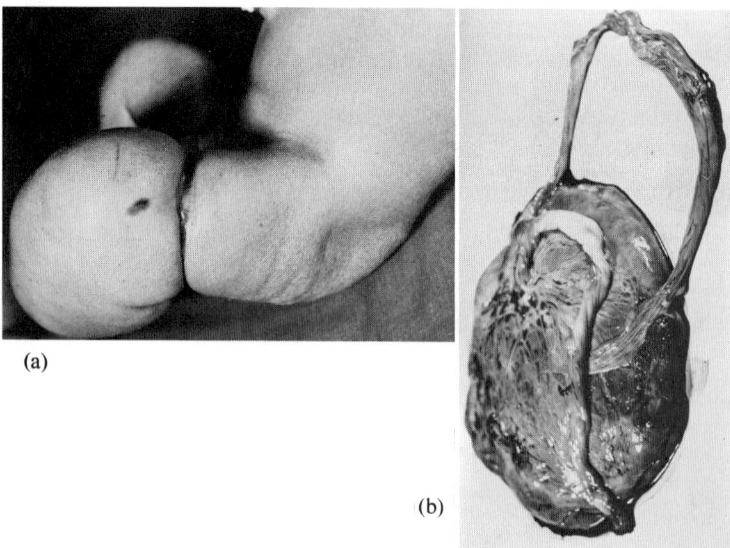

(a)

(b)

Figure 11.2 Constriction of thigh by amniotic band.

generations in whom this problem has been eliminated. For the mother who was not immunized naturally or artificially before pregnancy vaccine can be offered shortly after delivery. Vaccination must not be carried out during pregnancy and pregnancy should be avoided for three months after vaccination.

Drugs. Supervision of drugs being presented to pregnant women so

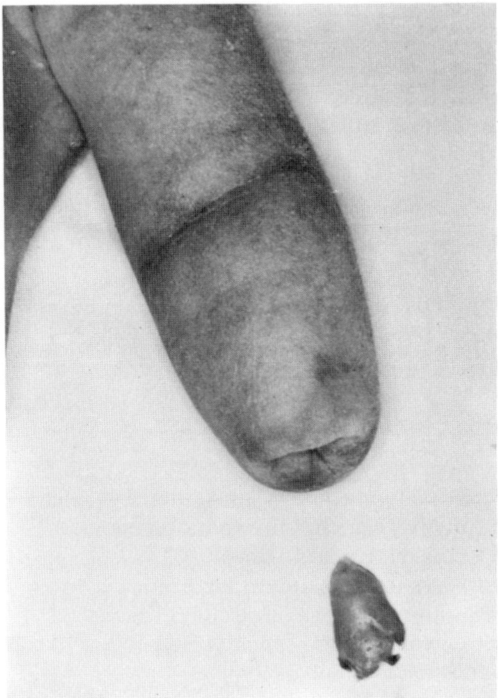

Figure 11.3 Intrauterine amputation of hand.

that no drug is given without good reason limits the risk from drug-induced abnormalities.

X-rays. Avoidance of exposure to X-rays during the first three months of pregnancy is essential.

GENETIC COUNSELLING

In families with a known high risk of abnormal offspring genetic counselling may help the family to decide whether they wish to have further children. If they do not, contraceptive advice should be given.

Therapeutic abortion. Where there has been proven exposure to harmful factors in early pregnancy or where there is a high risk of hereditary abnormality consideration has to be given in each situation to the justification for therapeutic abortion.

Amniocentesis. In some situations examination of the amniotic fluid or direct examination of the fetus by an endoscope passed into the amniotic cavity may be advisable before a decision can be reached (Chap. 4).

STERILIZATION

The ultimate preventive management is contraceptive advice or sterilization and this has to be accepted as the only suitable means of management in some situations of high risk.

ABNORMAL DEVELOPMENT

As in over half the cases of congenital abnormality we are not able to identify a cause and therefore to take preventive action we are still likely to be faced with problems of management of infants born with an abnormality. Most of these have resulted from a disturbance in embryological development. An understanding of the faults which occur in the early development of the embryo helps in the understanding of the deformities present at birth. In general terms abnormalities arise because of:

Failure of development, e.g. amelia, microcephaly
Failure to unite, e.g. cleft lip, spina bifida
Failure to divide, e.g. syndactyly
Failure to canalize, e.g. intestinal atresias
Failure to migrate, e.g. malrotation of bowel
Failure to atrophy, e.g. branchial clefts.
Excess division, e.g. polydactyly

The Embryological Basis

THE MOUTH AND FACE

The lips are developed from three processes—a midline central nasal process and the two wings of a branchial arch (the maxillary processes) which grow out on each side from dorsal attachments to the head to meet the nasal process ventrally in midline. When fusion does not take place a hare lip results (Fig. 11.4). The failure to fuse usually occurs between a maxillary process and the fronto-nasal process, resulting in a lateral hare lip. This may consist of a complete cleft extending up to the nostril or of only a slight notched depression of the lip margin. It may be single or double.

Cleft palate is another example of failure to fuse. The palate originates as two palatal processes from the same branchial arch as the lips and from other mesodermic processes (the nasal septum and the premaxilla) extending downwards, from the primitive head. Fusion begins between the premaxilla and the anterior edges of the palatal processes, and extends posteriorly along the opposed edges of those processes. Depending upon the exact nature of the failure to fuse, cleft palate can assume one of a variety of forms. Cleft palate

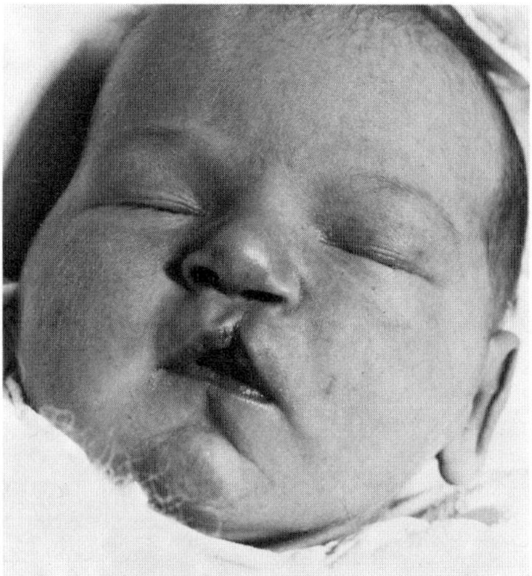

Figure 11.4 Hare lip.

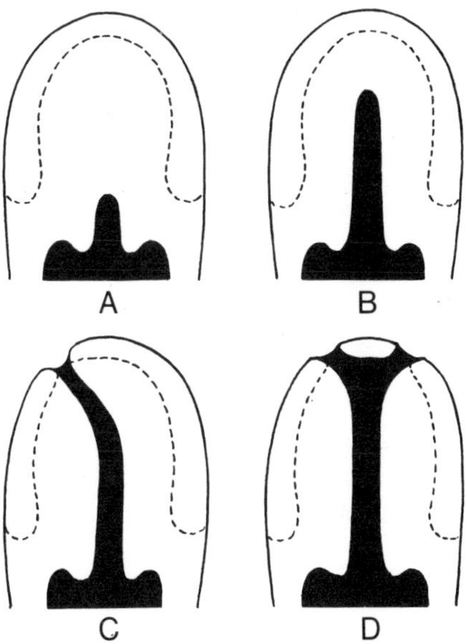

Figure 11.5 Forms of cleft palate and hare lip.

may exist alone or be associated with hare lip (unilateral or bilateral) (Fig. 11.5).

Micrognathia is smallness of the mandible, which is another structure derived from a branchial arch. It is an example of failure to develop.

Branchial arch abnormalities. Hare lip, cleft palate and micrognathia each represent a departure from normal in the embryological development of the first branchial arch. Other anomalies now

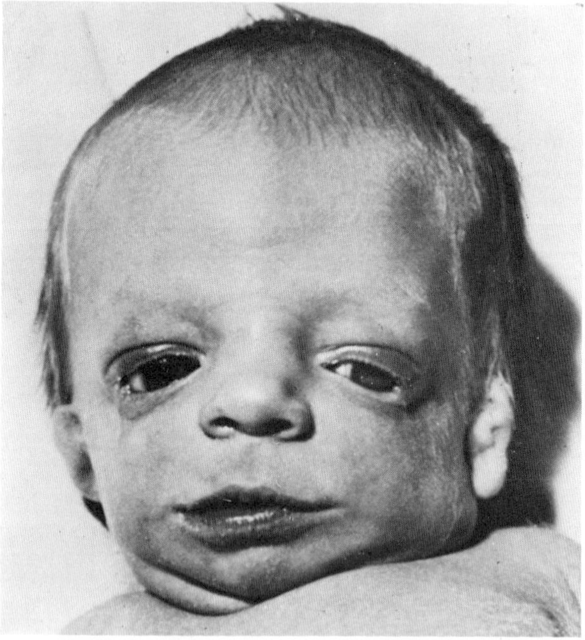

Figure 11.6 Mandibulofacial dysostosis.

generally considered to be variants of the same basic developmental error include mandibulofacial dysostosis (*Treacher-Collins syndrome*) (Fig. 11.6), mandibular hypoplasia and glossoptosis (*Pierre-Robin syndrome*), mandibular dysostosis, hypertelorism, and deformities of the external and middle ear (Fig. 11.7). The disorders mentioned above are collectively termed *the first arch syndrome* as they probably arise from inadequacy of blood supply to the first branchial arch.

GASTROINTESTINAL TRACT

The oesophagus. As the neck grows in length corresponding development of the oesophagus may be interrupted, giving rise to

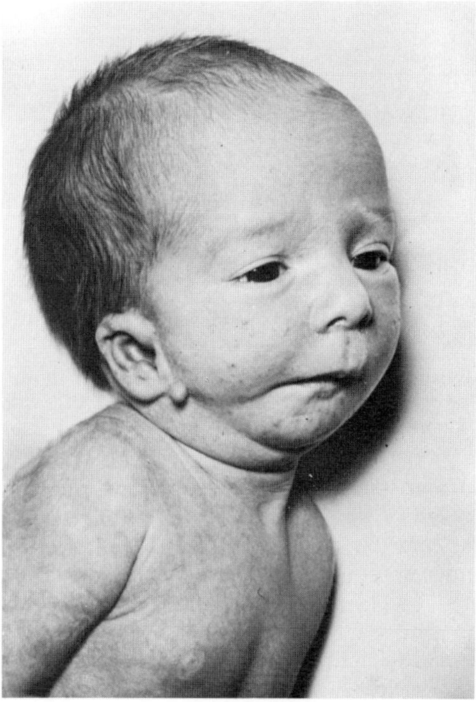

Figure 11.7 First arch syndrome showing unilateral deformity of the mandible and ear.

stenosis. Abnormal development may occur also during the time that the trachea is evolving from a pharyngeal pouch. A portion of the oesophagus may be completely absent or represented by a fibrous cord—atresia being present in either event. The anomaly is rare, but the most likely form to be encountered consists of a distally blind upper pouch and a lower pouch communicating with the trachea (by a persistent fistula) at one end and with the stomach at the other (Fig. 11.8).

Diaphragm. Errors in the development of the diaphragm may occur as failures of migration or fusion. Diaphragmatic anomalies are rare. When they occur they usually consist of persistence of one of the lateral openings which is a feature of early development. The deficiency is almost always on the left side and enables the intestines to herniate (diaphragmatic hernia) through the opening with the risk of strangulation.

The midgut. Any part of the midgut may be stenosed or occluded.

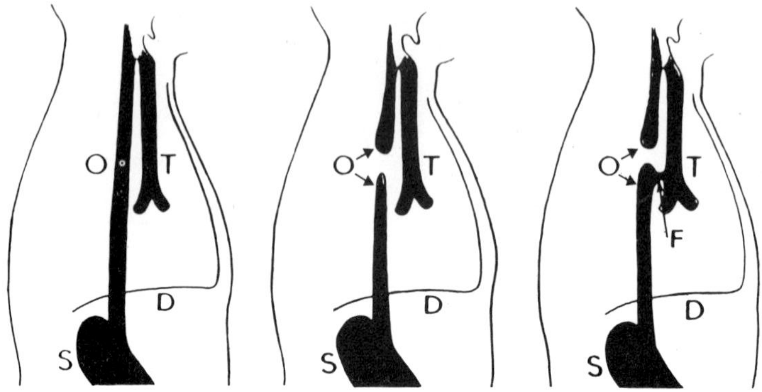

Figure 11.8 Oesophageal atresia. The figure on the left shows the anatomy in a normal baby. The other figures show two types of oesophageal atresia. O = oesophagus, S = stomach, D = diaphragm, F = fistula.

Duodenal atresia is the form most commonly encountered and is usually the result of local failure of the primitive gut to canalize.

Departure from the normal progressive rotation of the gut may result in the development of abnormal adhesions, the suspension of large and small intestine by a single short pedicle, or in the midgut having a notably narrow mesenteric attachment. These are all circumstances which favour the occurrence of acute intestinal obstruction due to volvulus.

Meckel's diverticulum is an uncommon anomaly related to early development of the intestine. It represents the part of the vitelline duct which opens into the ileum. The diverticulum may persist as a projection from the ileum, as a fibrous cord attached internally to the umbilicus, or as a sinus opening externally at the umbilicus (Fig. 11.9).

THE HINDGUT

Abnormalities of the anus and rectum may take several forms. An imperforate anus results when the anal membrane remains intact. Incomplete 'rupture' of the membrane accounts for partial atresia or anal stenosis. Rectovesical and rectourethral fistulae are attributable to failure of the cloaca to become completely separated into its alimentary and urogenital sections. Rectovesical fistulae are very rare in females but rectovaginal fistulae are encountered (Fig. 11.10).

ABDOMINAL WALL

Delayed development of the abdominal wall with excessively large development of the abdominal viscera and gut may result in the fetal

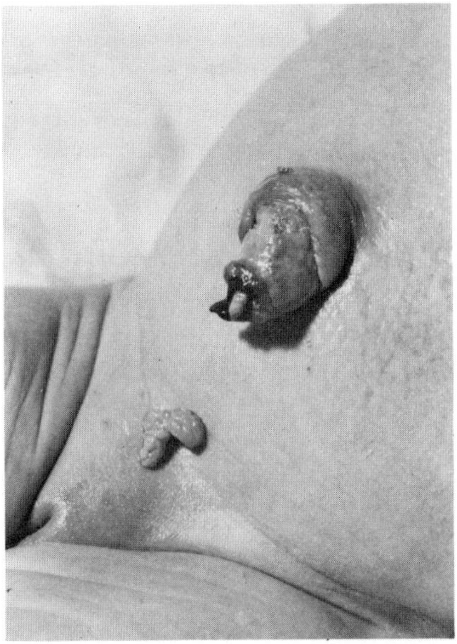

Figure 11.9 Persistent vitelline duct showing evacuation of stool.

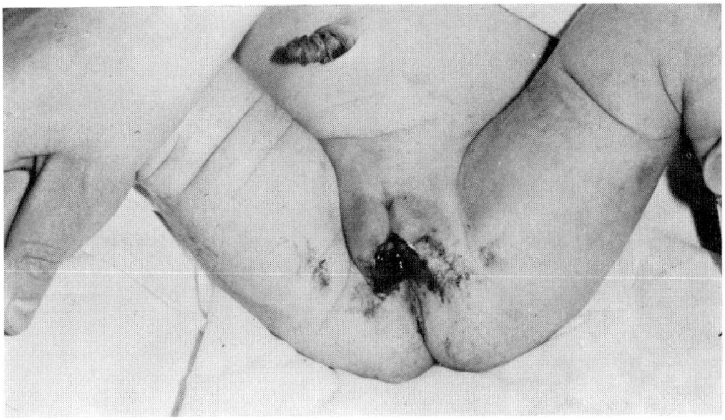

Figure 11.10 Rectovaginal fistula with meconium being passed through the vagina.

membranes and intestines, which normally extend temporarily into the base of the umbilical cord, not being able to return to the abdominal cavity. Should this persist exomphalos develops, the infant being born with abdominal viscera herniated through the abdominal wall and enclosed by peritoneum and amniotic membrane.

GENITOURINARY TRACT

The kidneys may be the site of polycystic disease which results from an abnormality of development of the nephrons. Abnormal fusion can give rise to a single horseshoe kidney.

The bladder. Developmentally the bladder is derived from a number of structures. Extroversion of the bladder (ectopia vesicae) (Fig. 11.11) is an anomaly consisting of imperfect closure of the anterior abdominal wall, absence of the anterior wall of the bladder, and failure of the pubic bones to unite anteriorly. The reason for the occurrence of the anomaly is not known, but the fact that the umbilicus is invariably situated in an unusually low position indicates that the disturbance of development has taken place early in fetal life.

Patent urachus is a persistent sinus extending from the bladder and opening to the exterior at the umbilicus which occurs if the urachus does not undergo complete obliteration. Alternatively a cyst may develop in the line of the urachus (Fig. 11.12).

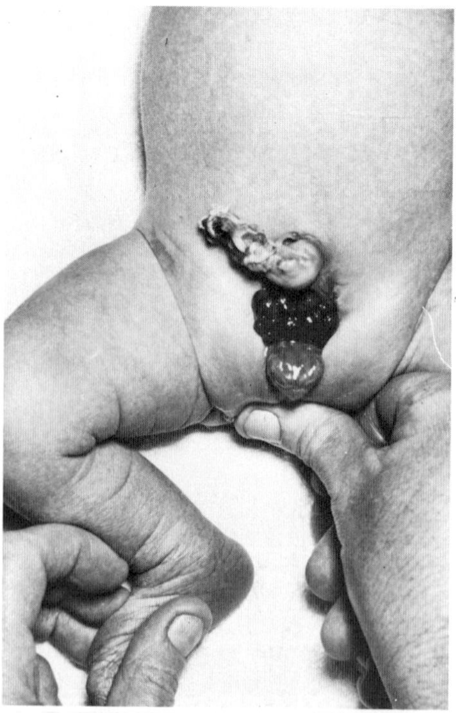

Figure 11.11 Ectopia vesicae with epispadias and low position of umbilicus.

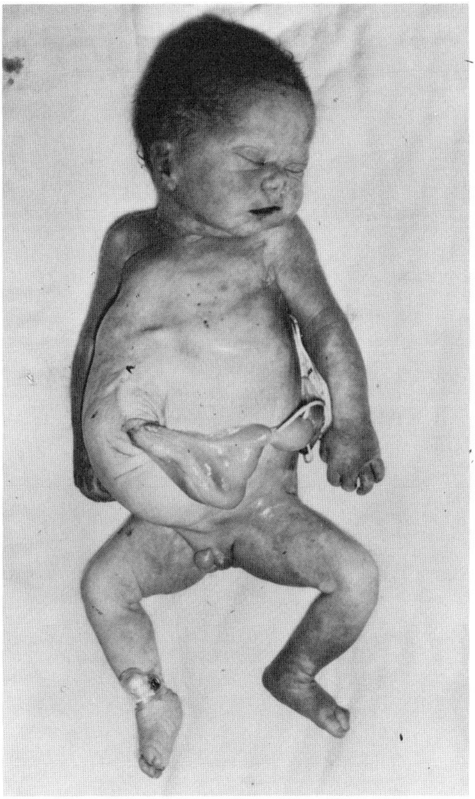

Figure 11.12 Urachal cyst extending into the umbilical cord.

The penis. At an early stage of the development of the penis a groove flanked by raised margins appears on the undersurface of the organ. The groove deepens and the overhanging margins meet, converting the groove into a patent tube. Closure of the ventral wall of the penis proceeds from behind forwards. Hypospadias results when ventral fusion is incomplete (Fig. 11.13). The nature of the hypospadias depends on the site of imperfect fusion, and may simulate the appearance of the external genitalia in the female.

The testes and inguinal canals. The testes form in the abdominal cavity and normally before birth they pass through the inguinal canals to reach the scrotum. In their descent into the scrotum the testes are contained in a sac of peritoneum. The sac becomes sealed off immediately above the testes and at the external inguinal ring, the

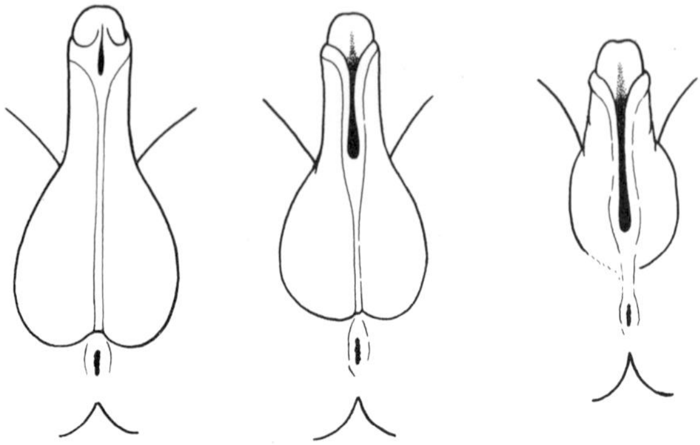

Figure 11.13 Degrees of hypospadias.

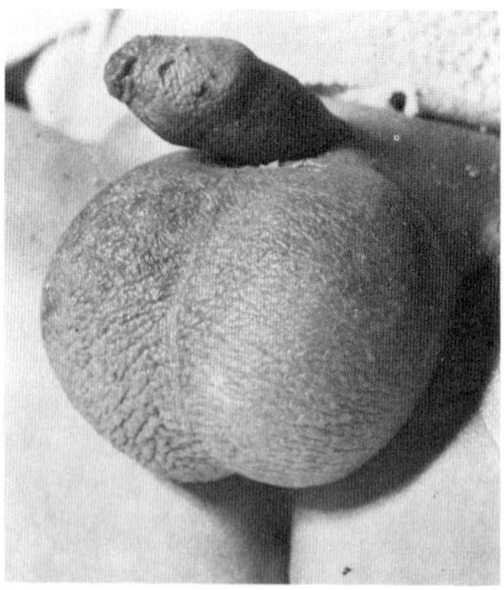

Figure 11.14 Bilateral hydrocele.

intervening portion becoming obliterated. The process of obliteration may not take place. If, as a result, the sac still communicates with the abdominal cavity, a hernia may develop—gut entering the sac. If on the other hand, despite sealing off of the sac from the abdominal cavity, the sac does not become obliterated, fluid may collect in it, forming a hydrocele (Fig. 11.14).

Exceptionally descent of the testes into the scrotum may be incomplete. The testis may remain in the abdominal cavity or inguinal canal (Fig. 11.15) or after passing through the inguinal canal it may take up an abnormal position (ectopic testis) in the upper thigh or lower abdominal wall (Fig. 11.16).

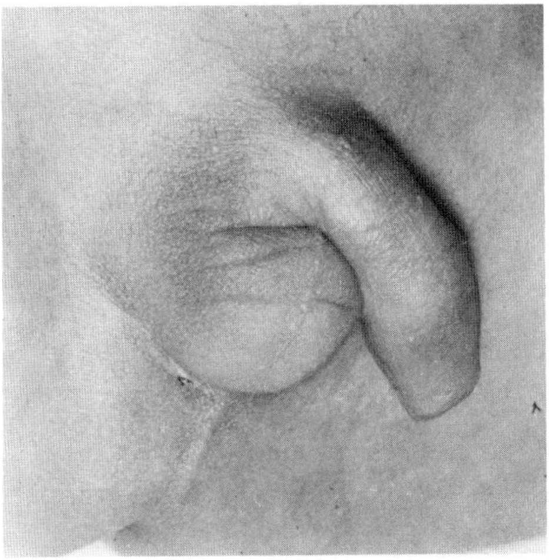

Figure 11.15 Undescended right testicle.

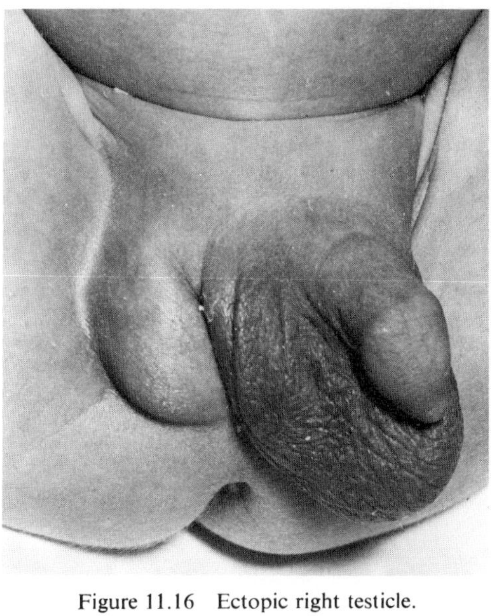

Figure 11.16 Ectopic right testicle.

THE SPINAL CORD AND COLUMN

The spinal cord develops from the neural tube, and the vertebral column from the mesodermal segments lying adjacent to the tube. Each vertebra is formed as a result of fusion of three processes. Of these, one represents the body of the vertebra and the other two the lateral halves of the neural arch and vertebral spine. Anomalies of the cord and column result from imperfect separation of the neural tube from the main ectodermal mass and from imperfect fusion of the two lateral sections of the neural arches.

Spina bifida is a defect in the vertebral column. The contents of the column are visible and may herniate through the defect. When the herniated structures consist of meninges only, the condition is known as meningocele.

Myelomeningocele. When nerve tissues are included in the sac, the condition is described as myelomeningocele. Occasionally there is no hernia despite defect of the vertebral column (spina bifida occulta). A localized depression of the skin or a hairy mole may be present over the site of the anomaly. Spina bifida may occur anywhere in the spine but is found most commonly in the lumbo-sacral region (Fig. 11.17).

Pilonidal sinus. At first the neural tube remains open at its caudal end, closure taking place with the fusion of the ectodermal layer of

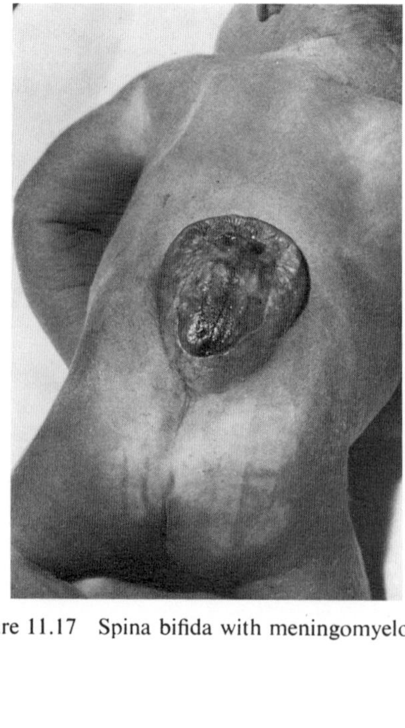

Figure 11.17 Spina bifida with meningomyelocele.

skin in midline. The distal end of the tube is converted into a delicate filament which remains attached distally in the region of the coccyx. A midline depression of the skin in the neighbourhood of the coccyx (pilonidal depression) sometimes indicates the point of attachment. Failure of the caudal end of the neural tube to become closed gives rise to a sinus (pilonidal sinus) which opens to the exterior (Fig. 11.18).

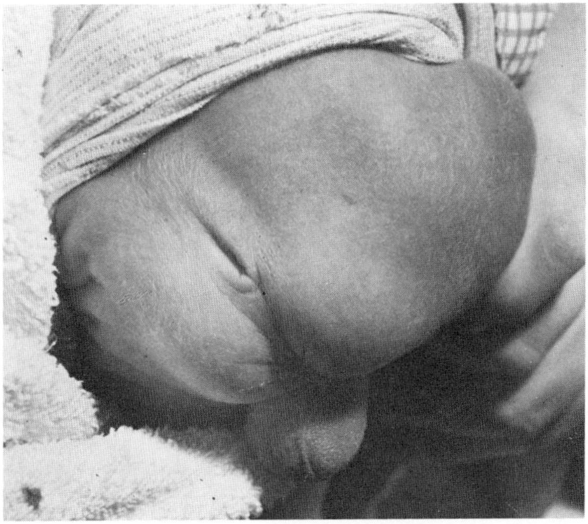

Figure 11.18 Pilonidal sinus.

THE BRAIN

The head end of the neural tube undergoes considerable elaboration to form the brain. Developmental errors analogous to those described in connection with the cord may involve the brain.

Anencephaly. Failure of the cephalic end of the cord to close gives rise to the condition known as anencephaly in which development of the vault of the skull and cerebral hemispheres is minimal.

Microcephaly, characterized by pronounced smallness of the skull and by an anterior fontanelle closed or almost closed at the time of birth, results from failure of the cerebral hemispheres to grow during intrauterine life (Fig. 11.19).

Hydrocephalus is another condition which is sometimes but not always the result of errors of development. Normally the cerebrospinal fluid is secreted by the choroid plexuses into the ventricles of the brain. The fluid circulates in the ventricular system and in the subarachnoid space of the spinal cord, but its main flow is directed

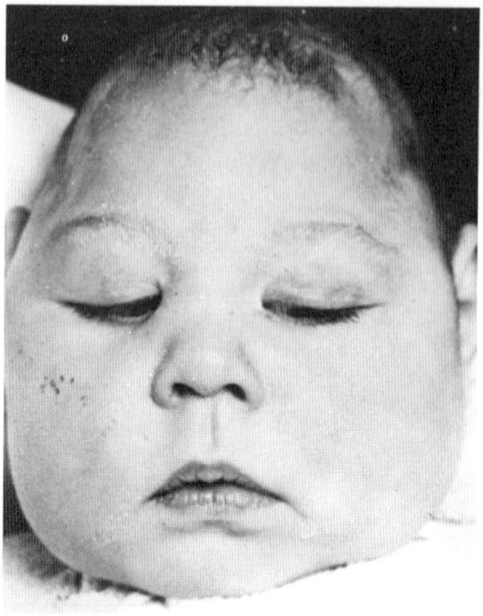

Figure 11.19 Microcephaly.

over the surface of the brain where it is absorbed. Any structural maldevelopment which interferes with the normal circulation or absorption involves the risk of excessive accumulation of cerebrospinal fluid within the skull and dilatation of the ventricles characteristic of hydrocephalus. The structural anomaly may be primarily developmental or secondary to intracranial infection or trauma *in utero*. Interference with absorption gives rise to communicating hydrocephalus, and interference with flow from the ventricles to obstructive hydrocephalus. Meningomyelocele is frequently associated with hydrocephalus resulting in lacunar skull. In these cases the spinal anomaly is accompanied by herniation of brain substance

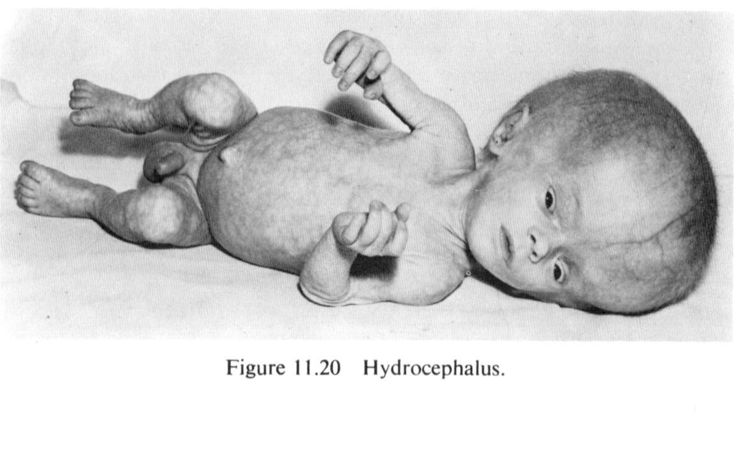

Figure 11.20 Hydrocephalus.

into the spinal canal (Arnold-Chiari malformation). The protruding brain substance is subjected to abnormal pressures which interfere with the circulation of the cerebrospinal fluid, leading to the subsequent development of hydrocephalus (Fig. 11.20). Encephalocoele is a protrusion of the meninges through a midline defect in the occipital bone. Parts of the brain may be present in the sac with resulting microcephaly.

THE HEART AND GREAT VESSELS

Arrest or interference with the normal development of the heart occurs at various stages of intrauterine life. The fifth to eighth week of fetal existence corresponds to a particularly important phase in the evolution of the heart and great vessels.

Septal defects. Development of the septa separating the chambers of the heart may be arrested before closure is complete. As a result, normal circulation within the heart may be interfered with and mixing of deoxygenated and freshly oxygenated blood occurs.

Transposition. Disturbance of the normal process of rotation of the embryonic heart and great vessels may result in the eventual malposition of certain structures. Thus the pulmonary artery may arise from the left instead of the right ventricle (transposition of the great vessels). In this event oxygenated blood is returned to the lungs while the poorly oxygenated blood in the right ventricle leaves the heart by the aorta to supply the body. Life is possible only if there is a shunt at septal level or patency of the ductus arteriosus.

Valve stenosis. Other deformities which occur include narrowing of the rings of the aortic and pulmonary valves and failure of the aorta and pulmonary arteries to develop normally in size.

Patent ductus arteriosus. Normally the ductus arteriosus undergoes spontaneous closure shortly after birth and becomes gradually converted into a fibrous cord. Where this does not occur, the ductus arteriosus remains patent—a remnant of a structure essential for intrauterine existence but unnecessary for healthy survival after birth.

Single chamber. A heart consisting of only one, two or three instead of the usual four chambers is sometimes seen at autopsy on a stillborn child or infant dying shortly after birth. In such an infant disturbance of cardiac development has occurred at an even earlier stage in fetal existence than in cases of septal defect or of transposition of the vessels.

THE URGENCY OF DIAGNOSIS

The urgency of diagnosis and treatment in infants with congenital abnormality depends upon the degree of risk associated with that abnormality. Those that produce the most marked abnormality of form may not be as urgent a problem as those with major abnormality of function. The following section therefore deals with congenital abnormalities liable to cause early neonatal death irrespective of their anatomical site. Subsequent sections will deal with abnormalities by the body system principally involved.

ABNORMALITIES LIABLE TO CAUSE EARLY NEONATAL DEATH

Atresia of the larynx is fortunately very rare but if recognized at birth, because of the extreme but ineffective inspiratory efforts, can be treated by immediate puncture of the web or by tracheotomy.

Laryngeal webs and *laryngeal stenosis* are also rare and produce immediate stridor when respiration begins. Tracheotomy may be required.

Choanal atresia when bilateral is a complete obstruction between the nose and the pharynx. Breathing is possible only through the open mouth (Fig. 11.21). If the mouth is closed, as during feeding, breathing is not possible and there is marked indrawing of the chest and cyanosis until the baby opens his mouth. There may be difficulty in establishing respiration or symptoms may be delayed if the infant learns to open his mouth frequently. Treatment is surgical by perforation of the obstructing plate. The symptoms are less marked in unilateral choanal atresia.

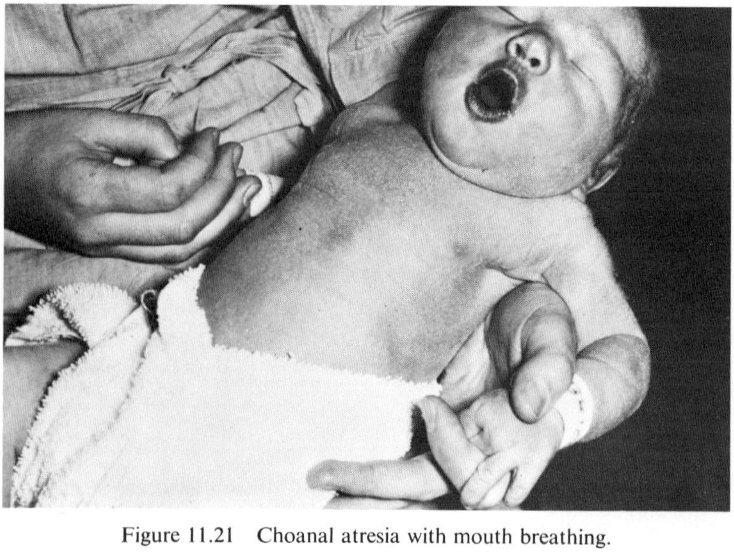

Figure 11.21 Choanal atresia with mouth breathing.

Glossoptosis in which the tongue rolls backward into the posterior pharynx obstructing the larynx is also a cause of respiratory obstruction. This is most likely to occur where there is hypomandibulosis and cleft palate as in the *Pierre-Robin syndrome* (Fig. 11.22). Immediate treatment is by holding the baby's face and head down and pulling the tongue forward. This position should then be maintained. A suitable frame is shown in Figure 11.23.

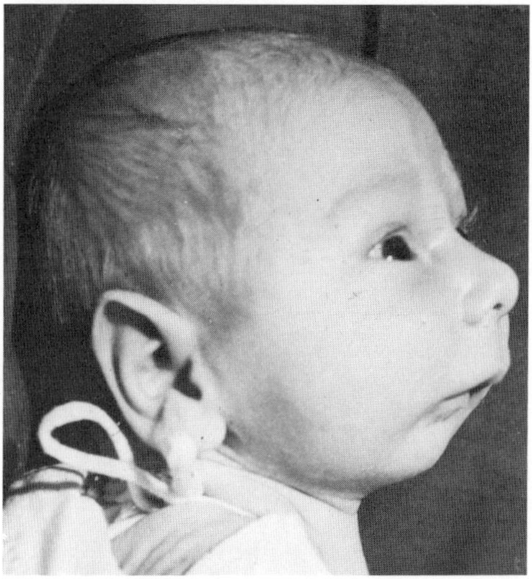

Figure 11.22 Hypomandibulosis.

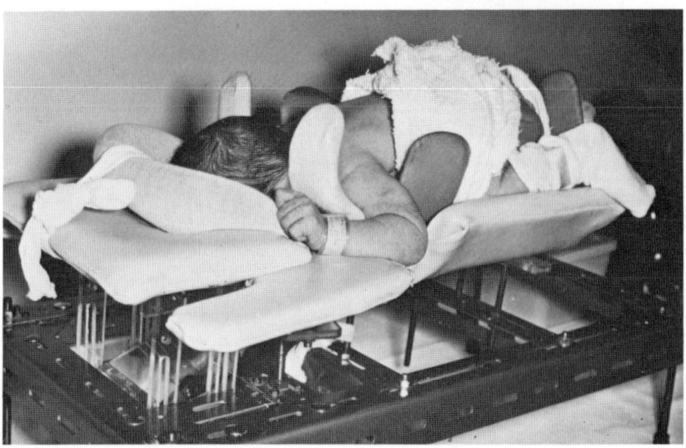

Figure 11.23 Frame for treatment of Pierre-Robin syndrome.

Macroglossia (a large tongue) may similarly obstruct the airway and require surgical treatment (Fig. 11.24).

OESOPHAGEAL ATRESIA

Oesophageal atresia may be recognized before birth. As the fetus cannot swallow amniotic fluid hydramnios occurs and oesophageal

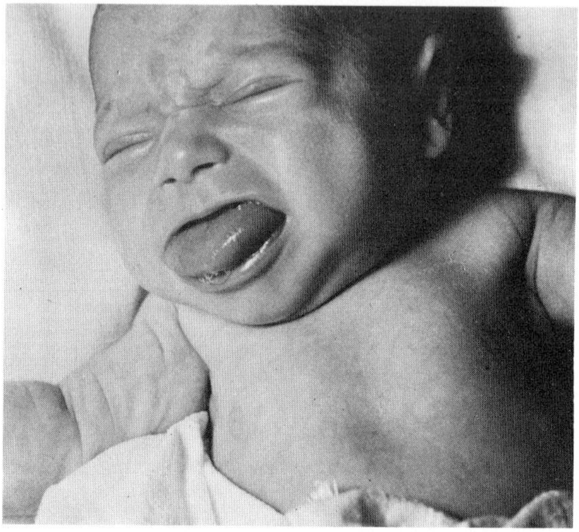

Figure 11.24 Macroglossia.

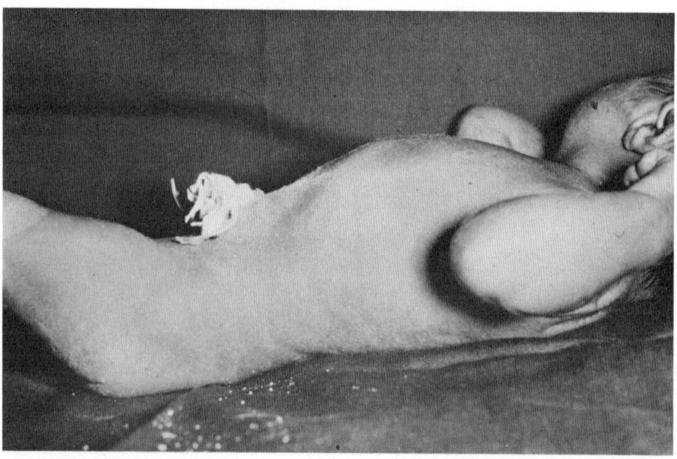

Figure 11.25 Flat abdomen with no air in the stomach or bowel. (In this baby this was due to oesophageal atresia *without* an oesophagotracheal fistula.)

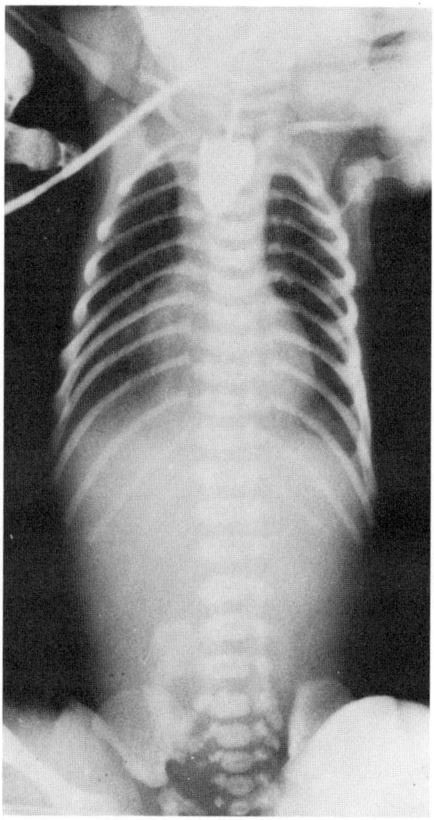

Figure 11.26 Radio-opaque material outlining upper oesophageal pouch in baby shown in Figure 11.25. Note the absence of air below the diaphragm.

atresia should always be looked for following maternal hydramnios. After birth the upper oesophageal pouch, which commonly ends at the level of the cricoid cartilage, fills with saliva and mucus. Respiration becomes bubbly and aspiration of oral fluid produces respiratory obstruction and cyanosis. The types of tracheo-oesophageal fistula associated with oesophageal atresia were shown in Figure 11.8. Where no air reaches the stomach the abdomen will remain flat (Fig. 11.25). The diagnosis can be confirmed by passing a radio-opaque and suitably large catheter into the upper pouch and taking an X-ray of the neck (Fig. 11.26). Immediate treatment is continuous aspiration of the upper oesophageal pouch to prevent overflow of mucus and the withholding of feeds. If the stomach is distended there is a risk of regurgitation of gastric contents into the lungs with resulting bronchopneumonia. Early gastrostomy and aspiration is the only adequate means of preventing this. Surgical repair of the fistula and anastomosis of the upper and lower oesophageal pouches may be preceded by the passage of bougies into both pouches to stretch them. As many of the babies affected are of low birth weight definitive operation may have to be deferred particularly if bronchopneumonia has developed. The prognosis is best in those infants diagnosed and treated early before chest complications develop.

DIAPHRAGMATIC HERNIA

Diaphragmatic hernia most commonly occurs through the left diaphragm where the left pleuroperitoneal canal has failed to close (Fig. 11.27). Abdominal viscera are present in the thorax and there is frequently underdevelopment of the lung. Symptoms of marked respiratory distress may occur from the moment of birth or be delayed for hours after birth. The symptoms occur earliest where there is most displacement of lung. The left chest may appear

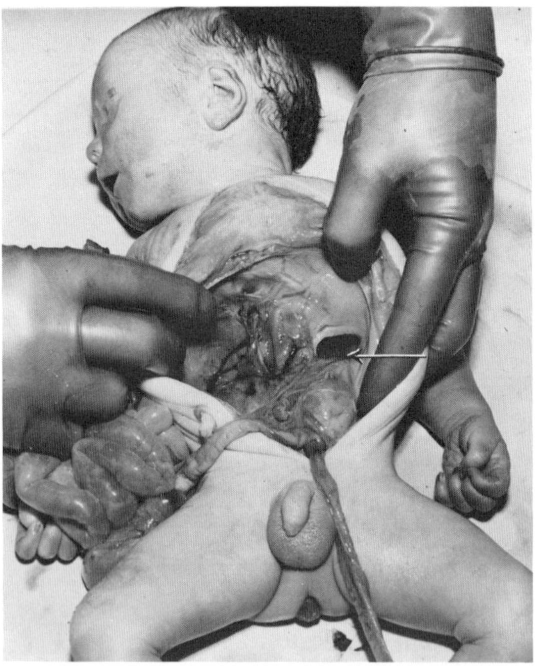

Figure 11.27 Diaphragmatic hernia. The arrow indicates the abnormal opening in the diaphragm through which the intestine passed into the thorax. The intestine, seen on the left, has been withdrawn.

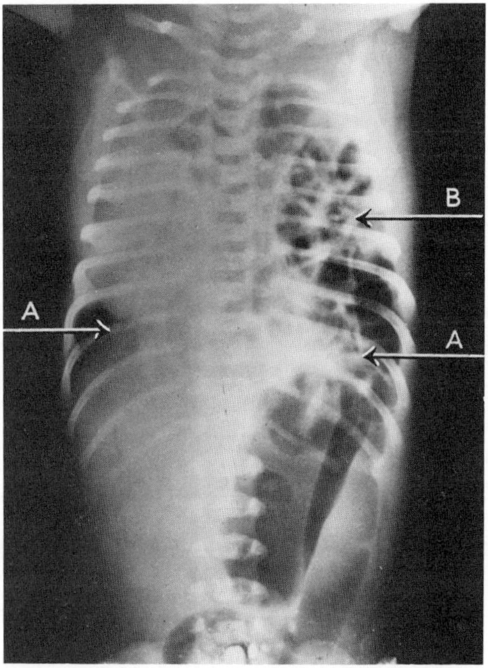

Figure 11.28 Diaphragmatic hernia. X-ray of patient shown in Figure 11.27 before withdrawal of the intestine. A, diaphragm; B, intestine in the left chest.

overfilled and the abdomen flat. Diagnosis is confirmed by X-ray, which shows air-containing bowel shadows in the chest (Fig. 11.28). The treatment is surgical. If this is not immediately available endotracheal intubation and artificial respiration may be required to maintain life until surgical treatment can be undertaken. With rapid recognition and treatment at least 50 per cent of affected infants should survive.

OTHER ABNORMALITIES

The majority of congenital abnormalities do not present quite such an urgent problem of diagnosis and treatment as those just discussed. It therefore seems more appropriate that these should be described under the heading of the anatomical region or the physiological system principally involved.

Face, Mouth and Neck

Many conditions such as Down's syndrome, achondroplasia, and some of the chromosomal abnormalities have characteristic facies which are a combination of a number of distinct features. These will be described under the heading of the principal system of the body involved. Apart from the recognized syndromes there are many infants with odd facies whom our American colleagues call funny-looking kids (or FLK syndrome) who cannot be allotted to any particular syndrome. Some of these infants will also have abnormalities such as hare lip or cleft palate, and when each of the individual abnormalities of the face, mouth and neck are mentioned it must be remembered that many of these abnormalities occur as one component of multiple abnormalities in the one infant.

Hare lip may be uni- or bilateral and can occur on its own or in combination with cleft palate. Isolated hare lip is commoner in boys and is often familial. Unless the failure of fusion is extensive there is little interference with sucking and breast feeding is possible (Fig. 11.29). The lip is repaired surgically at about 2 months of age. Mothers can be reassured by being shown photographs of the excellent results of good surgery.

Hare lip and cleft palate occur in several forms. In the most extensive form (Fig. 11.30) with bilateral clefts and distortion of the premaxilla the result is unsightly. As other abnormalities are frequently present a full and careful examination of the whole infant is

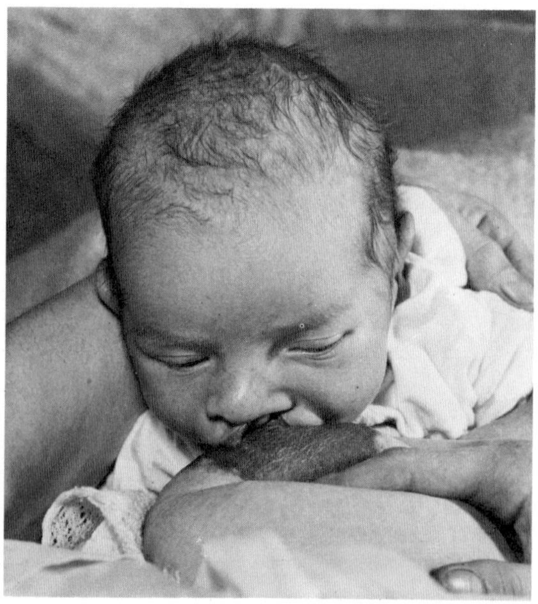

Figure 11.29 Baby with hare lip and cleft palate successfully feeding at the breast.

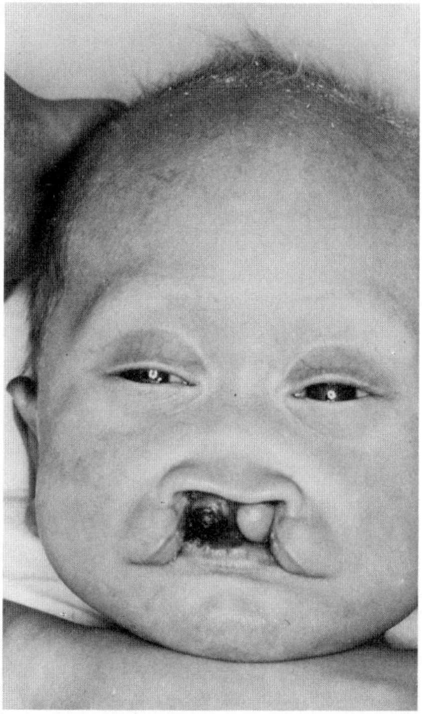

Figure 11.30 Bilateral hare lip and cleft palate with rotation of the premaxilla.

essential. Moulding of the maxilla into a more satisfactory shape can be achieved by plates specially prepared by orthodontists. This makes subsequent surgical repair simpler and more effective. Even with severe abnormalities feeding by normal bottle and teat is often possible particularly with an orthodontic plate in position. Middle ear infection is a constant risk and the ears should be examined regularly. Less extensive clefts may not require orthodontic preparatory treatment before surgery. It is advisable for infants with cleft palates to be examined and reviewed regularly by a team of paediatric physician and surgeon, orthodontic surgeon and ear, nose and throat surgeon—to decide the most appropriate therapy. This may require referral to a regional centre.

Other abnormalities of the facial bones give rise to characteristic facies by which some syndromes including those of the first arch syndrome are recognized. The Pierre-Robin syndrome has already been considered. Mandibulofacial dysostosis (Fig. 11.6) is less frequently a cause of difficulty with breathing and feeding but these may occur because of glossoptosis. The immediate treatment is as for Pierre-Robin syndrome. Later complications including hearing problems and repeated tests for hearing should be arranged.

True tongue tie is a very rare condition. This condition has been overdiagnosed in the past because of failure to recognize that the frenum passing from the tongue to the floor of the mouth is normally short in the newborn. In the healthy infant there is no indication for cutting the frenum at this age. The tongue becomes more mobile as the infant grows. Only in infants with severe limitation of tongue movement and inability to suck is division of the frenum indicated.

Teeth may be present at birth or erupt shortly afterwards. They are generally loose and either fall out or are readily removed.

Epulis is a projection from the gum (Fig. 11.31) most commonly of the upper jaw. It may interfere with feeding and should be removed.

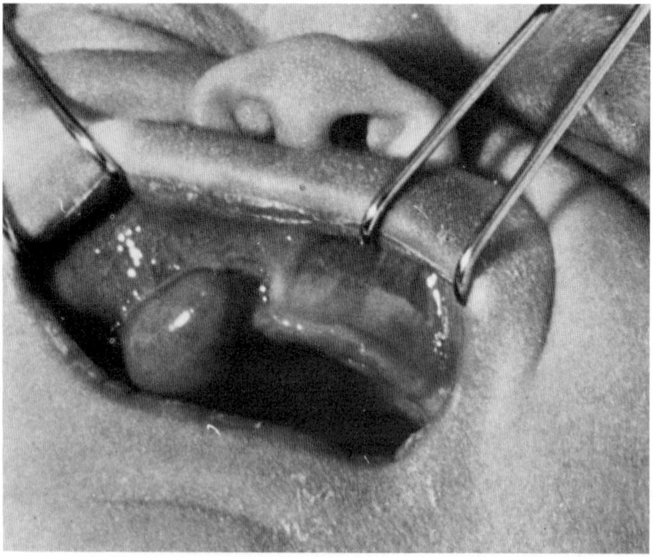

Figure 11.31 Epulis.

Ranula is a cystic swelling caused by obstruction of the sublingual duct. Most resolve without treatment but occasionally surgery is required if the cyst persists and interferes with feeding.

Branchial arch anomalies may present as skin tags (Fig. 11.32), cysts or sinuses. They may be found in the preauricular region or along the anterior border of the sternomastoid muscle. Surgical removal is generally required.

Cystic hygromas are most common in the neck (Fig. 11.33)

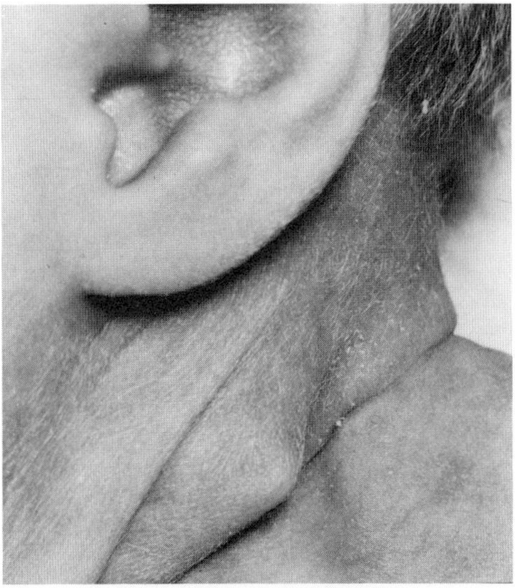

Figure 11.32 Branchial cyst.

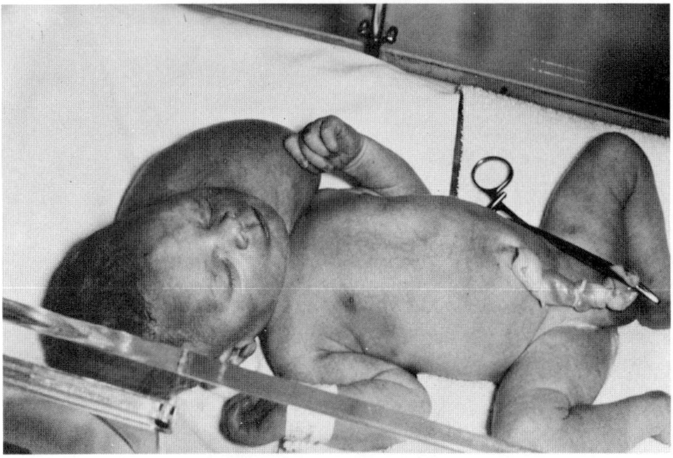

Figure 11.33 Cystic hygroma of neck.

although they may occur elsewhere (Fig. 11.34). They consist of a mass of proliferating lymph vessels and may cause pressure symptoms. Treatment is by surgical removal.

Goitre is rare in the newborn. Thyroid function may be normal as in simple goitre, decreased as in goitrous cretinism or increased as in the infant of a thyrotoxic mother.

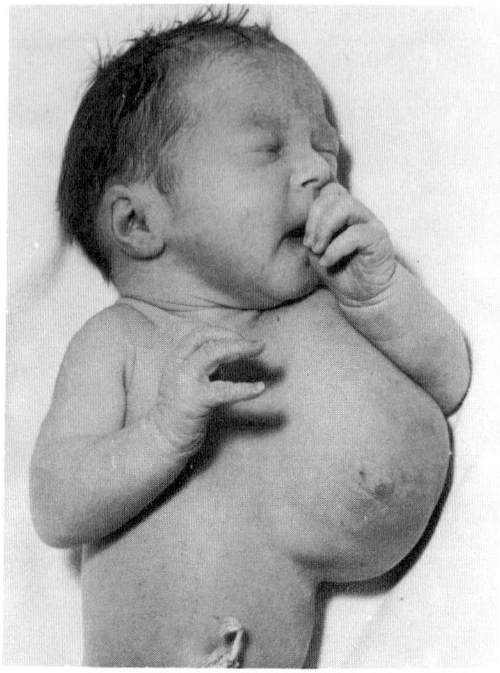

Figure 11.34 Cystic hygroma of axilla.

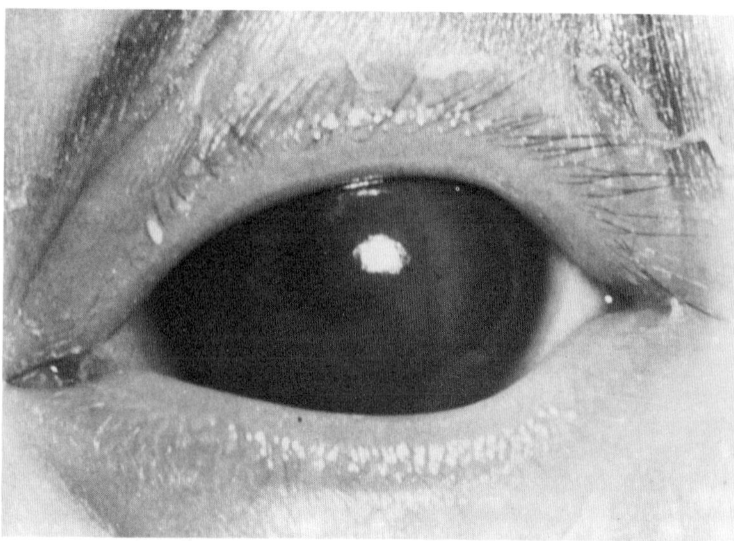

Figure 11.35 Congenital glaucoma.

THE EYE

Absence of the eye (anophthalmia) or a small eye (microphthalmia) are not always obvious at birth but should be looked for if the eye sockets are not normally filled.

Congenital glaucoma, enlargement of the eye, follows obstruction to drainage of the aqueous humour. Similar enlargement from other causes such as injury or infection is termed buphthalmos. Treatment depends on the cause and the opinion of an ophthalmologist should be sought (Fig. 11.35).

Congenital cataract may be evident at birth or become obvious during the following weeks. The cause in many cases is hereditary. Others follow maternal rubella in the first trimester of pregnancy or are associated with galactosaemia (Fig. 11.36).

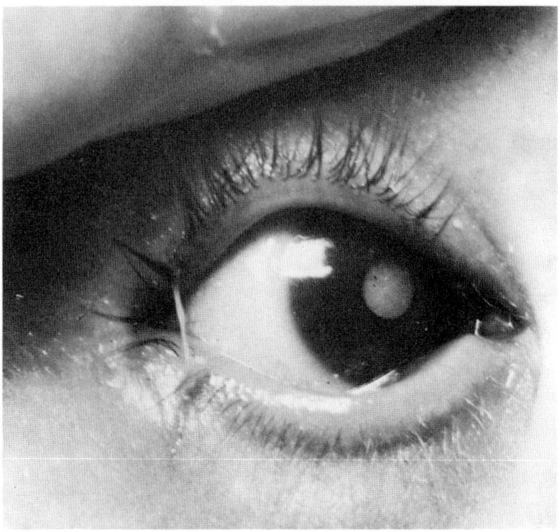

Figure 11.36 Congenital cataract.

The eyelids are occasionally partially fused at birth. In marked cases surgical separation is required (Fig. 11.37). Rarely the eyelids are everted after birth. This condition settles spontaneously. Obstruction of the nasolacrimal duct is sometimes misdiagnosed as prolonged conjunctivitis. Although there may be a slight yellow discharge there is no evidence of inflammation and tears can be seen trickling from the eye. Most ducts clear spontaneously and no treatment other than hygiene is required in the neonatal period.

Dermoid cysts are occasionally found overlying portions of both

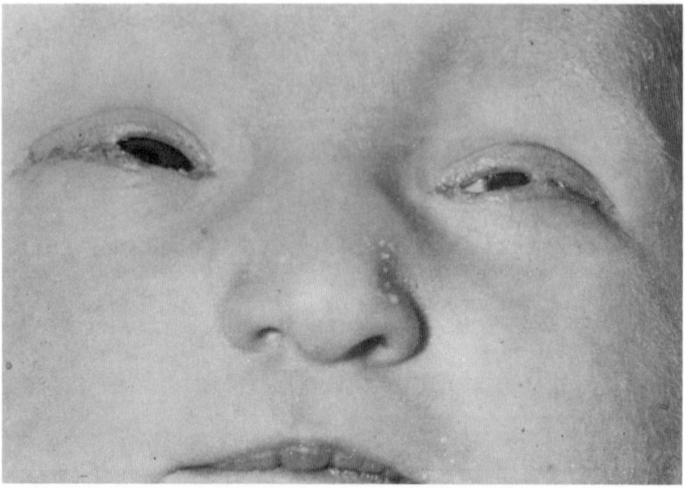

Figure 11.37 Partial fusion of eyelids.

cornea and conjunctiva. They are more commonly found at the outer end of the upper eyelid.

Retinoblastoma, which may be present at birth, is a potentially fatal tumour of the retina of the eye in which death can be prevented by early diagnosis and treatment. A greyish-yellow reflex is evident behind the pupil which may be dilated. Both eyes must be examined. In any case of doubt an ophthalmologist's opinion must be sought. Treatment is drastic by enucleation of one or both eyes. If this is not acceptable radiotherapy together with intra-arterial triethylene melamine is available as an alternative. As the condition is inherited as a dominant character genetic advice should be sought.

Central Nervous System

NEURAL TUBE DEFECTS

Neural tube defects, which include, anencephaly, myelomeningocele and hydrocephalus, constitute the largest single group of congenital abnormalities in most surveys. There is, however, a considerable geographical and seasonal variation in incidence; as mentioned earlier 'epidemics' of these defects appear to occur and it has been suggested that these may be related to environmental causes. One theory proposed is that in certain seasons potatoes and possibly other foods are more liable to blight, and it has been noted that epidemics of neural tube defects occur about two years after epidemics of blight in potatoes. The causative factor has not been positively identified but may be a chemical found in blighted potatoes. If confirmed this observation could lead to a reduction in the incidence of these serious abnormalities.

Anencephaly is the commonest of the neural tube defects. Because of the major malformation of the skull and brain affected infants are stillborn or die shortly after birth (Fig. 11.38).

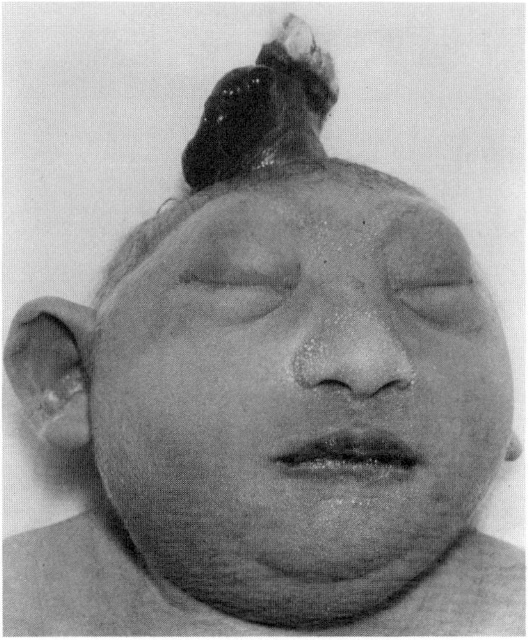

Figure 11.38 Anencephaly.

Spina bifida and myelomeningocele is less rapidly fatal and therefore constitutes the larger clinical problem. Eighty per cent of infants with myelomeningocele develop hydrocephalus.

The spinal defect most commonly occurs in the lumbar region (Fig. 11.17) but may occur elsewhere in the spinal column (Fig. 11.39). There is considerable variation in the degree of associated abnormality of the vertebral bodies. The presenting signs are generally the presence of the sac which if intact may protrude but if it has been punctured will lie flattened over the depression between the sides of the spina bifida. The sac may be a simple myelocele with no nervous tissue or a meningo-myelocele in which the spinal cord is exposed and enters the sac. Skin may cover the smaller sacs. If the sac has burst it should be covered with a non-adhesive sterile dressing.

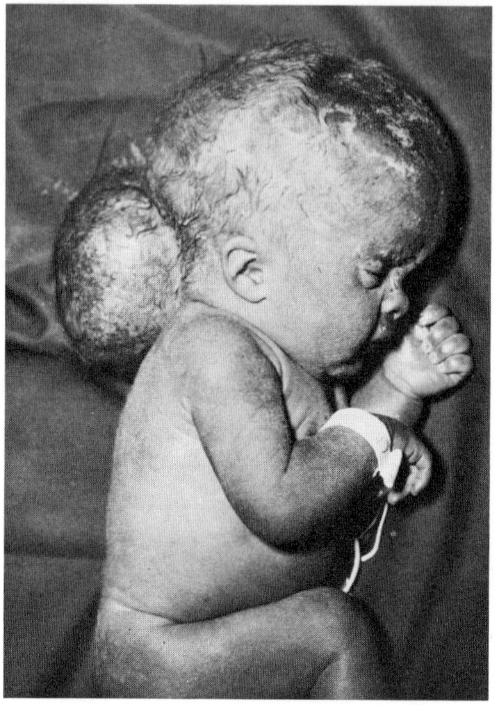

Figure 11.39 Cervical spina bifida and meningocele.

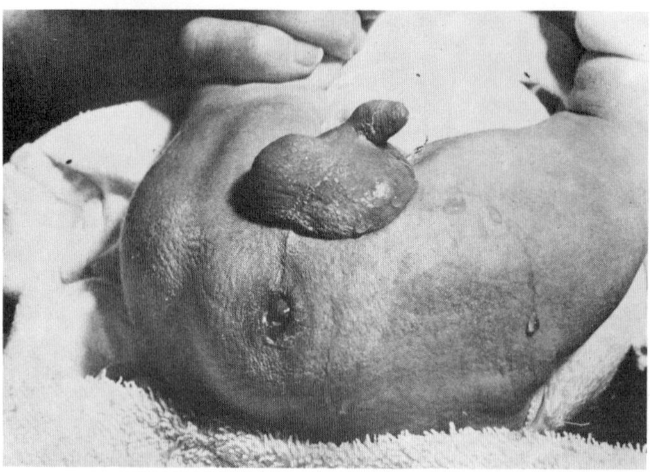

Figure 11.40 Patulous anus and dribble incontinence of urine because of lack of sphincter control in an infant with spina bifida.

The assessment of the degree of neurological involvement is not simple and examination at birth can be misleading. One or both lower limbs are commonly paralysed and there is often loss of sphincter control (Fig. 11.40).

Treatment is by the surgical introduction of a controlled drainage system to reduce the intracranial pressure. Opinions differ as to the need for immediate surgical treatment to cover an exposed sac with skin. Without this treatment even very severely affected infants may survive and subsequent management is made more difficult. Surgical treatment while limiting the risk of infection and of further deterioration in neurological function is not of course curative and may precipitate the onset of hydrocephalus and the need for further operations.

Hydrocephalus may have been recognized during delivery but more commonly is evident later as widely spread skull sutures even although the occipito-frontal circumference (o.f.c.) is normal. Repeated measurement of o.f.c. will show a rapid increase in size and the classical, clinical and radiological features of hydrocephalus will become more obvious (Fig. 11.41).

The longer term complications of spina bifida are principally renal and orthopaedic. Many question whether the quality of life achieved by the procedures required to correct these features justifies the considerable expenditure of skill and time involved, particularly when society at the same time allows large numbers of healthy fetuses to be aborted.

Policy in relation to spina bifida therefore varies from centre to centre. If all the staff concerned are not aware of or disagree with local policy parents may be given conflicting advice and it is important that this should be avoided. Referral to a regional assessment centre where available allows more detailed neurological and other assessment. Policy with regard to an individual infant can then be decided on the basis of objective findings taking into account the parents' wishes.

Microcephaly is not amenable to treatment unless the small skull size is due to premature fusion of the cranial sutures (craniosynostosis) in which case surgical treatment is possible. Other forms of central nervous system (CNS) abnormality are seldom obvious as such at birth but may present in the first month of life as abnormalities of behaviour such as convulsions.

Some CNS abnormalities may be suspect because of associated physical abnormality as in Down's syndrome (mongolism) which is considered later. A limited number of potential causes of mental abnormality can be recognized by specific testing for biochemical abnormality as in the case of phenylketonuria.

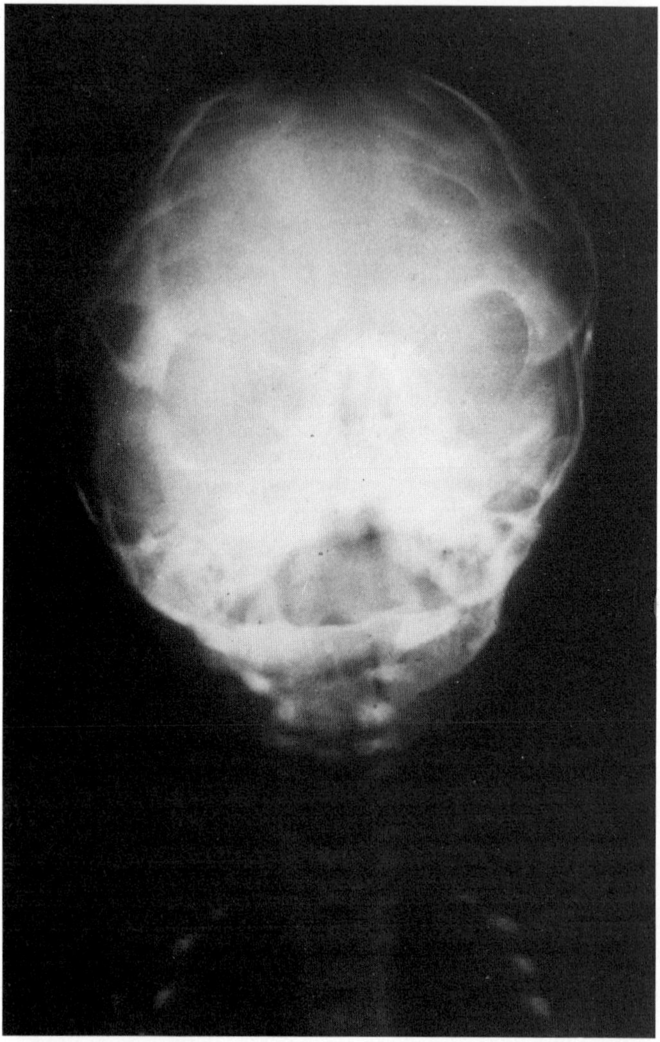

Figure 11.41 X-ray of skull in hydrocephalus. (Lacunar skull.)

Cardiovascular System

With the development of new techniques of investigation and surgical treatment it is now possible to save the lives of some infants with serious cardiac abnormalities who would otherwise have died shortly after birth. It is therefore more important now to recognize such conditions early and to have a planned policy of investigation.

Cardiac abnormalities occur in 1 to 2 per cent of liveborn infants. About half of these will die within the first weeks or months of life. This is therefore a serious and relatively common form of congenital abnormality.

Plan of management. The detailed investigation of the more serious anomalies is complicated and will not be referred to here. It is essential however that doctors and midwives dealing with the newborn should be able to recognize the earliest signs which might indicate a cardiac abnormality and arrange for further investigation and treatment without delay. How this is done will vary according to the facilities available in any particular unit. In all units an agreed plan of action is vital and this will generally involve consultation with cardiologists skilled in the management of such problems in the newborn.

COMMONER ABNORMALITIES

Although there are a large number of individual abnormalities which can occur in the cardiovascular system nine of these account for about 85 per cent of the total. These nine are shown in Table 11.2 grouped according to their principal interference with function. The remaining 15 per cent of cardiac abnormalities include a wide range of abnormalities which are individually rare and for further details about these reference should be made to textbooks of paediatric cardiology.

CYANOTIC GROUP

The abnormalities shown in Table 11.2 are compatible with varying lengths of life if not corrected by surgery. The first group are

Table 11.2 The common types of congenital cardiac abnormality

Anatomical abnormality	Functional disorder
Hypoplastic left heart syndrome Transposition of the great vessels Fallot's tetralogy	Hypoxaemia
Aortic stenosis Pulmonary stenosis Coarctation of the aorta	Obstruction and pressure overload
Ventricular septal defect Atrial septal defect Patent ductus arteriosus	Shunting and circulatory overload

characterized by early onset of cyanosis—the earlier the onset the worse the prognosis.

Hypoplastic left heart syndrome which includes hypoplasia of the left ventricle, aortic valve and aortic arch is the commonest cause of cardiac death in the neonatal period. No treatment is available.

Transposition of the great vessels is the second most common cause of death. The anatomy is very variable and complex. In the commonest form the aorta arises from the right ventricle and the pulmonary artery from the left ventricle, life being made possible by a shunt at ventricular or atrial level and by patency of the ductus arteriosus. This shunt can be increased in some cases by atrial septostomy using a balloon catheter. By this means life may be preserved until the infant is large enough for corrective surgery to be undertaken.

Fallot's tetralogy is pulmonary stenosis associated with ventricular septal defect, overriding of the right ventricle by the aortic valve and hypertrophy of the right ventricle. Although cyanosis is a common finding in older children it is less commonly found in the neonatal period unless the pulmonary stenosis is of severe degree.

OBSTRUCTIVE GROUP

Valve stenosis. Obstructive lesions as in severe stenosis of the pulmonary or aortic valves or coarctation of the aorta throws an extra burden on the associated ventricle and heart failure may follow. Cyanosis is an early feature in severe pulmonary stenosis. Diagnosis may first be suspected by the presence of a cardiac murmur on first day examination.

Coarctation. Absent or delayed femoral pulses point to the likelihood of coarctation of the aorta. Heart failure frequently develops within the first week or two.

Surgical treatment is possible for each of these conditions following medical treatment for the heart failure.

SHUNT LESIONS

Patent ductus arteriosus, ventricular septal defect and atrial septal defect are generally first discovered because of the presence of a cardiac murmur. This may not be present on the first day examination but may be detected later in the first week of life.

Reversal of the shunt from a left to right to a right to left shunt will cause cyanosis. This is most likely to occur where there is increased resistance to pulmonary blood flow and increase in pulmonary blood pressure. The shunt increases pulmonary blood flow to a varying extent according to its size and heart failure is commonest where there is the largest increase in flow.

CARDIAC FAILURE

During the first month of life cardiac failure is a common complication of congenital cardiac abnormality. The commonest of the abnormalities likely to precipitate failure are coarctation of the aorta, transposition of the great vessels, patent ductus arteriosus and aortic atresia. Other acquired abnormalities such as myocarditis, endocardial fibroelastosis or profound anaemia, as in hydrops fetalis, also cause heart failure.

Clinical manifestations. An abnormal weight gain, increase in pulse and respiratory rates and difficulty in feeding are the first clinical signs of failure likely to be noticed. Each or all may be attributed to other causes, and the presence of cardiac failure may not be recognized until signs such as dyspnoea, moderate cyanosis and hepatosplenomegaly occur. Peripheral oedema is a late sign and cardiac failure should be diagnosed and treated before it is present. Pulmonary signs are variable and not a reliable indication of the presence or absence of failure.

Medical management. The treatment of cardiac failure in infants in the first month of life differs only in detail from management at later ages. Dosages of the drugs used must be calculated carefully by the doctors concerned and the nursing staff must pay particular attention to the measurement of the doses given. This applies particularly to drugs such as digoxin.

The digitalizing dose of digoxin is of the order of 50 to 60 μg per kg of body weight and is normally given in three or four doses over a period of 12 to 24 hours according to the severity of the signs of failure and the rapidity of the infant's response. The initial doses may be given intramuscularly or intravenously. A daily maintenance dose of 20 to 25 per cent of the digitalizing dose divided into two doses can generally be given by mouth. Treatment with digoxin should be withheld if the heart rate falls below 100 per minute.

Frusemide 1.0 mg per kg per dose can be used in the early stages of treatment to promote diuresis and repeated in four to six hours if indicated. Maintenance diuretic therapy can be continued orally with bendrofluazide in a dose of 2.5 mg every day or every second day. Potassium supplements are generally required.

In addition to drug therapy the infant should be propped up and nursed in 30 per cent oxygen. Tube feeding may be required. It is not generally necessary to use a low sodium milk but suitable preparations such as Edosol are available if required.

INVESTIGATION

Of the nine abnormalities listed in Table 11.2 three are responsible for almost half of the neonatal deaths due to cardiac abnormality.

The three are hypoplastic left heart syndrome, coarctation of the aorta and transposition of the great vessels. Surgical treatment is available for the last two. It is important therefore that accurate clinical observations are made and where a potentially lethal heart abnormality is suspect investigation in a suitably equipped centre is called for. This will generally include cardiac catheterization, which should be carried out on all infants who have been in cardiac failure or who have been persistently cyanosed because of a cardiac cause. The number of infants requiring such investigation in any one maternity unit is small and it is only by the referral of infants to a regional centre that we can hope for an improvement in the present high

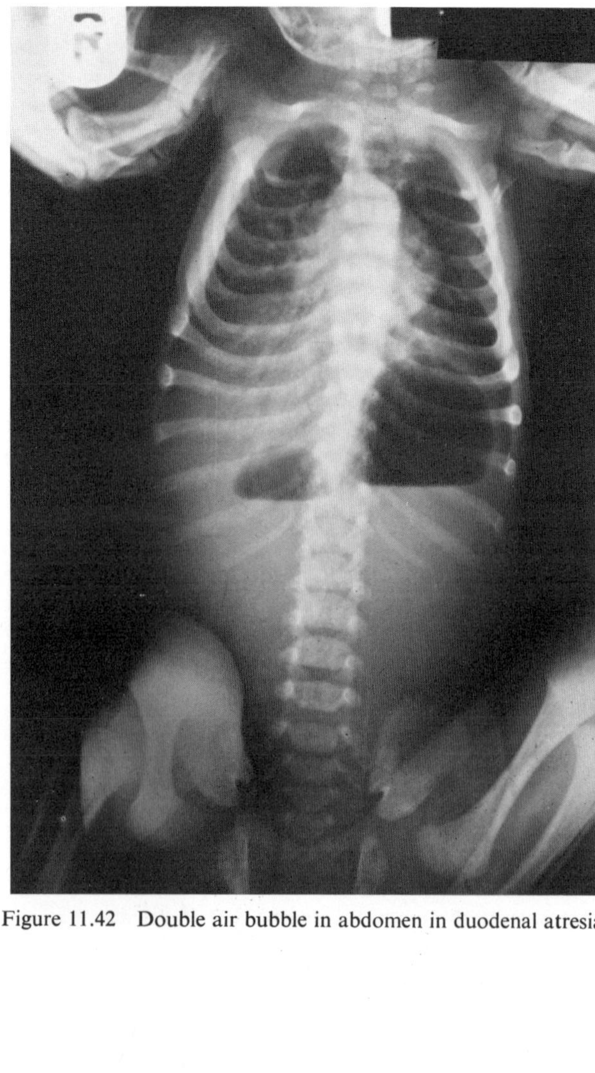

Figure 11.42 Double air bubble in abdomen in duodenal atresia.

mortality from serious cardiac abnormalities. Where this policy is in force there is already evidence of improvement in the situation.

Alimentary System

Consideration has already been given to diaphragmatic hernia and oesophageal atresia which are a threat to life because of interference with respiration.

Duodenal atresia or severe stenosis presents as vomiting occurring shortly after the first feed. Bile may or may not be present according to the site of the stricture. The lower abdomen is flat as opposed to the distended upper abdomen. X-ray of the abdomen shows the characteristic double bubble sign (Fig. 11.42). Treatment is surgical.

Intestinal atresia may occur at any level. The further down the bowel the site of the obstruction the later will be the onset of symptoms of vomiting which becomes bile-stained and then faecal in type. Obstruction of the small intestine may be due to atresia, stenosis, volvulus or meconium ileus.

Anal atresia should be recognized at the first examination (Fig. 11.43) but other abnormalities in this region are not so easily

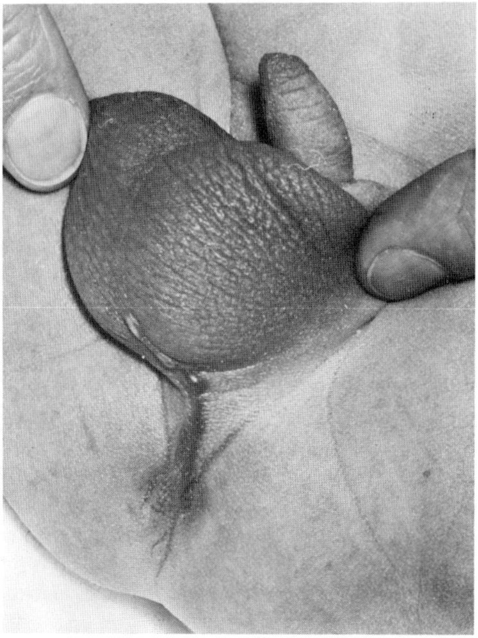

Figure 11.43 Covered anus with intradermal sinus passing along the median raphe.

diagnosed but are noted as delay in passage of meconium, passage of meconium from an abnormal site (Fig. 11.44) or difficulty in inserting a rectal thermometer. Treatment of bowel obstruction at any level in the neonate is surgical.

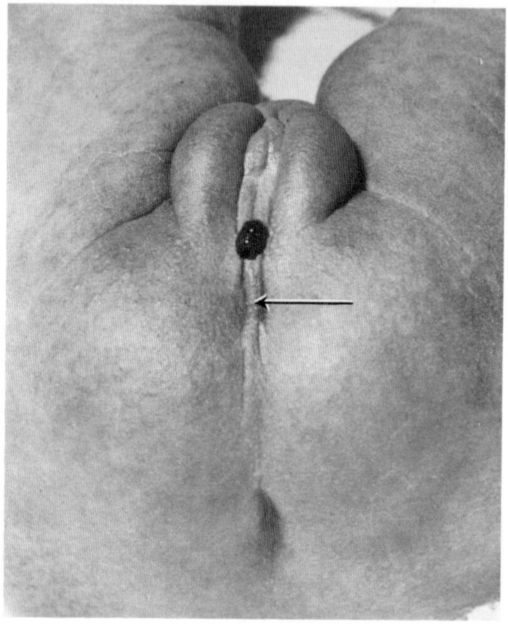

Figure 11.44 Ectopic anus. The arrow indicates the normal site of the anus. (Compare Fig. 11.10.)

Meconium ileus is obstruction of the intestine by thick viscid meconium and is the earliest manifestation of cystic fibrosis with absence of pancreatic trypsin. The meconium contains unaltered albumin which can be recognized in a suspension of meconium by its positive reaction with Albustix. Rupture of the bowel may have occurred *in utero* resulting in meconium peritonitis. Areas of calcification may be seen on abdominal X-ray.

Hirschsprung's disease is due to absence of ganglion cells of Auerbach's plexus in a segment of bowel in which peristalsis ceases, causing obstruction. There is delay in the passage of meconium but after the passage of a 'meconium plug' normal bowel movements may be present for a period of days, weeks or months before obstruction recurs. Diagnosis is by demonstration of the aganglionic area on biopsy and treatment is surgical. A similar situation may be caused by a meconium plug which is not associated with Hirschspung's disease. After a finger has been inserted into the rectum the plug is often passed and the obstruction relieved.

For more detailed discussion of the rarer causes of intestinal obstruction in the newborn reference should be made to a textbook of neonatal surgery.

Vomiting later in the neonatal period may be due to hiatus hernia or pyloric stenosis.

The Umbilicus

The umbilical cord normally contains two arteries and one vein.

A single umbilical artery is associated with an increased incidence of other congenital abnormalities.

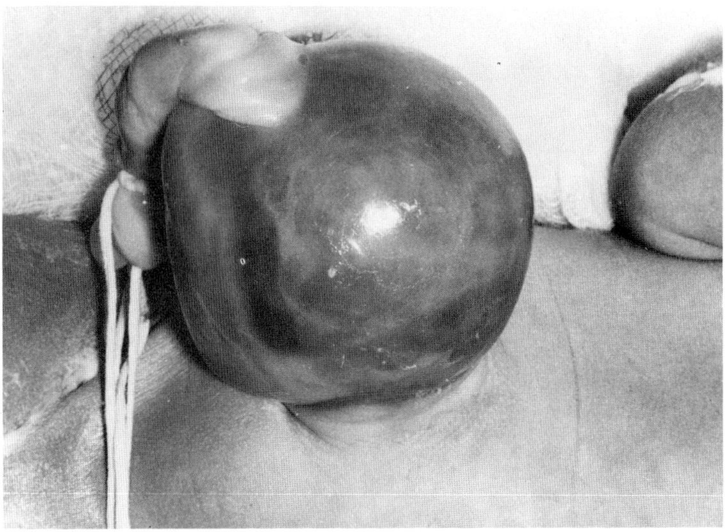

Figure 11.45 Exomphalos.

Persistence of the allantois results in the discharge of urine from a patent urachus opening at the umbilical stump or the formation of a urachal cyst or sinus. These have to be distinguished from similar persistence of the omphalomesenteric duct from which faecal matter may be discharged at the umbilicus.

Exomphalos (Fig. 11.45) with protrusion of the bowel into a sac of peritoneum and amnion follows failure of closure of the anterior abdominal wall. The covering of the sac may rupture during labour exposing the bowel (Fig. 11.46) and early surgery is required. Meanwhile the bowel should be covered with sterile moistened swabs.

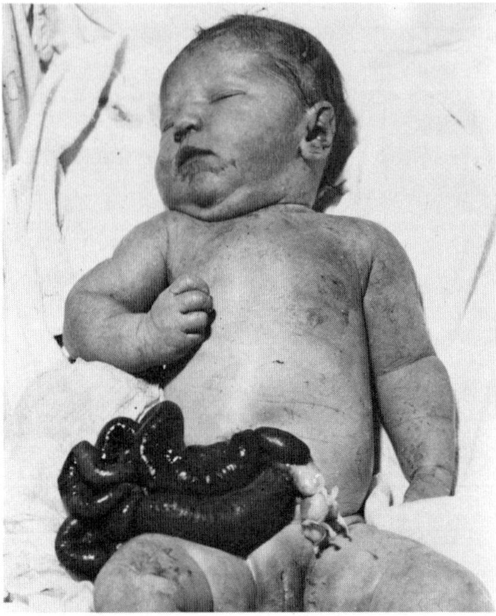

Figure 11.46 Exomphalos after rupture of the covering sac.

Conservative treatment of the intact sac (with local application of one per cent mercurochrome) is now recommended when there is no evidence of other abnormality in the bowel. Hernia into the cord is a minor degree of exomphalos. The cord must be clamped distal to any bowel present to avoid intestinal obstruction.

Urogenital System

RENAL AGENESIS

Failure of the fetus *in utero* to pass urine results in oligohydramnios and a 'squashed baby' with large floppy ears and hands, deformities of the feet and characteristic facies. The membranes of the placenta show fine nodules, amnion nodosum (Fig. 11.47). The commonest cause is failure of development of both kidneys—renal agenesis, but a similar picture follows complete obstruction to the flow of urine from, for example, urethral stricture (Fig. 11.48).

Obstructive uropathy. Infants with obstructive uropathy will have an enlarged bladder and kidneys. In either case there is insufficient functioning renal tissue to support life, no urine is passed and death occurs at or shortly after birth.

Cystic kidneys. Large renal masses at birth may also be due to multicystic disease which is generally unilateral and polycystic

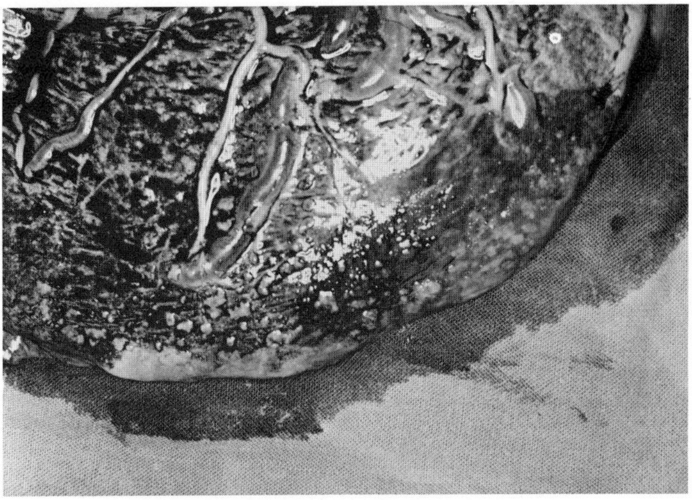

Figure 11.47 Amnion nodosum.

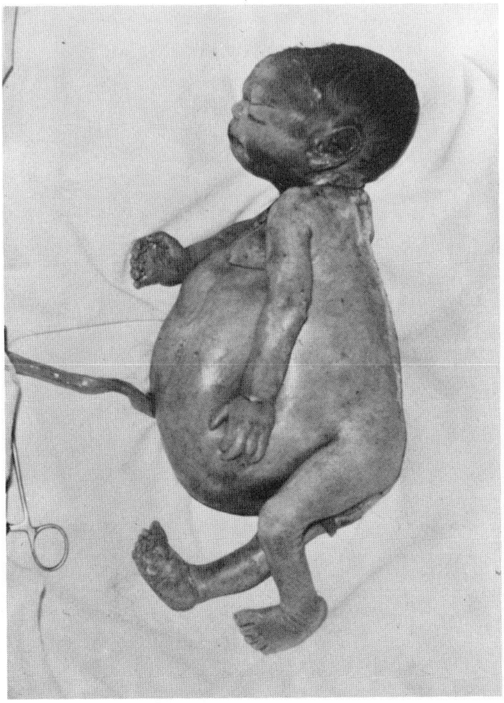

Figure 11.48 Gross enlargement of kidneys, ureters and bladder secondary to complete obstruction of the urethra.

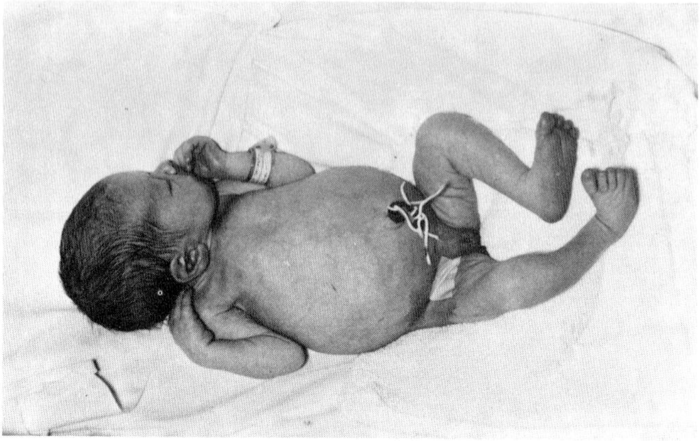

Figure 11.49 Abdominal distension due to polycystic disease of the kidneys.

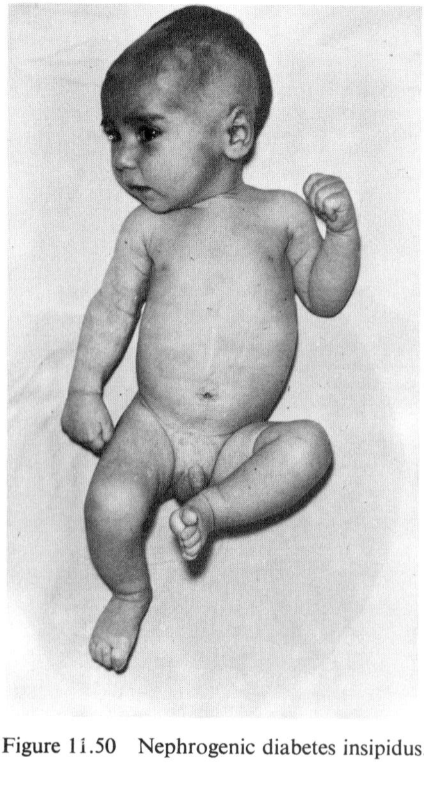

Figure 11.50 Nephrogenic diabetes insipidus.

disease which is bilateral (Fig. 11.49). Survival is possible only if there is sufficient functioning renal tissue.

Exstrophy of the bladder is commoner in boys and is associated with epispadias, wide divarication of the recti abdominis muscles and the symphysis pubis (Fig. 11.11). Although unsightly it is not an immediate threat to life and surgical closure may be possible after a few years. Other abnormalities of the renal system may present at any age of infancy or childhood because they have predisposed to urinary tract infection.

Polyuria may be due to diabetes mellitus or to nephrogenic diabetes insipidus (Fig. 11.50).

DOUBTFUL SEX

The most urgent problems likely to arise in the genital system at birth are connected with the diagnosis of sex. In any infant where there is doubt about the external genitalia expert advice should be sought immediately so that a decision can be made as to which sex to announce to the parents.

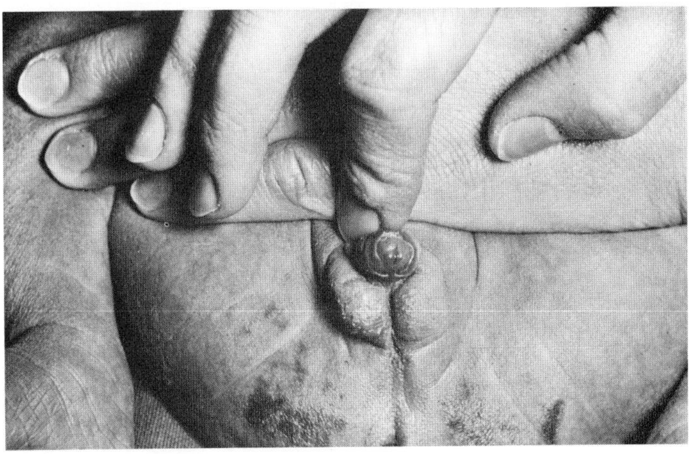

Figure 11.51 Virilization of female infant in adrenogenital syndrome.

Adrenogenital syndrome. Female infants suffering from the adrenogenital syndrome may have undergone virilization *in utero* and, as in the case of the girl shown in Figure 11.51, the urethra may pass through the clitoris and resemble a penis. Although the labia majora are fused and resemble a scrotum no gonads are palpable. Rapid help can be obtained from suitable staining of cells from the buccal mucosa. The presence of a chromatin body in the nucleus

(Fig. 11.52) indicates that the infant has two X chromosomes and is probably female. Fluorescent staining can indicate the presence or absence of a Y chromosome, but chromosome karyotype analysis, which takes two to three days, is essential for a firm sex chromosome diagnosis. As some infants with adrenogenital syndrome also have adrenal failure examination of serum electrolytes is an essential early

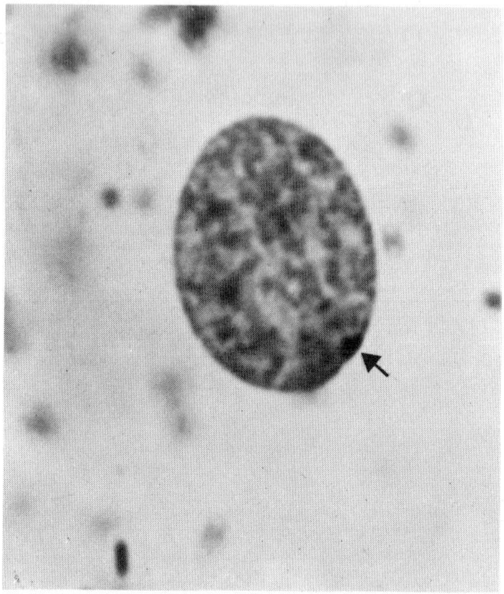

Figure 11.52 Single chromatin (Barr) body in nucleus of buccal cell of a female infant. (Photograph by courtesy of the MRC Clinical and Population Cytogenetics Unit.)

investigation. If there is a raised potassium and lowered sodium and chloride the infant is at serious risk of early death unless given corticosteroids.

Intersex. Other forms of intersex (Fig. 11.53) will require detailed investigation, which often includes laparotomy, to examine the gonads. As such infants can often not function as either males or females and as the fetus is fundamentally female until acted upon by male hormones it is sensible when in doubt about the sex of a newborn infant to announce that it is female. Where no sexual function exists it is easier for the patient and parents if the infant is brought up as a female. The asexual individual is more 'feminine' in character and is generally happier as a female.

Less serious minor abnormalities of the external genitalia are more common and occur mainly in male infants.

Hypospadias results from failure of closure of the urogenital

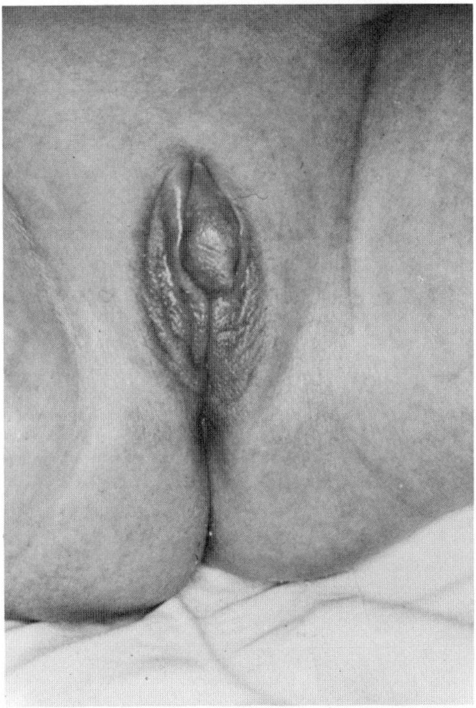

Figure 11.53 External genitalia of an infant with a vestigial testis on one side and a vestigial ovum on the other side.

groove leaving the meatal opening at the base of the glans penis or more proximally on the penis or scrotum (Fig. 11.54). No treatment is required in the neonatal period unless stricture of the meatus prevents the normal passage of urine.

Epispadias. Less commonly the urethra may open on the dorsal surface of the penis (epispadias). Treatment is surgical at a later stage of infancy.

Absence of testes. Failure of descent of one or both testes into the scrotum does not require treatment in the first month of life but is an indication for arranging regular follow-up examination. If neither testis is palpable buccal smear examination for sex chromatin should be undertaken.

Torsion of the testis. The presence of a hard reddish blue mass in the scrotum is suggestive of torsion of the testis and is an indication for immediate operation.

Hydrocele. A translucent swelling in the scrotum around the testis is indicative of a non-communicating hydrocele which will clear

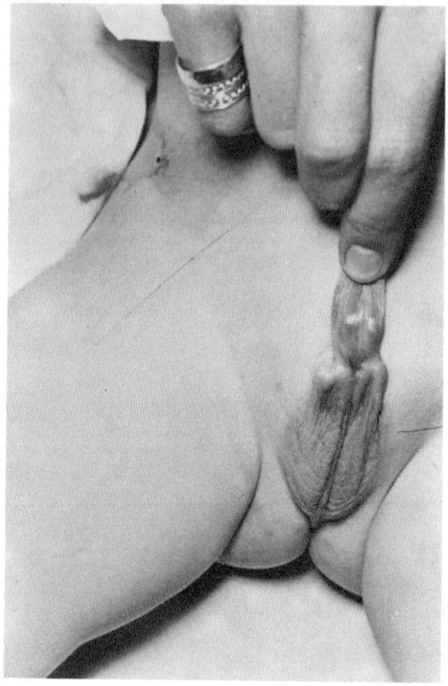

Figure 11.54 Hypospadias.

spontaneously (Fig. 11.55). A similar scrotal swelling extending upwards towards the inguinal ring and which alters in size is suggestive of a communicating hydrocele which is often associated with an inguinal hernia. Surgical treatment is required.

Foreskin. The foreskin in the newborn is not fully retractable and attempts at retracting it may cause adhesion and the development of phimosis. Circumcision is only indicated medically if there is obstruction to urine flow by a narrow meatus, a rare occurrence.

Labial adhesions in the female can often be separated by simple traction.

Imperforate hymen. Bulging of the perineum in female infants occurs where there is obstruction by an imperforate hymen and an abnormal collection of vaginal fluid. Incision of the hymen relieves the situation.

Abnormalities of the sex chromosomes are considered later in this chapter.

Endocrine Disorders

Hypothyroidism. The physical signs of athyrotic cretinism (hypothyroidism) are rarely evident at birth but may be suspected later in

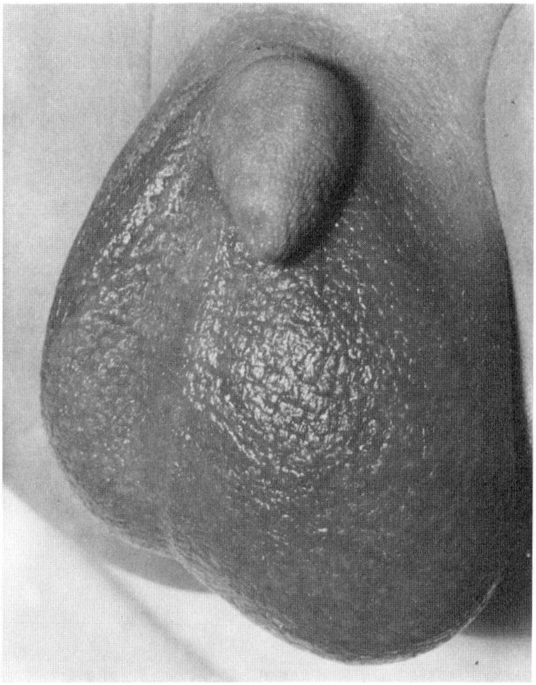

Figure 11.55 Hydrocele.

the first month of life because of sluggish movements and feeding difficulties including choking episodes. Prolongation of 'physiological' jaundice beyond the 10th to 14th day may be due to hypothyroidism and is often the first sign to suggest this possibility. The characteristic picture of the cretin is seldom evident until after one month of age. Diagnosis can be confirmed by the demonstration of a low and falling level of protein-bound iodine, a level below 2 μg per 100 ml being diagnostic. X-ray shows delayed epiphyseal development, and epiphyses present show stippling due to multiple centres of ossification. The ECG shows low voltage waves. Treatment is by a thyroid preparation such as sodium L-thyroxine beginning with 0.02 mg daily. In some families with an inherited disorder of thyroid metabolism a goitre may be present at birth with evidence of hypothyroidism. Goitre may also appear in the infants of mothers treated with thiouracil during pregnancy.

Hyperthyroidism. Some mothers with present or past thyrotoxicosis have infants with transient hyperthyroidism who are flushed and over-active and who may develop heart failure. Such infants should be treated temporarily with Lugol's iodine solution 0.1 ml three times daily. Sedation and digoxin may be necessary.

Adrenal failure. The frequency of haemorrhage into the adrenal glands is difficult to assess but it is seen at postmortem examination on infants who have collapsed suddenly. Occasionally a mass may be palpable in the flank. The differentiation from haemorrhage into the brain or lungs is difficult and all are liable to occur in infants with birth injury or a bleeding disorder (Chap. 17).

Congenital adrenal hyperplasia is most evident in female infants who have evidence of a virilizing effect *in utero*. Both male and female infants may present as vomiting with biochemical evidence of adrenocortical failure in that the serum potassium is high and the sodium and chloride low. Treatment with sodium chloride by mouth or intravenously and fludrocortisone is life-saving. Urine collection for 17 ketosteroid, 17 OH steroid and pregnanetriol output should be started. Raised levels confirm the diagnosis and treatment with cortisone or prednisolone will be required. Such treatment is best controlled in a regional centre but the control of the electrolyte disorder is an urgent matter and should not be delayed.

Cushing's syndrome is rarely seen in the newborn period.

True diabetes mellitus is uncommon in the first month of life but must be remembered in an infant with polyuria and weight loss.

A transient form of diabetes mellitus with glycosuria and hyperglycaemia occurs in the newborn period. After a period when treatment with insulin may be required the infant appears to make a spontaneous recovery.

Skeletal System

ACHONDROPLASIA

The infant with classical achondroplasia (Fig. 11.56) presents little diagnostic problem at birth and can be recognized by X-ray examination *in utero*. The limbs are relatively short particularly in their proximal segments. Head size is a little larger than normal and although hydrocephalus is self-arresting in most infants with achondroplasia in others it is progressive and requires treatment. The bridge of the nose is flattened, the forehead prominent and the mandible may protrude. Lumbar lordosis makes the buttocks and abdomen prominent. Mentality is unaffected and parents often require firm reassurance on this point. Many cases arise from sporadic mutation but a dominant form of inheritance also occurs. No treatment is available for the skeletal abnormality in infancy.

Dyschondroplasias. There are several forms of abnormal growth of cartilage resulting in other forms of dyschondroplasia some of which,

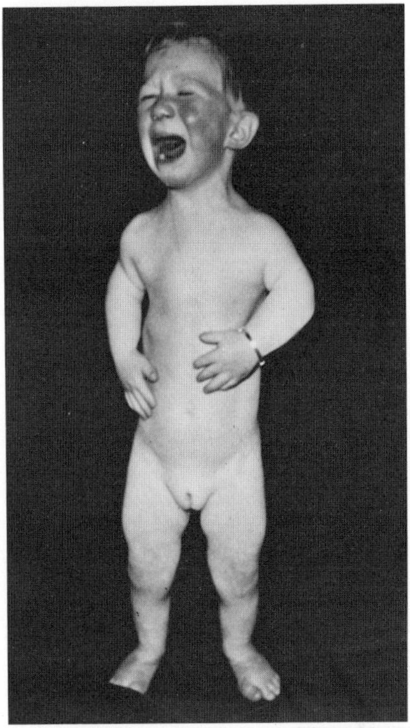

Figure 11.56 Achondroplasia showing short proximal segments of the limbs.

such as Conradi's disease (Fig. 11.57), are recognizable at birth. Others such as Morquio's disease and the various forms of gargoylism do not become evident until later infancy or early childhood. Others may present at birth with respiratory difficulty because of the small chest syndrome.

Osteogenesis imperfecta results in extremely fragile bones. In its severe form it affects the fetus *in utero* where fractures occur and the infant is born with shortened deformed limbs and X-ray shows multiple fractures. Many are stillborn. In those less severely affected survival may be possible but frequent fractures occur (Fig. 11.58). No treatment other than protection and gentle handling is possible.

Cleidocranial dysostosis is inherited as a dominant character and causes abnormalities in the clavicles and skull. The cranial sutures are widely open and parts of the clavicles are missing. Treatment is not available and is not required as the condition causes no disability. The importance of this condition lies in the differential diagnosis from other conditions. This is generally clear when the family history is known.

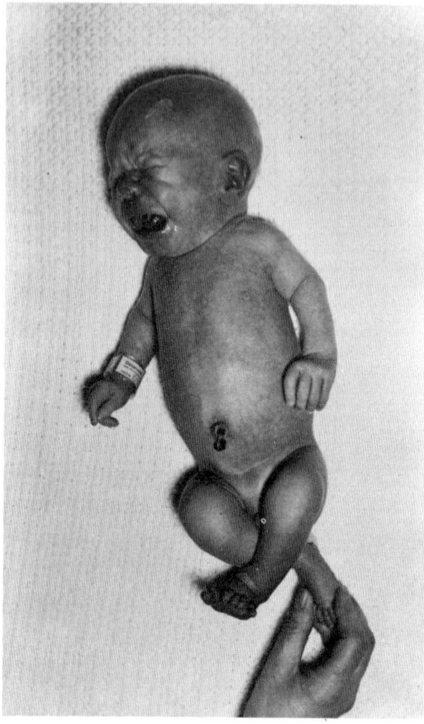

Figure 11.57 Conradi's disease.

THE LAX HIP

Laxity of the hip joint with partial or complete subluxation on suitable testing (Chap. 7) can be detected at birth relatively frequently. Subluxation or dislocatability is more common in females and in breech deliveries. A few infants whose hips later dislocate when weight-bearing is started may not show evidence of subluxation at birth, and in these the abnormality is in the structure of the acetabulum rather than in laxity of the joint. Lax hips can recover if diagnosed early and treated by being kept in a position of abduction. In the first few days of life this can most easily be done by nursing the infant prone with a roll of napkin holding the legs widely apart and held in place by another napkin pinned tightly. This is of no use after the first four or five days when a more rigid splint of the type shown in Figure 11.59 is indicated. Regular follow-up of infants with lax hips is essential and in most centres this is arranged by the orthopaedic service. As there is an increased risk in the siblings of affected infants particular care must be taken in the initial examination and

(a)

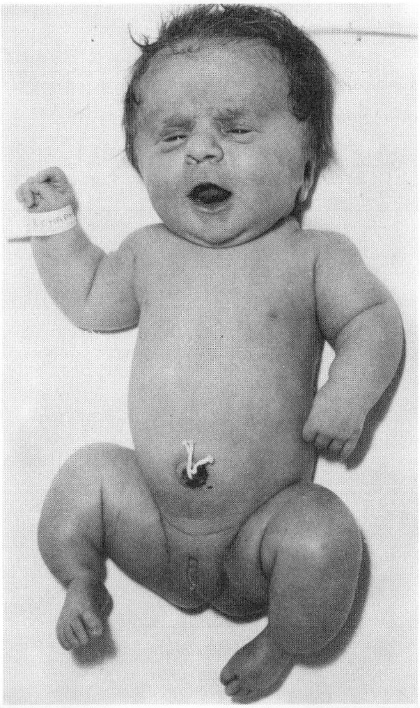

(b)

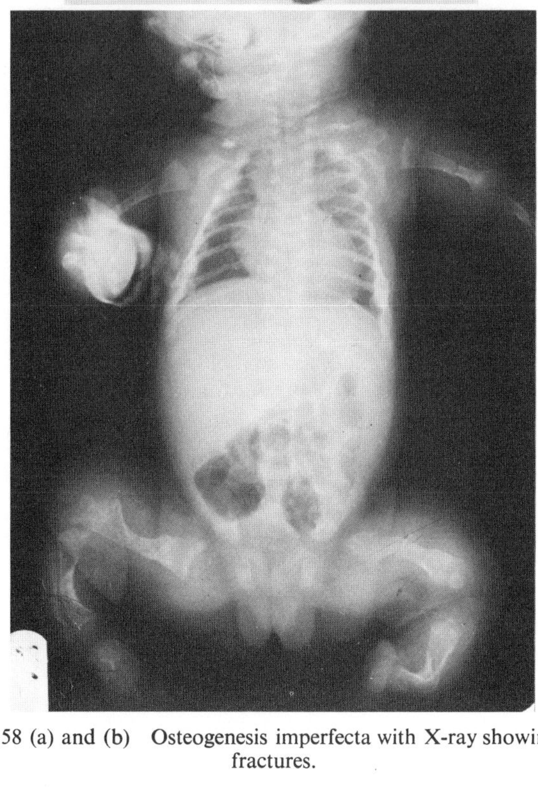

Figure 11.58 (a) and (b) Osteogenesis imperfecta with X-ray showing multiple fractures.

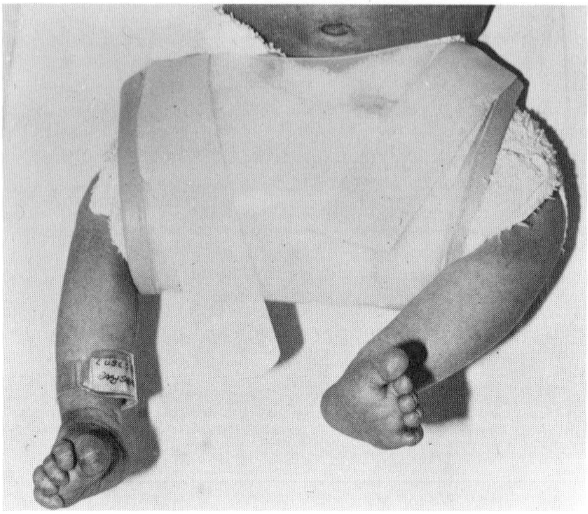

Figure 11.59 Light plastic splint over napkin to hold hips in abduction.

follow-up of infants in whose family there is a history of dislocation of the hip.

Dislocation of the hip at birth, which may be unilateral or bilateral, is uncommon in the absence of other major abnormalities such as spina bifida. Careful splinting and long-term follow-up are essential.

TALIPES

The pressure of the uterine wall frequently produces positional abnormality of the feet at birth which can be corrected by passive movements. As with the true club foot which cannot be corrected by passive movement the abnormality may be in equinovarus with the foot pointing downward and inward, calcaneus with the foot pointing upward and outward, or metatarsus varus in which the forefoot only is angulated inwards. One or both feet may be affected.

Positional talipes is treated by frequent manipulation and stimulation of active movement of the stretched muscles.

Fixed club foot requires orthopaedic management with progressive splinting.

Scoliosis. Abnormalities of the vertebral bodies such as hemivertebrae produce scoliosis.

The Skin

Abnormalities of the skin are readily discernible by parents and are frequently the cause of concern.

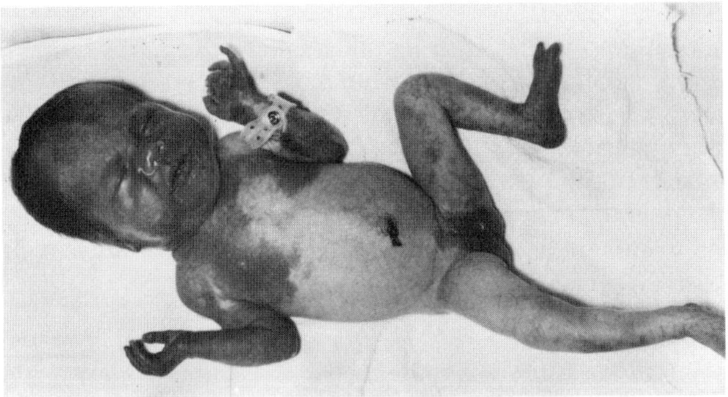

Figure 11.60 Extensive port wine naevi.

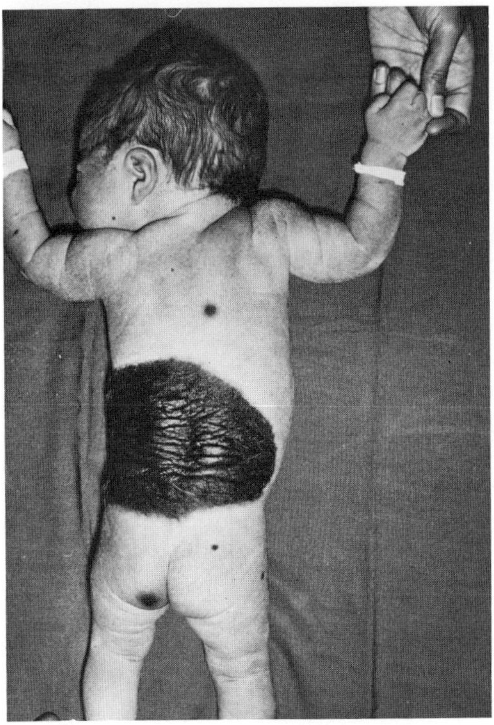

Figure 11.61 Pigmented naevi.

BIRTHMARKS

Minor abnormalities such as the smaller birthmarks (mongolian) blue spots and urticaria neonatorum have been considered in Chapter 6. Larger naevi are most commonly of the port wine type (Fig. 11.60) or are pigmented (Fig. 11.61). Treatment is not required in the neonatal period.

Epidermolysis bullosa (Fig. 11.62) is a rare inherited condition in which pressure on the skin produces bullae which rupture leaving raw

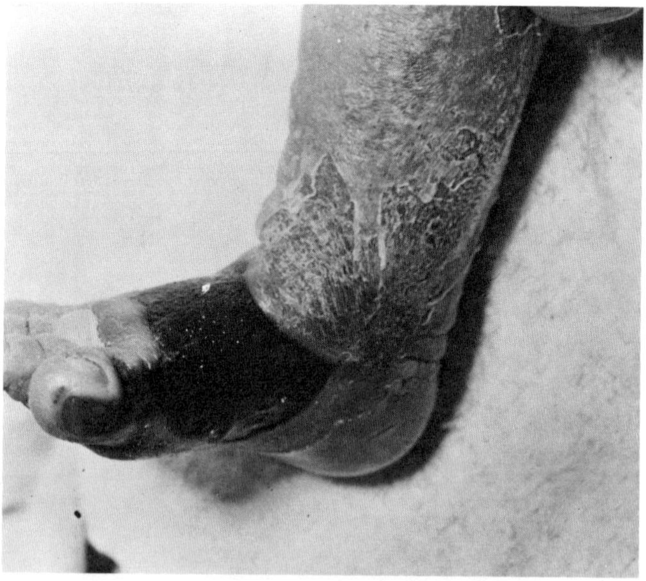

Figure 11.62 Raw area over dorsum of foot following rupture of bulla in epidermolysis bullosa.

red areas which are readily infected. The mucous membranes are similarly affected in some infants making feeding very difficult. Treatment is palliative by gentle handling and prevention of infection. The prognosis is poor in severe cases.

Collodion skin is evident at birth. The skin has a varnished appearance and cracks readily. As the abnormal skin is desquamated it is replaced either by normal skin or by skin showing signs of ichthyosis.

Ichthyosis, in which the skin is papery, dry and scaly, may also occur independently (Fig. 11.63).

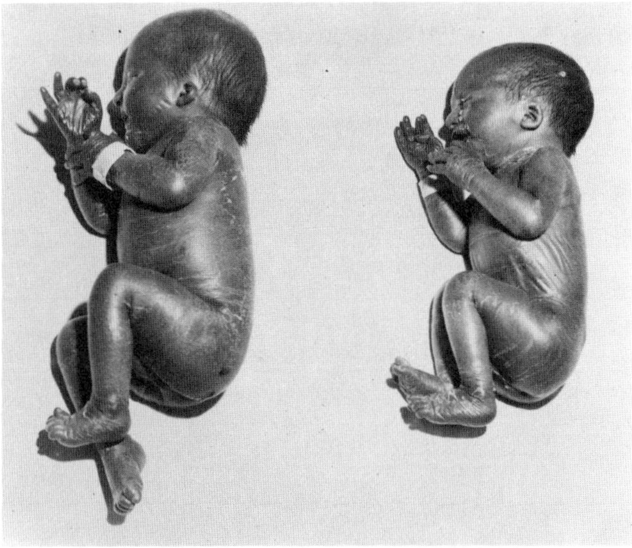

Figure 11.63 Severe congenital ichthyosis in twins.

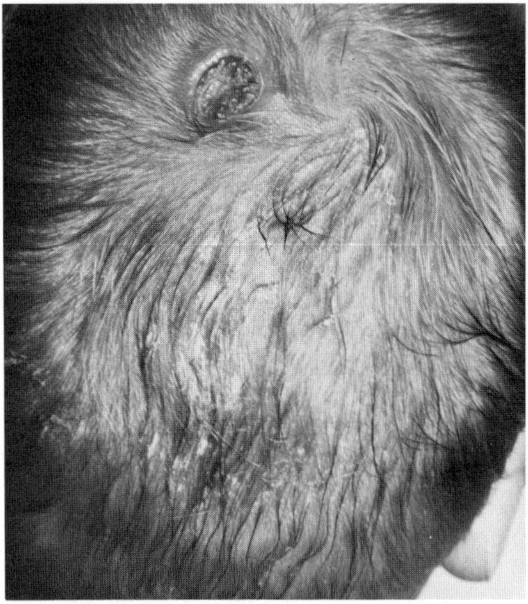

Figure 11.64 Cutaneous defect of the scalp.

Scalp defects. Defects of the skin, particularly over the scalp (Fig. 11.64), may be found at birth. These heal in a few weeks leaving a fibrous scar (Fig. 11.65).

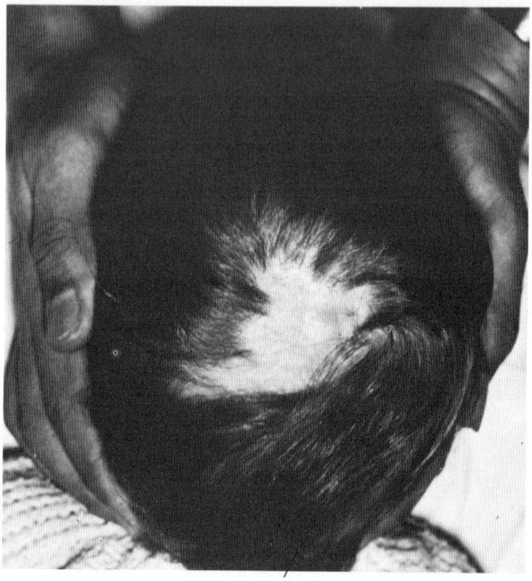

Figure 11.65 Bald area following healing of cutaneous defect of the scalp.

Chromosome Abnormalities

BUCCAL SMEARS

Since 1959 it has been possible to examine cells for their sex chromatin content. The presence of a chromatin particle, made visible in the nucleus by suitable staining, indicates a 'resting' X chromosome. The number of X chromosomes present in a cell is one greater than the number of chromatin bodies. Normal females have one chromatin body and males have none. A female is said to be chromatin-positive and a male chromatin-negative. The relative simplicity and cheapness of the buccal cell examination for sex chromatin has allowed large-scale surveys of newborn populations to be carried out and the frequency of abnormalities of the X chromosome has been well established.

The Y chromosome. In 1971 it also became possible to recognize the Y chromosome in buccal smears using a fluorescing stain (Fig. 11.66). The incidence of abnormalities of the Y chromosome had by then been established by chromosome karyotype surveys of newborn male populations.

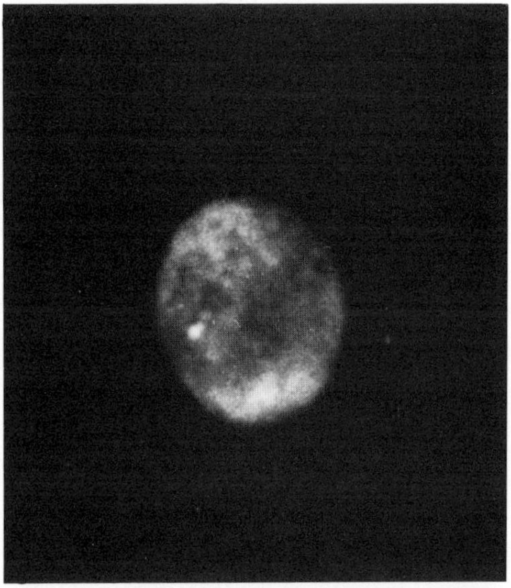

Figure 11.66 Y chromosome demonstrated in buccal cell by fluorescent staining. (Photographs of Figures 11.66, 11.67 and 11.68 by courtesy of MRC Clinical and Population Cytogenetics Unit.)

CHROMOSOME KARYOTYPE ANALYSIS

Chromosome karyotype analysis is now carried out on capillary blood specimens (Fig. 11.67). Improvements in staining technique now allow the 'banding' of individual chromosomes (Fig. 11.68). This increases the ease with which individual chromosomes can be recognized. Surveys of newborn populations using this technique are costly and at present routine chromosome karyotype analysis of all newborn infants cannot be justified other than for research purposes. Initially such surveys were limited to infants with a congenital abnormality and it soon became evident that the great majority of abnormal infants had no recognizable chromosomal abnormality.

Most of the infants with a sex chromosome abnormality are apparently normal at birth but infants with the X0 constitution can be diagnosed clinically. The presence of an additional autosome or deletion of part of an autosome results in physical abnormality. Screening of infant populations also reveals apparently normal infants in whom the chromosome pattern is rearranged without gain or loss of chromosome material (balanced translocations). Some infants show a mosaicism with a mixture of cells, some normal some abnormal. The incidence of the commoner chromosome

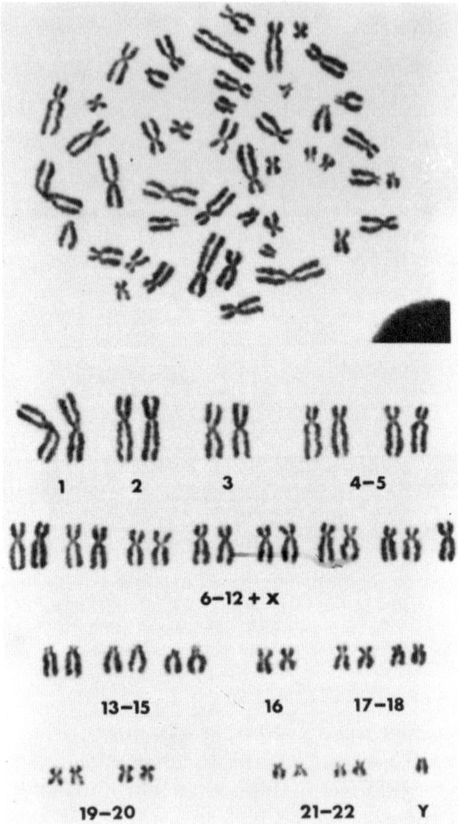

Figure 11.67 Chromosome karyotype 46 XY of normal male infant.

abnormalities in infants in an Edinburgh hospital is shown in Table 11.3.

SEX CHROMOSOME ABNORMALITIES

Infant Turner's syndrome. Infants with a single X chromosome and no Y chromosome have 45 chromosomes, have female external genitalia but, because of gonadal dysgenesis, do not develop sexually. At birth there is oedema of the extremities, abnormal nails, loose folds of skin in the neck and widely spaced nipples. Buccal cell testing shows them to be chromatin-negative. Associated abnormalities include coarctation of the aorta. The incidence of 45 X fetuses who are aborted is very much higher than the incidence of 45 X females at

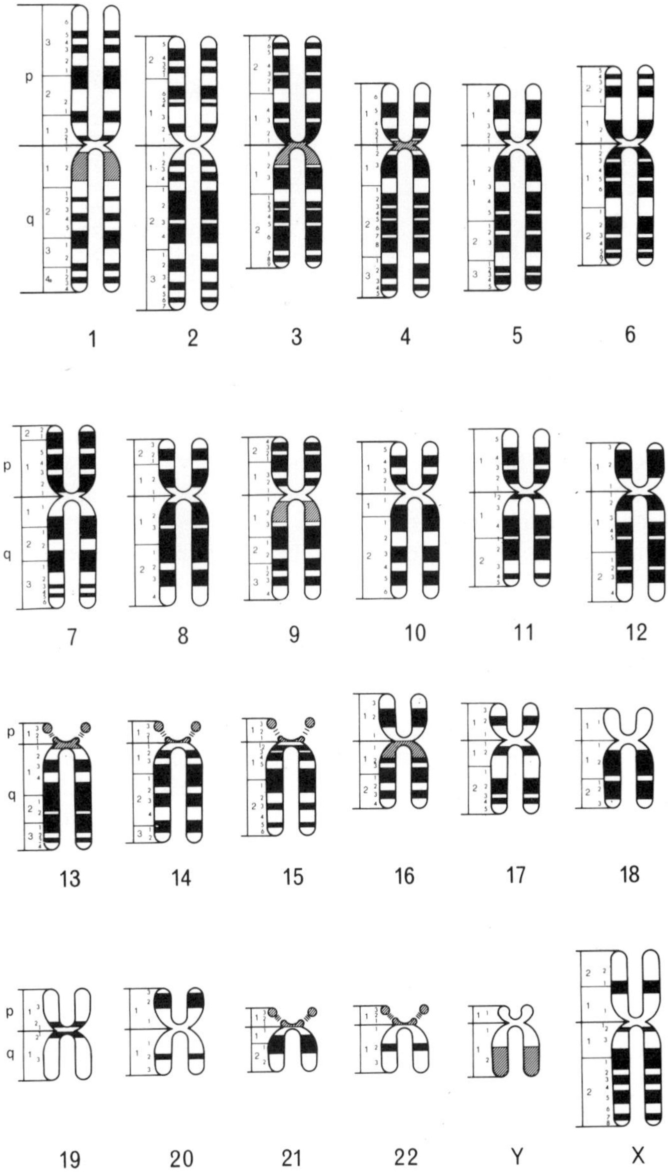

Figure 11.68 Diagrammatic representation of band patterns of individual chromosomes.

Table 11.3 Incidence of abnormalities of chromosome karyotype occurring more frequently than 1 per 1000 live births in a survey of 11 129 infants in Edinburgh

Karotype	Incidence (per 1000 live births)	
Sex chromosome abnormality		
47, XYY (extra Y)	1.58	1 in 664 males
47, XXY (Klinefelter's syndrome)	1.45	1 in 689 males
47, XXX (triple X)	1.41	1 in 709 females
Autosome abnormality		
47, 21+ (Down's syndrome)	1.53	1 in 654 both sexes

birth and this condition therefore occurs much more frequently than appears from the number diagnosed at birth.

Klinefelter's syndrome. Other sex chromosome abnormalities such as XXY males (Klinefelter's syndrome) and XXX females can only be recognized at birth by routine buccal cell examination or by chromosome karyotype testing.

Although the XYY male can now be recognized by modifications of the buccal cell technique he has until recently only been recognized by routine chromosome karyotype screening. No physical abnormality is evident at birth.

Down's Syndrome

Mongolism (Down's syndrome) had been diagnosed by the physical characteristics present for nearly 100 years before it was known to be associated with an extra chromosome number 21. At meiosis when the gamete is formed the 21 chromosome pair fails to separate and two instead of one go to one gamete.

Non-disjunction. This separation is termed non-disjunction and results after fertilization in a trisomy, the presence of three chromosomes instead of the usual pair. Non-disjunction occurs more frequently the older the mother and Down's syndrome is more commonly found in older mothers.

Translocation. Rarely the extra chromosome results from the translocation of a 21 chromosome to another chromosome, e.g. number 15 of the parent who therefore has the genetic material from two 21 chromosomes but only 45 chromosomes in all. If the infant inherits a 15/21 translocation and a normal 21 chromosome from one parent and a normal 21 chromosome from the other parent he will have 46 chromosomes but the genetic material from three 21 chromosomes and thus will have Down's syndrome. This type of inheritance is irrespective of parent's age. It accounts for less than 5 per cent of cases of Down's syndrome.

CLINICAL FEATURES

The clinical features of Down's syndrome are recognizable at birth.

Birth weight is low for gestational age.

The head is round with a short antero-posterior diameter and the face is flat. The nose is small with forward-facing nostrils and a poorly formed bridge.

Epicanthic folds may be present bilaterally and the palpebral fissures are slanting with the inner end below the outer.

The tongue tends to protrude and there may be a double alveolar margin resulting in a narrow palatal arch. Ear folds are poorly developed (Fig. 11.69).

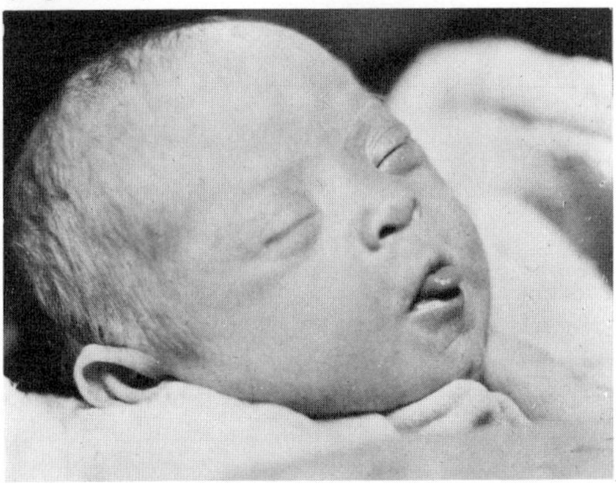

Figure 11.69 Down's syndrome showing protruding tongue.

The hands may show a single transverse palmar crease (simian line) and the little finger is often short and incurved (Fig. 11.70).

Feet. A gap may be evident between the big and second toes.

Muscular hypotonicity is a very characteristic finding.

It must be emphasized that each of the features mentioned may be present in a normal infant and not all the features are present in every infant with Down's syndrome. It is the number of these features present in one infant which arouses suspicion. In cases of doubt chromosome karyotype analysis should be carried out.

Mental retardation. The significance of the diagnosis is in the associated abnormalities likely to be present, principally mental retardation. This cannot be diagnosed at birth but it can be inferred from the physical features present. There is considerable variation in

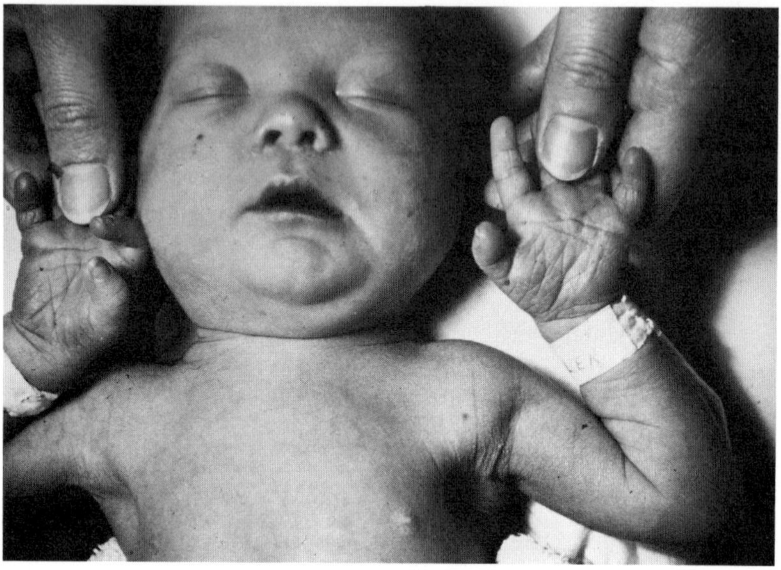

Figure 11.70 Down's syndrome showing epicanthic folds and incurved fifth finger.

the ultimate level of intelligence and this is not related to the number of physical stigmata present at birth.

Other complications include congenital heart disease, particularly ventricular septal defect, duodenal atresia and leukaemia. Infants with Down's syndrome are particularly susceptible to upper respiratory infections.

THE PARENTS

As Down's syndrome is one of the few conditions in which mental deficiency can be forecast from birth it is most important that great care is taken in informing the parents of the diagnosis and explaining its significance. This subject is discussed later in this chapter in more detail but it is appropriate to mention it in this section as many mothers, particularly if elderly, are well aware of the increased risk of having a 'mongol'. They are eager to have their own suspicions allayed if the infant is normal. If the infant has Down's syndrome, and mother suspects this, she may be afraid of voicing her suspicion. She may decide that she was wrong because she is certain that she would have been told but no one has said anything to her. Most mothers of affected children who have not been told feel let down by the staff whom they had previously trusted.

RISK OF RECURRENCE

The risk of recurrence after the birth of an infant with Down's syndrome to a mother with normal chromosomes is no greater than the risk to other women of the same age bearing in mind that the risk rises rapidly after 40 years of age. If mother has a balanced translocation involving a 21 chromosome the risk of further infants being affected is very high. Expert genetic advice is advisable to define the precise degree of risk which varies with the type of translocation. As translocations are not age-dependent it is important that the chromosomes of both infant and parents are examined when a young mother has an infant with Down's syndrome.

Other Trisomies

TRISOMY 18

Trisomy 18 may be suspect in infants with low-set abnormal ears, flexed and overlapping fingers, small jaw and mouth, rocker bottom

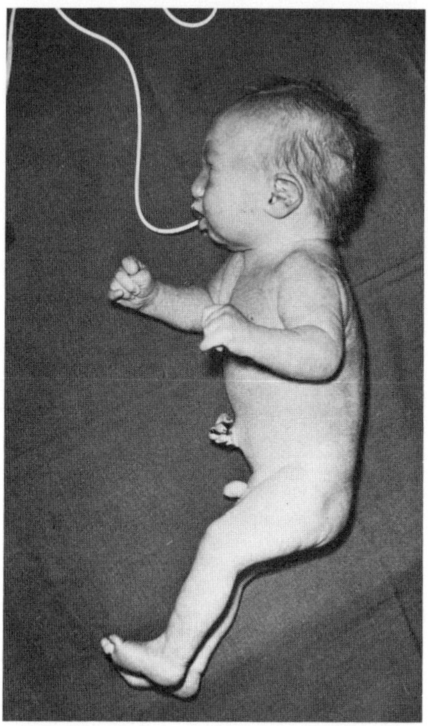

Figure 11.71 Trisomy 18 showing low-set ears, micrognathia, flexion of middle digits with overlapping of fifth digit.

feet, evidence of congenital heart disease and low birth weight (Fig. 11.71). No treatment is available and most die in infancy.

TRISOMY 13–15

Trisomy 13–15 presents as multiple abnormalities including cleft palate, cerebral and cardiac defects, microphthalmia (Fig. 11.72). The prognosis is poor.

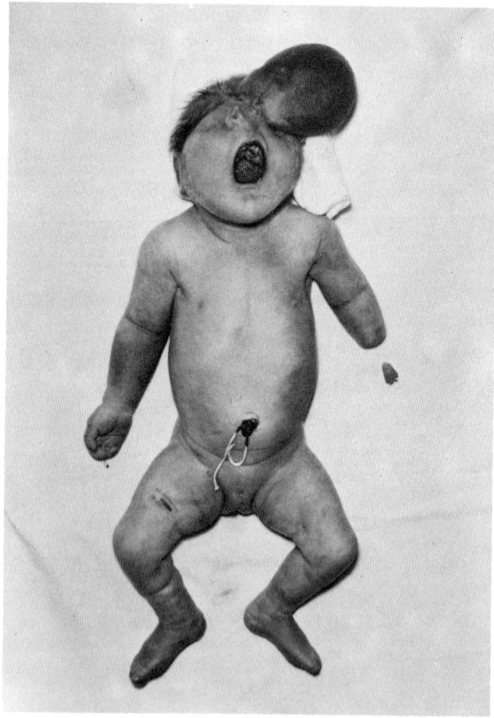

Figure 11.72 Trisomy 13–15 showing multiple abnormalities. This infant also had intrauterine amputation of the left hand.

CRI DU CHAT SYNDROME

The only well-recognized syndrome in which there is deletion of part of an autosome is termed cri du chat syndrome after the mewing cry evident in such infants. They have oblique palpebral fissures with widely spaced eyes, low-set ears, a small jaw and may be mentally retarded.

METABOLIC DISORDERS

RECOGNITION

Most metabolic disorders are present at birth and are therefore congenital abnormalities but they are not evident unless special investigations are carried out. Simplifications in the techniques involved have now made it possible to screen whole newborn populations for a number of biochemical abnormalities.

Guthrie test. The Guthrie technique uses bacterial inhibition to detect such disorders as phenylalaninaemia, histidinaemia, tyrosinaemia, maple syrup urine disease and galactosaemia. Capillary blood is collected on prepared blotting paper and sent to a central laboratory which can carry out hundreds of examinations simultaneously. The test is normally carried out on the sixth day of life (Fig. 11.73).

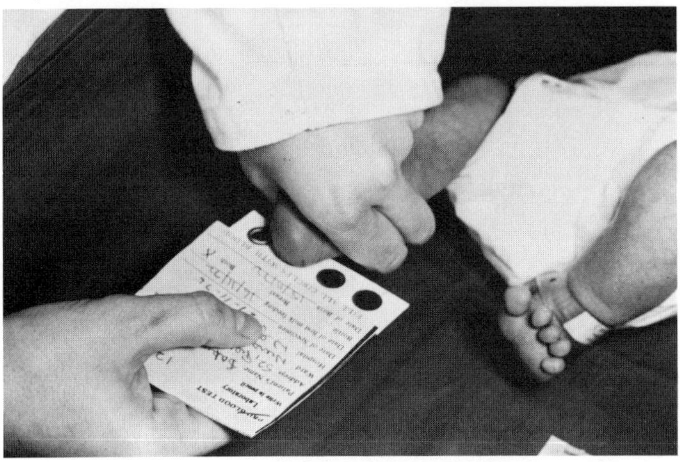

Figure 11.73 Collecting blood for Guthrie test.

Chemical and chromatographic tests on urine are more accurate in some conditions but less easy to apply in large numbers.

Transient tyrosinaemia. Low birth-weight infants may show a transient tyrosinaemia which is probably benign and which responds to treatment with ascorbic acid (vitamin C) 25 mg daily.

Other metabolic disorders are best managed in central units specializing in such conditions and referral is indicated.

GALACTOSAEMIA

Special mention must be made of the need for early diagnosis and management of the severe form of galactosaemia which presents as enlarged liver and jaundice shortly after either human or cow's milk feeding is introduced (Fig. 11.74). It is due to deficiency of an enzyme which converts galactose, one of the monosaccharides of lactose, to

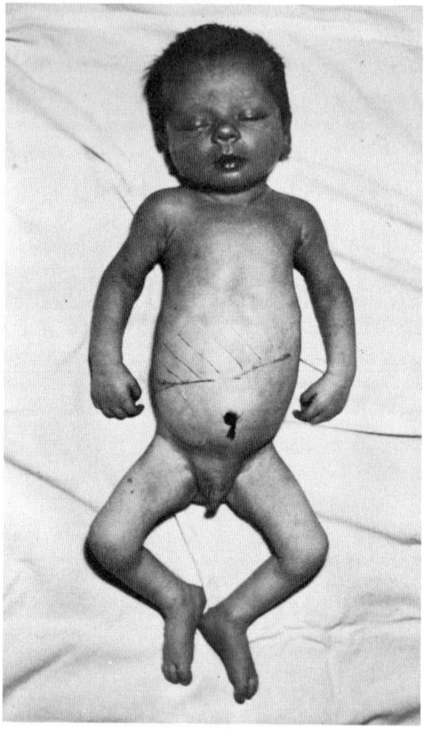

Figure 11.74 Enlarged liver in galactosaemia.

glucose. Treatment is the withdrawal of all feeds containing lactose. With satisfactory dietary control the later severe complications of this condition can be prevented.

Telling the parents

It is no longer believed that abnormal infants should be separated from their families and nursed in special institutions. Home-care benefits the handicapped child and families have to be helped to accept deformed children into their homes and be given support by the medical and social services. This support has to be given from birth if the abnormality is obvious and from the time when the diagnosis is confirmed if investigations have been indicated.

Trust. Parents are being asked to accept a considerable responsibility and it is essential that a trusting relationship is established with them from the beginning. This implies truthfulness and the willingness to answer direct questions. Absence of questions by parents about their infant does not necessarily indicate lack of concern or unawareness of the possibility of abnormality. Many parents expect doctors or midwives to take the initiative in explaining any abnormality present.

Early explanation rarely results in rejection but much depends upon the way in which the information is given. A terse announcement that a baby is abnormal will clearly distress and annoy parents. Similarly a false reassurance that all is well can be equally harmful. The procedure to be adopted in an individual situation has to suit the need of the moment.

A general policy for dealing with this problem should, however, be made in every nursery for the newborn. Whoever is to speak to the parents must have sufficient experience and authority to convince the parents that he understands the situation and is capable of advising them. The significance of the abnormality, the likely prognosis, the facilities available for management and the probability of recurrence in further pregnancies must be known before the parents are approached.

Family doctor. It is often very helpful for the situation to have been discussed with the family doctor, the social worker and physiotherapist before the interview is arranged.

Father. In some cases father is best approached on his own before anything is said to his wife.

Support for mother. Whichever approach is made it is essential that mother is given support during the hours and days after the original news has been given as her initial reaction may not indicate the true state of her anxiety. Opportunity should be given for further interviews to answer questions and to confirm arrangements for home care and follow-up examinations.

Responsibility. Telling parents is clearly a matter of considerable responsibility and not one which should devolve on the most junior members of the team. Even the most junior student midwife, however, must appreciate that she may be asked crucial questions. If in doubt as to the answer always explain that you will arrange for a more senior person, whether nurse or doctor, who has the necessary information to answer the question as soon as possible.

FURTHER READING

BECK, F. (1971). Aetiology of congenital heart disease. *British Journal of Hospital Medicine*, **6**, 409–418.

BECK, F., MOFFAT, D. B. & LLOYD, J. B. (1973). *Human Embryology and Genetics*. Oxford: Blackwell.

BRITISH MEDICAL JOURNAL (1971). Congenital dislocation of the hip. ii, 6–7.

BUTLER, N. R. & ALBERMAN, E. D. (editors) (1969). *Prenatal Problems. The Second Report of the 1958 British Perinatal Mortality Survey*. Edinburgh: Livingstone.

CARTER, C. O. (1971). Genetics of common malformations. In *Recent Advances in Paediatrics*, 4th ed. Edited by D. Gairdner and D. Hull. London: Churchill.

LANCET (1971). The birth of an abnormal child: telling the parents. Special article, ii, 1075–1077.

LIGHTLOWER, C. D. R. (1971). Meningomyelocele: the price of treatment. *British Medical Journal*, ii, 385–387.

LORBER, J. (1972). Spina bifida cystica: results of treatment of 270 consecutive cases with criteria for selection for the future. *Archives of Disease in Childhood*, **47**, 854–873.

NELSON, M. M. & FORFAR, J. O. (1971). Associations between drugs administered during pregnancy and congenital abnormalities of the fetus. *British Medical Journal*, i, 523–527.

SMITH, D. W. (1970). *Recognizable Patterns of Human Malformation*. Philadelphia: Saunders.

SMITHELLS, R. W. (1970). The epidemiology of congenital malformations. In *Modern Trends in Paediatrics*, vol. 3. Edited by J. Apley. London: Butterworths.

TUCKER, S. M. (1971). Clinical presentation of congenital heart disease. *British Journal of Hospital Medicine*, **6**, 421–427.

WARKANY, J. (1972). *Congenital malformations*. Chicago: Year Book Medical Publishers.

12

Birth Injuries

Trauma may arise from causes operating before, during or after birth and may be the result of mechanical injury or of deprivation of oxygen.

DECLINE IN BIRTH INJURY

There has been a progressive and considerable decline in the incidence of 'mechanical' birth injuries within the last two or three decades. More recently we have happily witnessed a corresponding decline in the incidence of hypoxic brain injury which may leave surviving infants permanently physically or mentally handicapped. This decline in the incidence of hypoxic brain damage has followed prompt and efficient treatment of hypoxia at birth based on an improved understanding of perinatal physiology. Hypoxia and subsequent brain damage are not always easily preventable and this type of birth injury still remains a considerable problem.

Although intracranial injury in the newborn presents a dramatic clinical picture the doctor and midwife must not neglect the potential danger in every bruise, abrasion, laceration, haematoma and fracture. Damage to tissues increases the risk of infection.

PREVENTION

Trauma widely interpreted is an inevitable accompaniment of the mechanics of birth even when delivery is spontaneous and uncomplicated. The nature of the injury varies greatly and, depending upon the site and severity, may be of minor or major significance. A doctor or midwife must therefore always be on the alert to reduce to the minimum the risk of an infant being seriously injured and to recognize damage to tissues without delay. This can be done by exercising the maximum care when undertaking antenatal supervision, when conducting a delivery and when carrying out subsequent nursing procedures.

CAUSES OF BIRTH INJURY

Fetal Hypoxia

Fetal hypoxia is likely to occur where there is interference with maternal oxygen uptake and distribution, interference with the normal function of the placenta or interference with fetal circulation and oxygenation.

Maternal hypoxia. Any condition which lowers the maternal blood oxygen will cause fetal hypoxia. Such conditions include environmental factors, such as high altitude or a smoke-filled atmosphere after a fire, pulmonary dysfunction, as during infection, cardiovascular failure, severe anaemia and some poisonings. Temporary apnoea as may occur during a prolonged fit may cause hypoxia.

Placental dysfunction. Poor development, premature separation and early degeneration of the placenta will reduce maternofetal blood gas exchange and cause fetal hypoxia. These conditions are more likely to occur when the mother suffers from pre-eclamptic toxaemia or hypertension.

Obstruction to the cord. Interference to the fetal circulation through the cord can be caused by external pressure on the cord, by the cord being tightly stretched because it is too short or is looped round a part of the fetus, commonly the neck, or because there is a true knot in the cord.

Fetal anaemia. If the fetus is severely anaemic because of haemolysis or external blood loss serious hypoxaemia of vital organs may occur.

Mechanical Trauma

ANTENATAL

Induction of labour. Antenatally superficial trauma, generally of minor degree, can occur following the use of a catheter for the rupture of membranes (Fig. 12.1).

Caesarean section. Occasionally the incision during caesarean section will include some part of the fetus.

DURING DELIVERY

Mechanical birth injury during delivery is most likely to be severe in the presence of one or more of the following situations:

Disproportion of the size of the fetal head for the maternal pelvis
Excessive uterine contractions
Abnormal presentations
Low birth weight
Instrumental delivery

The following situations further contribute to the risk of injury:

Firstborn infant
Elderly mother
High parity mother

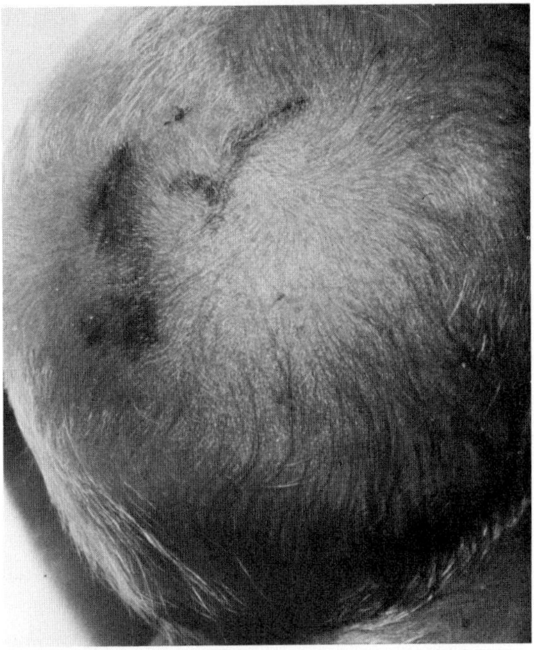

Figure 12.1 Superficial trauma of scalp. Caused by catheter during artificial rupture of membranes.

POSTNATAL INJURY

Successful delivery is not an assurance that the newly born infant is no longer exposed to the risks of trauma. As the factors causing postnatal injury differ from those causing ante- and intrapartum injury they will be considered separately at the end of this chapter.

TYPES OF BIRTH INJURY

It is important to consider trauma according to the structures involved and according to whether it is of temporary or of long-term significance.

Injury to the Superficial Tissues

Damage to the superficial tissues of presenting parts may take the form of simple bruising or the skin may be abraded.

A caput succedaneum consists of oedematous swelling and bruising in the superficial tissues of the presenting part of the fetus. In vertex presentations the caput is not sharply defined and it may extend across the lines of the sutures (Fig. 12.2). If the presentation is abnormal the 'caput' will be formed elsewhere (Fig. 12.3, 4). It 'pits' on pressure, is present at birth and disappears in the course of a day or two. The tissues involved are those encircled by the 'girdle of contact' formed by the maternal soft passages, and the oedema is the result of interference with local venous return.

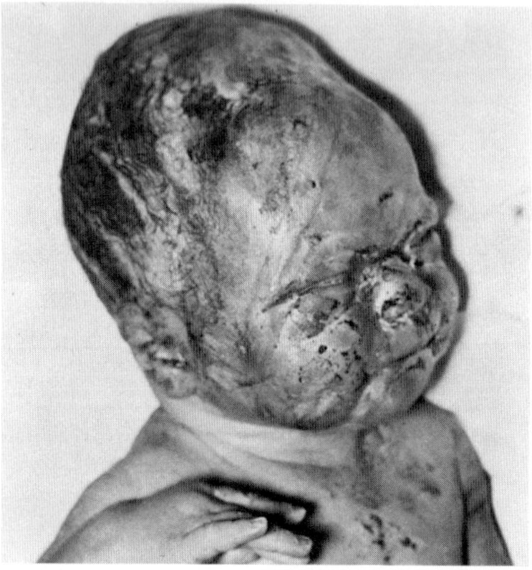

Figure 12.2 Caput succedaneum over vertex.

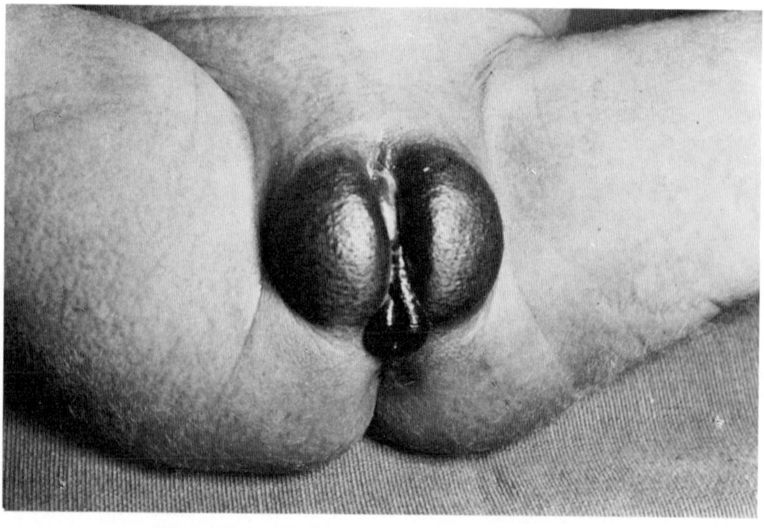

Figure 12.3 Bruising of vulva in breech delivery.

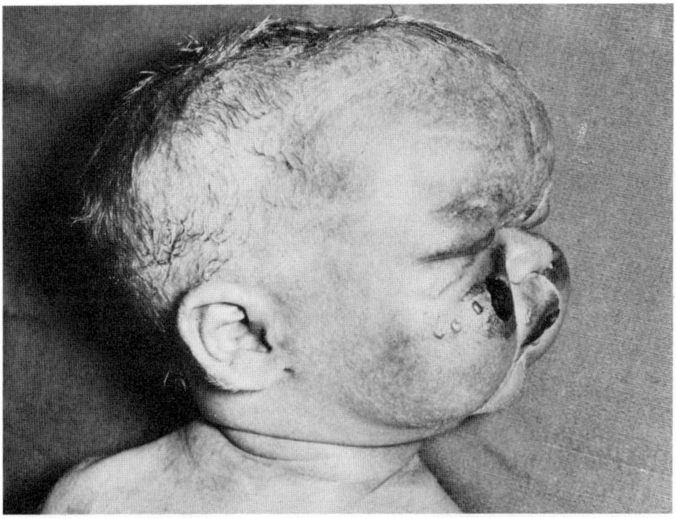

Figure 12.4 Bruising of face with excoriation of skin in face presentation.

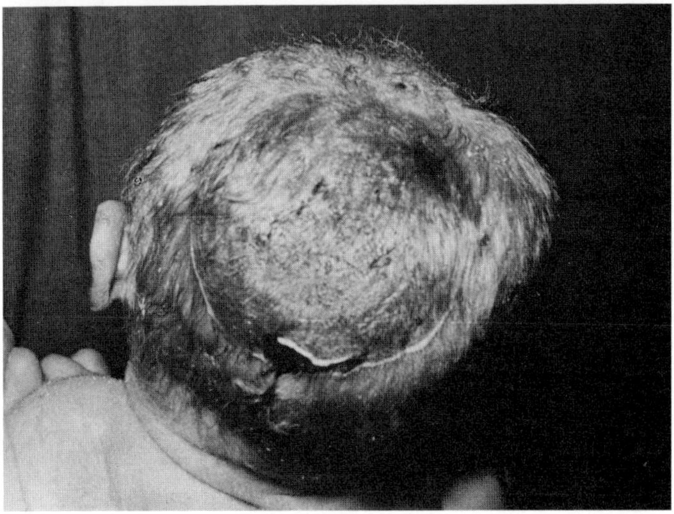

Figure 12.5 Bruising of scalp with abrasions following use of vacuum extractor.

Abrasions are sometimes present in the skin over a caput succedaneum and unless particular care is taken may allow the entry of organisms leading to infection and suppuration.

Bruising and minor abrasions of the scalp not infrequently result from applications of a vacuum extractor (Fig. 12.5). Tissues within the encircling site of application tend to be oedematous.

Cephalhaematoma is a swelling consisting of blood situated more deeply between the periosteum and the underlying skull bone. A cephalhaematoma is evidence of the escape of blood from capillaries damaged as a result of the separation of periosteum from the bone. The swelling may cover a part or the whole of one or other of the parietal bones (Fig. 12.6) or the occiput (Fig. 12.7) but does not

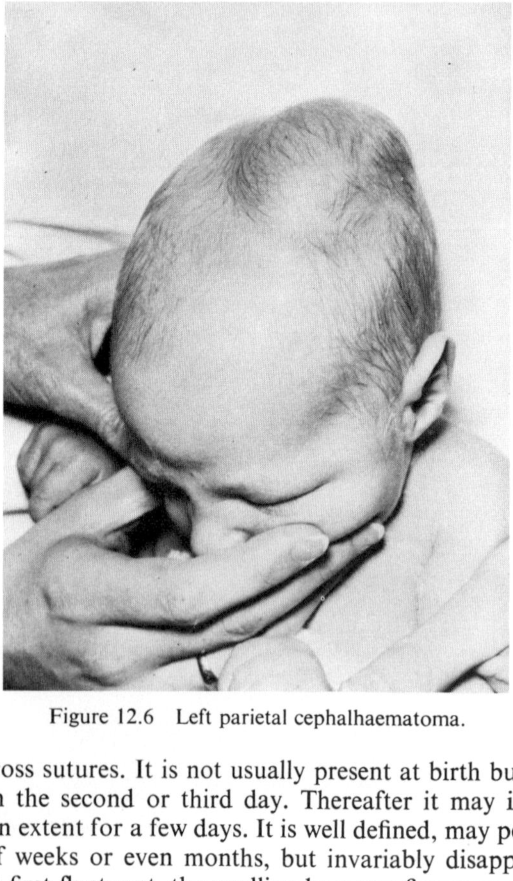

Figure 12.6 Left parietal cephalhaematoma.

extend across sutures. It is not usually present at birth but becomes evident on the second or third day. Thereafter it may increase in bulk and in extent for a few days. It is well defined, may persist for a number of weeks or even months, but invariably disappears completely. At first fluctuant, the swelling becomes firmer as absorption of fluid due to osmosis takes place. In the course of a few days a firm ring may be felt surrounding the swelling. This is evidence of commencing calcification which sometimes extends to form a localized hard elevation around the site of the original tumour. A cephalhaematoma may be unilateral or bilateral (Fig. 12.8).

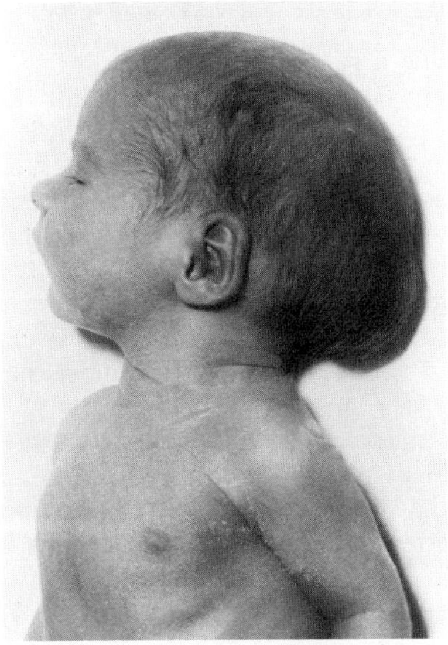

Figure 12.7 Occipital cephalhaematoma.

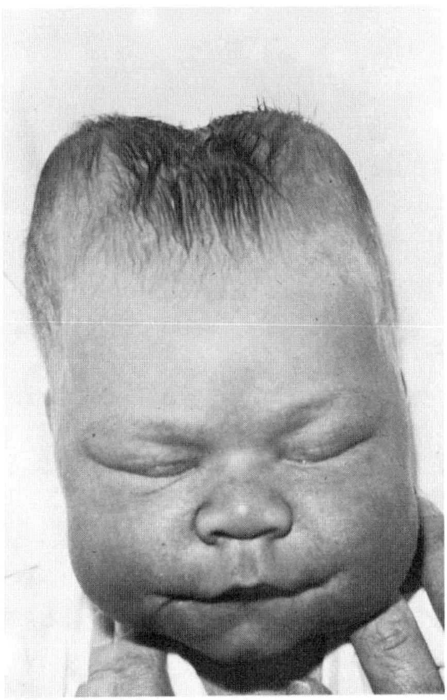

Figure 12.8 Bilateral parietal cephalhaematomas.

In general neither a caput succedaneum nor a cephalhaematoma need cause concern. They do not distress the infant. There is no need to place the baby in any special position, and it is sufficient to keep the scalp clean. Localized swelling of the scalp, especially if large and unsightly, may distress the mother. She can be confidently assured that the swelling will disappear completely and (should she raise the question) that it will most certainly not interfere with the baby's normal development. Active treatment is seldom required and the need for a blood transfusion is exceptional. Aspiration may introduce infection and is contraindicated. Jaundice may follow lysis of the contained blood.

Subaponeurotic haemorrhage occasionally results from application of a vacuum extractor. This may be confused with a caput succedaneum as the swelling extends across the lines of the sutures. Deaths have been reported as a result of excessive blood loss.

Forceps marks. Inevitably superficial trauma of some degree accompanies the application of forceps (Fig. 12.9). The injury may be scarcely perceptible and consists only of indentation, hyperaemia or minimal abrasions. On the other hand there may be comparatively deep laceration.

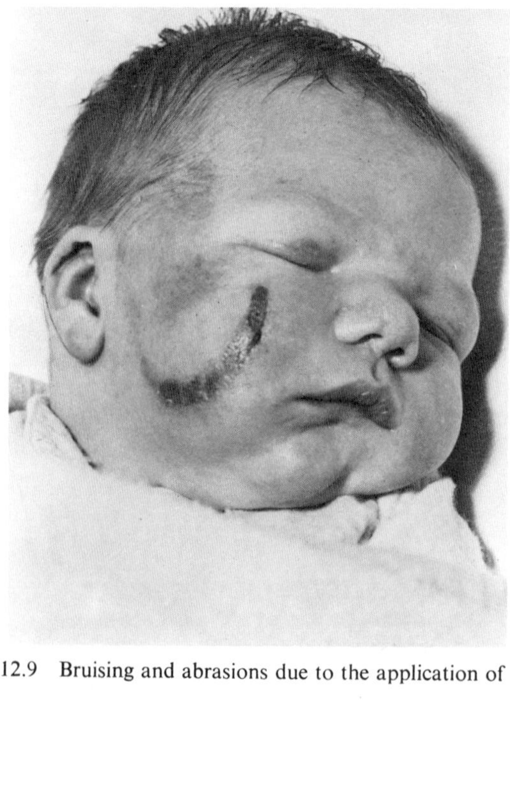

Figure 12.9 Bruising and abrasions due to the application of forceps.

Accidental incision (Fig. 12.10) of the face or buttock occasionally occurs during caesarean delivery. Such injuries are easily overlooked in a hurried initial examination following delivery only to be discovered later as the cause of severe blood loss.

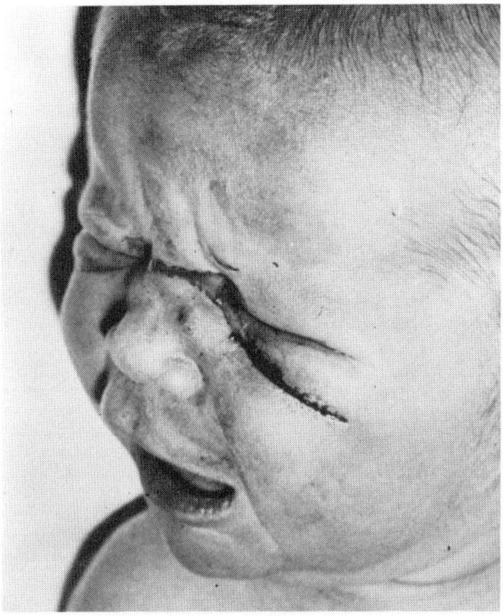

Figure 12.10 Accidental incision of left cheek during emergency caesarean section.

Subcutaneous fat necrosis takes place in areas subjected to undue pressure or along the line of forceps pressure, appearing a week or two after delivery as small areas of induration.

Injury to the Eyes

Subconjunctival and retinal haemorrhages occur most frequently after a difficult delivery and almost always disappear spontaneously within a month. Temporary blockage of the nasolacrimal duct by a small haematoma can occur after abnormal local pressure by forceps blades. Injury accounts for a small proportion of cases of glaucoma.

Injury to Muscle

Sternomastoid tumour sometimes appears in the body of a sternomastoid muscle when delivery has involved excessive rotation or gross lateral extension of the neck. The tumour appears a number of days after birth, and among babies born in hospital is frequently first discovered after and not before discharge home. It is usually situated in the lower half of the muscle, and may be relatively small or as large as a marble (Fig. 12.11). Extending the neck by gently pulling into the sitting position makes the swelling more obvious. Hard and painless, the tumour does not fluctuate, occurs most commonly after a breech delivery and eventually disappears spontaneously. There are doubts concerning the exact nature of the pathology. Some authorities regard the swelling as a haemorrhage into torn muscle, whilst others believe that it is a desmoid or fibrous tumour being completely unrelated to injury.

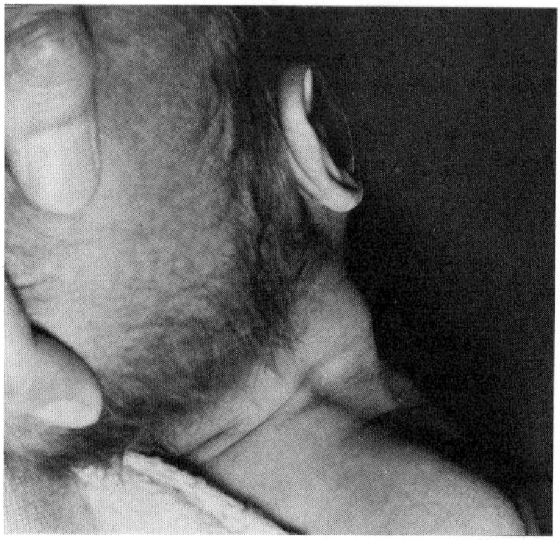

Figure 12.11 Sternomastoid tumour.

Treatment commonly consists of daily passive movements of the head and neck to maintain a full range of movement.

Injury to Peripheral Nerves

PARALYSIS

Paralysis as a result of damage to a peripheral nerve may be temporary or permanent.

Temporary loss of function occurs following damage by local pressure effects, particularly where the nerve is superficial and lying over bone. In most cases such injury is the equivalent of bruising. Normal function is restored within a few days as the bruising subsides.

More prolonged loss of function occurs if the axon is torn but the neurolemmal sheath remains intact, as may happen in the lesser traction injuries. Function will be restored as the axon regrows inside the sheath and reaches the motor end-plate.

Permanent paralysis follows complete division of axon and sheath as may occur with accidental incision or after a severe traction injury.

INJURY LEADING TO TEMPORARY PARALYSIS

Facial paralysis follows pronounced pressure on the facial nerve beyond the point where it leaves the skull at the stylomastoid foramen. Most commonly the damage is due to pressure by the blade of forceps but it can occur during normal delivery, possibly due to excessive pressure on the ramus of the mandible while the head is being held. Evidence of facial paresis consists in diminished movement of the affected side of the face. The mouth is drawn over to the uninjured side when the infant cries. Although milk may 'dribble' out of the dependent angle of the mouth there is no interference with sucking. On the injured side the eye frequently, but by no means always, remains partly open (Fig. 12.12). Restoration of

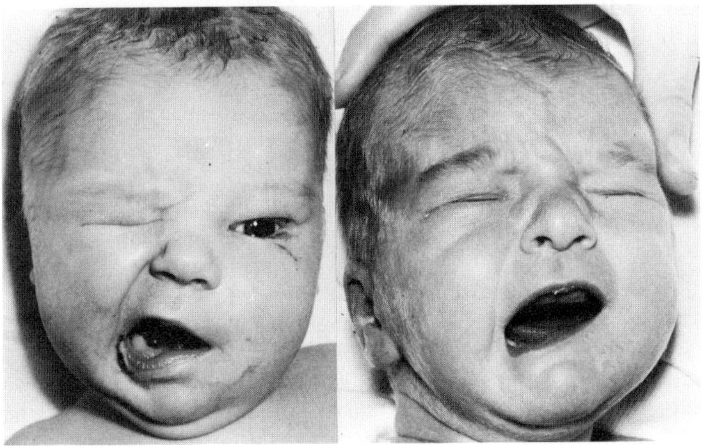

(a) (b)

Figure 12.12 Left facial palsy: (a) complete; (b) partial.

normal function and disappearance of the paresis may be complete in a few days, and in any event are usually complete within two or three weeks of birth.

In the mild case no treatment is required. Where the eye of the affected side remains open it is customary to lay the infant down with the injured side uppermost. This is intended to prevent secretions draining into the affected eye. The affected eye should be kept clean and drops of sterile normal saline instilled to prevent corneal ulceration.

Radial palsy (Fig. 12.13) is characterized by wrist drop, ability to grip with the fingers and voluntary extension of the fingers with the wrist in the dropped position. Palsy is usually detected within a few hours of birth. Spontaneous recovery in the course of days, weeks or several months takes place. The condition is probably due to interference with blood supply to the nerve as a result of abnormal compression or traction. Bruising or later fat necrosis over the antero-lateral aspect of the upper arm is sometimes present. Difficult labour accounts for the majority of cases. Exceptionally the palsy may be bilateral as when pressure on both arms has been exerted by a uterine contraction ring.

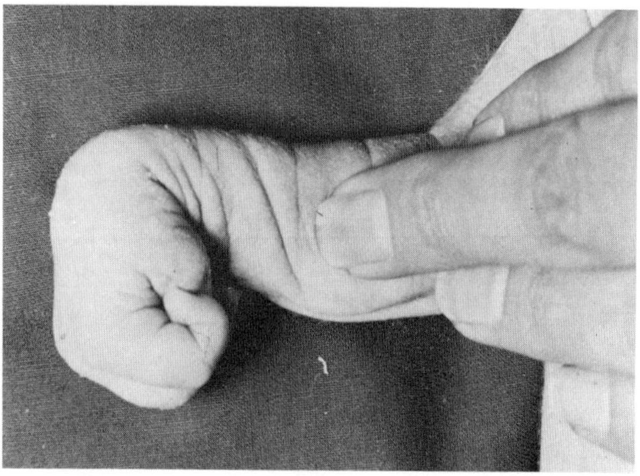

Figure 12.13 Wrist drop due to radial nerve palsy.

Obturator and external popliteal palsies (Fig. 12.14) are uncommon findings and are examples of nerve damage caused by sustained traction on the nerve involved consequent upon the intrauterine position of the limb. The palsies are detectable at birth and according to their severity disappear spontaneously within days or a few weeks.

Sciatic palsy is usually the result of unskilled intramuscular injections into the buttocks but can follow the injection of drugs into the umbilical artery.

INJURY LEADING TO PROLONGED OR PERMANENT PARALYSIS

Brachial palsy. The nerves forming the brachial plexus pass from the spinal cord to supply the upper extremities. Damage to the plexus may follow excessive rotation, stretching or lateral flexion of the neck during delivery of the shoulders in a vertex presentation, or of the aftercoming head in a breech presentation. The clinical picture of brachial palsy varies according to the nerves of the plexus which have been damaged.

Erb's palsy. In Erb's palsy (Fig. 12.15), which results from damage

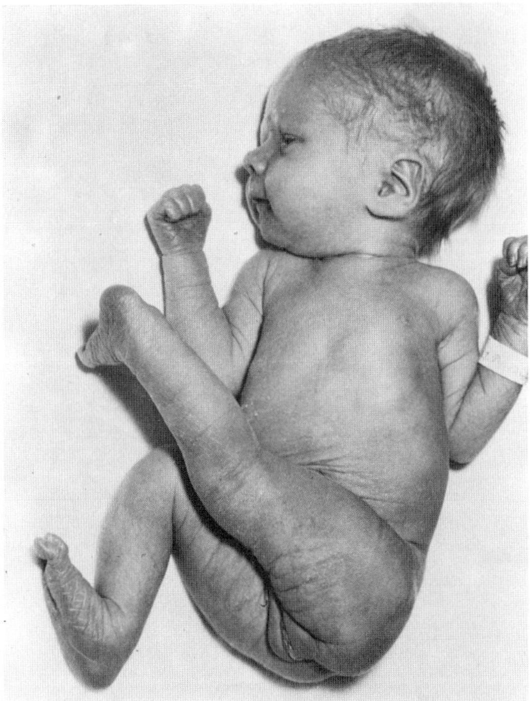

Figure 12.14 Left obturator palsy.

to cervical nerve roots 5 and 6, the arm is rotated internally and hangs limply from the shoulder, the elbow is extended, and the hand is partially closed with the palm directed outwards and posteriorly. Although movements of the hand and fingers are possible, the infant cannot raise the arm. Flexing a deflexed head to allow delivery may damage the spinal cord resulting in a bilateral palsy. The majority of cases recover completely, some in the matter of weeks and others after a number of months. Where damage has been particularly severe, paralysis may persist permanently and be accompanied by wasting of muscles.

Treatment requires specialist orthopaedic advice. Until this is obtained, and as a temporary measure, a padded bandage is applied to the wrist and pinned to the pillow with the object of maintaining abduction, external rotation and supination of the arm. Methods of orthopaedic treatment differ. One consists in the application of a light splint designed to keep the arm at right angles to the trunk, the elbow flexed at 90 degrees, and the forearm externally rotated.

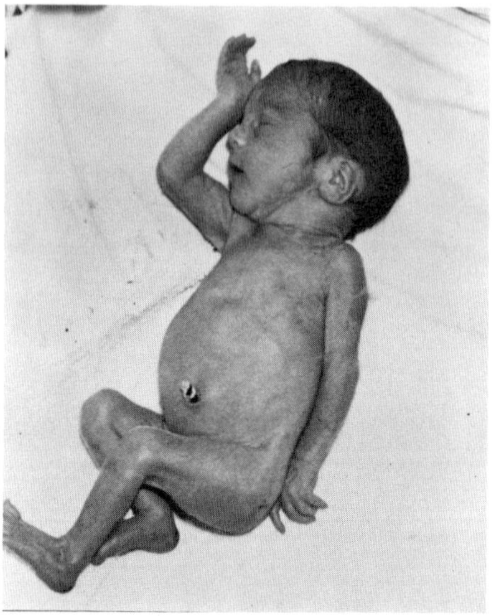

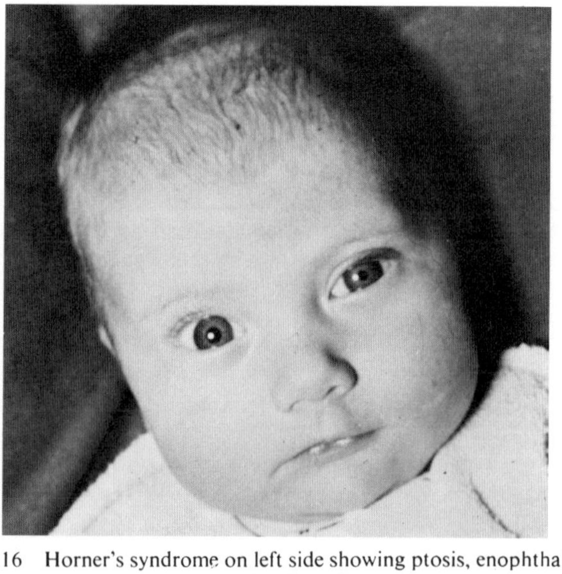

Figure 12.16 Horner's syndrome on left side showing ptosis, enophthalmos and constricted pupil.

Some surgeons are opposed to elevation of the arm, and where damage is minimal would favour encouragement of free movement of the limb rather than strapping or splinting. Passive movements are commenced two or three weeks after birth.

Klumpke's paralysis is a rare condition involving nerve roots cervical 8 and thoracic 1. The clinical features are wrist drop, flaccid paralysis of the hand with absence of the grasp reflex and sometimes local swelling and redness. A splint is applied which extends the wrist at the same time as keeping the hand flat. Complete recovery is rare.

Horner's syndrome (Fig. 12.16) with ptosis, enophthalmos, constriction of the pupil and absence of sweating on the affected side of the head and face is caused by damage to the cervical sympathetic nerves.

The *entire brachial plexus* may be ruptured following excessive traction and results in a permanent flaccid paralysis of the arm with wasting of all muscles.

Phrenic nerve paralysis causes paralysis of half of the diaphragm on the side concerned. As the phrenic nerve arises from the same cervical nerve roots as are affected in Erb's palsy the two conditions may coexist (Fig. 12.17).

OTHER CAUSES OF PARALYSIS

Although not due to injury it is important to recognize that permanent paralysis of the angle of the mouth may be due to congenital absence of the labial branch of the seventh cranial nerve, which has been associated with congenital heart disease. Möbius' syndrome is permanent bilateral paralysis of the facial and swallowing muscles due to agenesis of cranial nerve nuclei.

Injuries to Internal Organs

Recognition. Injuries to internal organs are much less common than superficial injuries. Because they are, in general, less obvious on external inspection and as their diagnosis relies on the correct interpretation of a number of clinical signs which may also arise from other causes, the recognition of internal injuries requires constant awareness of the possibility of their occurrence and alertness and good observation to recognize the presenting signs.

ABDOMINAL ORGANS

The organs most likely to be involved are those least well protected by a covering of bone. Abdominal organs are therefore particularly prone to injury.

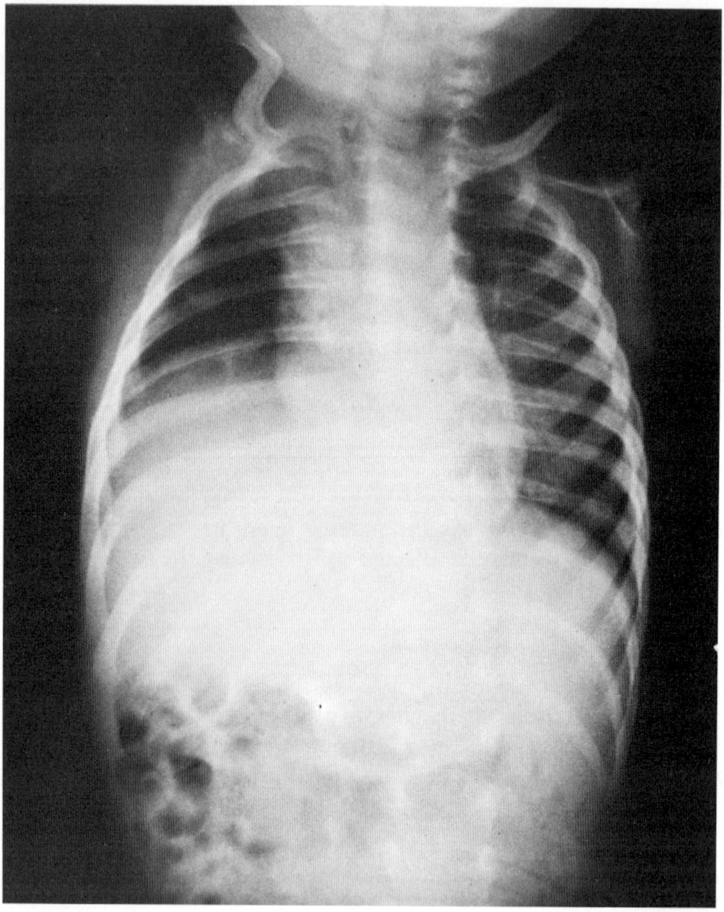

Figure 12.17 Elevation of right diaphragm due to right phrenic nerve palsy.

THE LIVER

Occasionally difficulty in delivery results in bleeding from veins on the surface of the liver with the subsequent formation of a subcapsular haematoma. If bleeding persists the capsule ruptures and haemorrhage into the peritoneal cavity takes place. The liver may be ruptured in the course of a breech delivery if the infant's trunk is grasped to firmly. Similar injury can take place during mismanaged artificial respiration using techniques of manipulating the infant which have now been abandoned.

THE SPLEEN

The spleen may be injured at the same time as the liver for the same reasons. Occasionally the spleen only will be ruptured.

Subcapsular haematoma. Injury to the liver or spleen or both may result in haemorrhage below the capsule without rupture of the capsule. Suspicion should be aroused if, in the absence of external haemorrhage, there are increasing pallor, restlessness and dyspnoea, a low body temperature and slight fullness of the abdomen. Local swelling in the neighbourhood of the liver or spleen with local tenderness may be detectable. Examination of the infant must be reduced to a minimum. Treatment consists in immediate blood transfusion and operative intervention.

Rupture of liver or spleen may occur immediately during trauma or follow development of a subcapsular haematoma and will then not occur until several hours after birth. The infant shows signs of collapse and unless given a blood transfusion and operative repair of the tear within a short period death will ensue.

ADRENAL GLANDS

These glands are normally congested at birth and if subjected to local stress are liable to be the site of a fatal haemorrhage.

Adrenal haemorrhage is most likely to occur in large infants following a difficult delivery particularly where there has been fetal hypoxia. If both glands are involved in a massive haemorrhage death follows rapidly. Unilateral or smaller bleeds are compatible with survival if the appropriate supportive therapy has been given.

The Skeleton

Almost any bone in the body may be the site of a fracture, but the incidence of fractures in relation to the number of difficult deliveries is notably small.

THE CLAVICLES

The clavicles (Fig. 12.18) are fractured with greater frequency than is generally supposed. Such fractures are sometimes found unexpectedly after an apparent normal delivery, cause no trouble and require no special treatment.

THE LONG BONES

The long bones (Fig. 12.19) of the limbs are liable to fracture when difficulty is experienced in bringing down extended limbs in the course of delivery. Healing is invariably rapid because of the speed with which callus formation takes place (Fig. 12.20), and there is

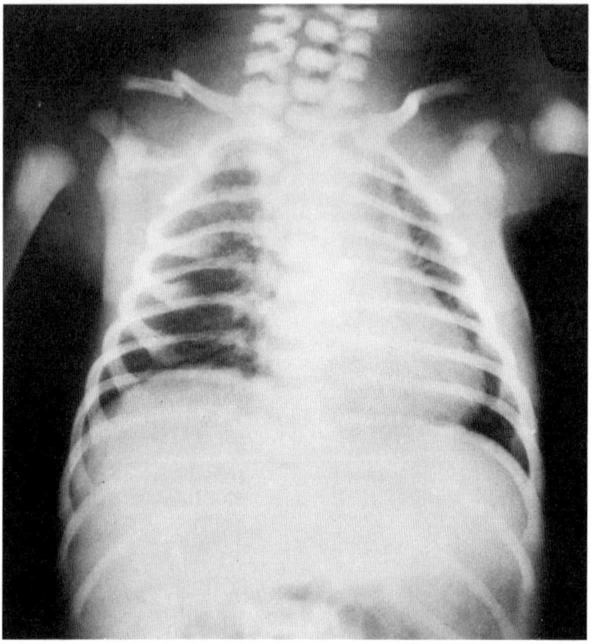

Figure 12.18 Fracture of right clavicle.

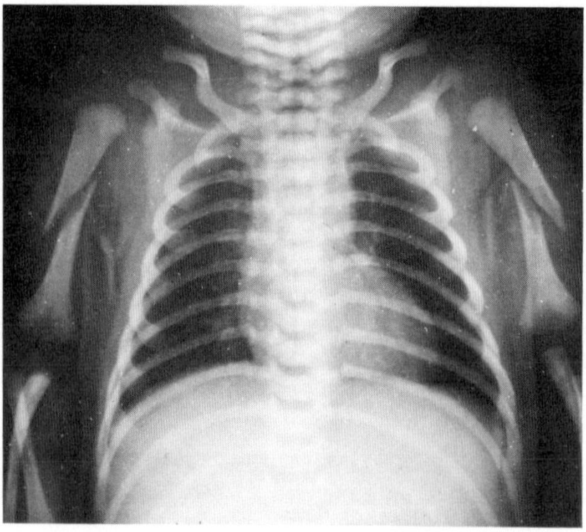

Figure 12.19 Fracture of both humeri.

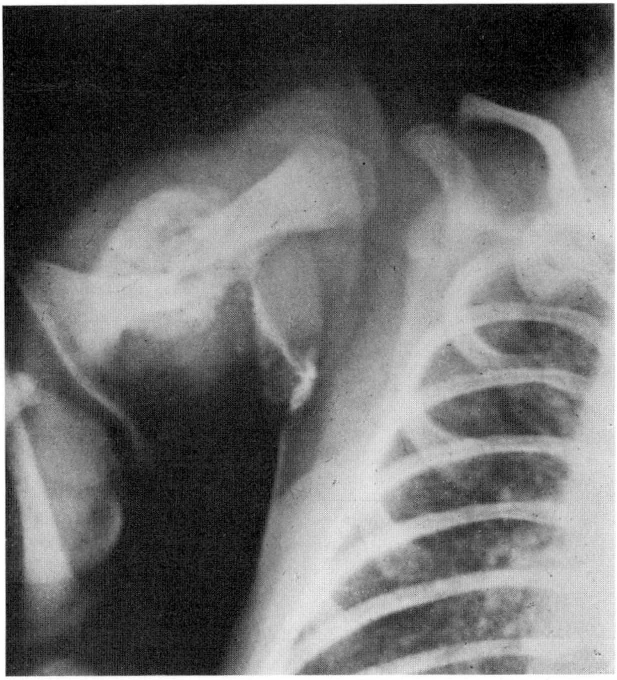

Figure 12.20 Fractured humerus showing massive callus formation three weeks after birth.

rarely permanent deformity. The occurrence of a fracture is sometimes suspected by the obstetrician during delivery. Fractures can result from inexpert handling of babies.

Apparent paralysis, more especially if associated with deformity of a limb in a newly born baby, should always raise the question of fracture.

Suspicion of a fracture at delivery is an indication for a medical opinion to be obtained at once. During the time that the doctor's arrival is waited, only the baby's face and eyes should be cleaned. Handling should be minimal, and instead of being dressed the infant should be covered with a warm blanket. Movement of the trunk and limbs must be avoided. If there is unavoidable delay in obtaining a medical opinion and the infant is in obvious distress, the affected limb may be lightly bandaged to the trunk or the other leg.

Epiphyseal injuries (Fig. 12.21) are uncommon, usually occur in the course of breech delivery, and on clinical examination may be indistinguishable from fracture. The upper epiphyses of the femur

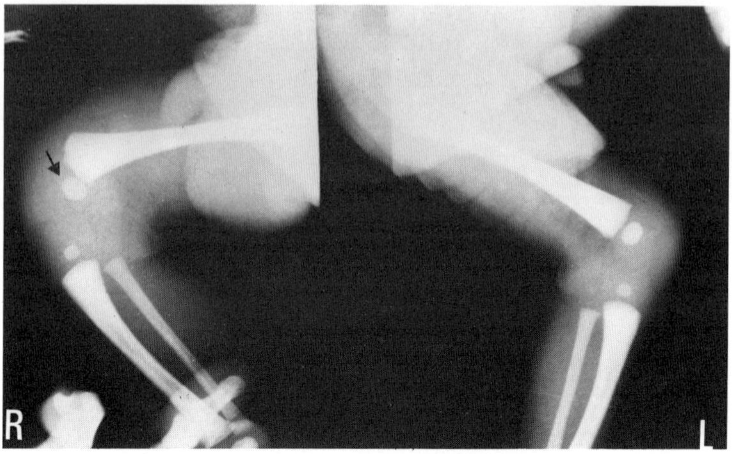

Figure 12.21 Displaced epiphysis. Lateral views of knee joint showing displaced lower right femoral epiphysis. Delivery was by the breech. Clinical signs consisted of swelling of the thigh and immobility of the limb. (By courtesy of Mr J. M. Fitton, F.R.C.S.)

and humerus are the most commonly affected. Separation of the epiphyses may be accompanied by dislocation in which event application of a splint is necessary.

THE SKULL

The skull is rarely the site of fractures.

Stellate fractures without displacement are the most common.

A depressed fracture (Fig. 12.22) may occur where labour has been allowed to proceed despite a maternal pelvic deformity and where excessive pressure has been exerted by the sacral promontory. The depression usually disappears spontaneously and operative elevation is seldom required. Where delivery has been precipitate the cranium should be examined for any obvious damage (Fig. 12.23). Should injury to the head be suspected, a doctor's opinion is essential and, pending his arrival, the baby must be observed for clinical evidence of intracranial irritation. Circumstances such as delivery into a lavatory pan and falls onto the floor make this especially necessary.

THE SPINE

Fractures of the spine are rare, result from excessive traction during breech delivery and are usually fatal.

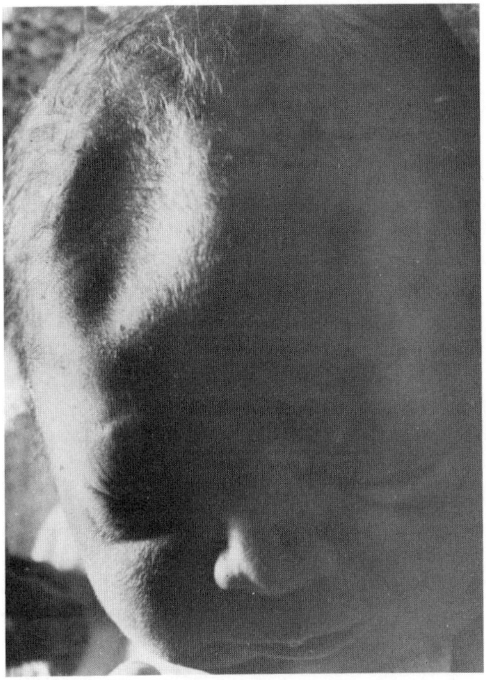

Figure 12.22 Depressed fracture of the skull which disappeared spontaneously in six months.

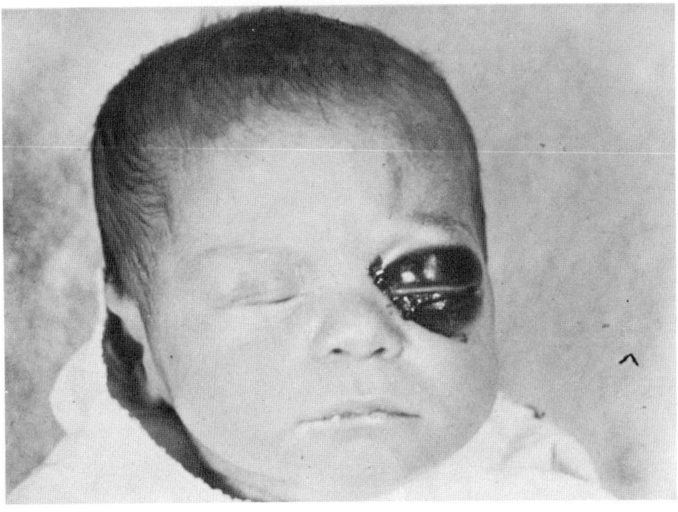

Figure 12.23 Orbital haematoma following fracture of the roof of the orbit during forceps delivery.

INTRACRANIAL INJURY

Intracranial injury may result from mechanical causes or from hypoxia. In the introduction to this chapter reference was made to the relatively greater importance of hypoxic brain damage now that improved standards of midwifery and obstetric care have reduced the incidence of mechanical injury. It must not be forgotten, however, that where standards of care are not high mechanical injury will still occur.

Mechanical Brain Injury

MOULDING

Moulding of the fetal head is a necessary accompaniment of vaginal delivery, but the structural adaptability of the skull to varying pressures and tensions protects the skull and its contents from damage. This adaptability depends upon the normal elasticity and partial mobility of the fetal skull bones, the fact that the cranial sutures are not closed, and upon the detailed structure and attachments of the supporting falx cerebri and tentorium cerebelli. Damage occurs when the moulding is of unusual degree, is excessively rapid or is applied in an abnormal direction.

Excessive moulding occurs in a variety of circumstances, including disproportion between the fetal head and the maternal pelvis or

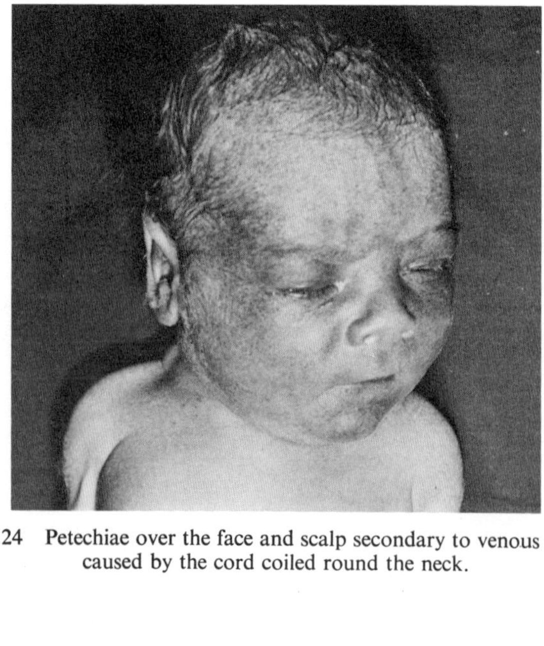

Figure 12.24 Petechiae over the face and scalp secondary to venous congestion caused by the cord coiled round the neck.

birth passages, rigidity of the pelvic floor and prolonged or violent uterine contractions. Instrumental delivery and certain obstetrical manipulations entail the application of abnormal forces. Moulding may be excessive in an occipito-posterior position, and may develop rapidly in precipitate deliveries and in a proportion of breech deliveries. It must be emphasized, however, that the severest degree of moulding can occur without there being any clinical evidence of intracranial damage.

Falx cerebri. Where damage does occur it may assume one of a number of forms. The actual rupture or tearing of structures is not invariable. There may be no more than oedema or congestion of the skull contents. The falx cerebri and tentorium cerebelli are the structures most liable to tearing, and when this occurs there is always a serious risk of fatal haemorrhage from involvement of one of the large veins or sinuses. If copious and not arrested, the bleeding may spread over the surface of the cerebrum giving rise to clinical signs, or it may spread down and around the brain stem, threatening death from the pressure exerted on vital centres.

SUBDURAL HAEMATOMA

In the event of a baby surviving extensive bleeding into the subdural space there is the possibility that organization may lead to the formation of an encysted haematoma. Unrelieved pressure from a subdural haematoma involves risk of necrosis and atrophy of the underlying brain tissues.

VENOUS CONGESTION

It is important to remember that disproportion is not essential to intracranial trauma. Successful delivery depends upon a balance between the stresses involved and the ability of the fetus to withstand those stresses. Where this does not obtain birth trauma occurs. This serves to explain the occasional occurrence of haemorrhage where delivery has been normal and spontaneous, or by caesarean section. Venous congestion consequent upon breech delivery may lead to cerebral bleeding—as the trunk is subjected to pressure during its passage through the maternal canal, the contents of the aftercoming skull become congested and the combination of congestion and cranial distortion increases the possibility of damage.

The cord may become coiled round the infant's neck. Descent of the fetus into the pelvis may then tighten the cord and strangle the fetus. At the same time cord circulation is impaired. Both venous congestion and hypoxia will contribute to the ensuing haemorrhage (Fig. 12.24).

INTRAVENTRICULAR HAEMORRHAGE

The low birth-weight baby (Chap. 9) is more liable to intracranial injury than the child born at term. This is due to the extreme mobility of his skull, to vulnerability of the tissues in general and the capillaries in particular, and to a greater tendency to bleeding. Intraventricular haemorrhage (Fig. 12.25) is a relatively common finding at postmortem examination in low birth-weight babies.

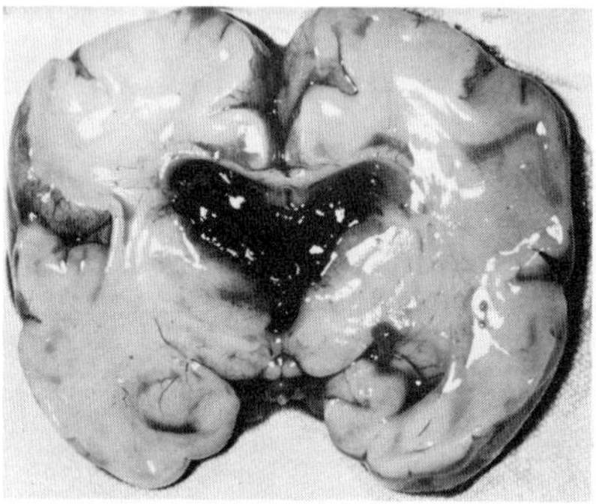

(a)

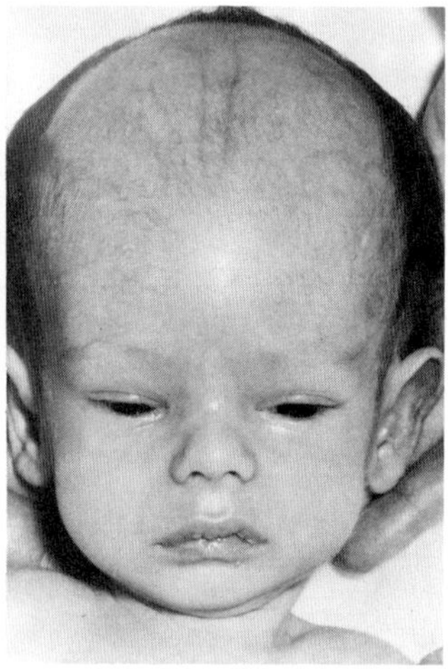

(b)

Figure 12.25 Intraventricular haemorrhage. Enlargement of head three days before death.

HAEMORRHAGIC DISEASES

Defective coagulation of the blood (Chap. 17) can aggravate the severity of bleeding from injured tissues in low birth-weight babies and in infants born at or after term. The likelihood is particularly great in the case of low birth-weight babies in whom impaired clotting is frequently associated with intrapartum hypoxia and low blood-glucose level.

Hypoxic Brain Injury

FETAL HYPOXIA

This has been considered in Chapter 4.

The onset of respiration at birth is stimulated by a lowering of the oxygen saturation of the blood, a concomitant rise in carbon dioxide tension and by external sensory stimuli. The brain stem respiratory centres are stimulated by oxygen lack which is mediated through the carotid and aortic chemoreceptors. Once the lungs have been expanded by the first few breaths the Hering-Breuer reflex maintains normal rhythmical respirations as in the adult. Sensory impulses from the skin, muscles and joints raise the general sensitivity of the central nervous system and so make the brain stem respiratory centres more sensitive to lack of oxygen.

NEONATAL HYPOXIA

Hypoxia is a natural consequence of neonatal respiratory failure for which several causes can be recognized.

Central nervous system depression may involve depression of the respiratory centres. This may be caused by malformations of the brain or depression from trauma or infection, by intrauterine hypoxia due to dysfunction and premature separation of the placenta, by umbilical cord compression, by inadequate oxygenation of the maternal blood during eclamptic convulsions or during a general anaesthetic, and by the effects of drugs given to the mother.

Failure of aeration and alveolar ventilation may be caused by airways obstruction at any level. This can be from intrinsic or extrinsic causes. A common cause is failure to drain the respiratory passages of amniotic fluid contaminated by mucus and meconium. Diaphragmatic hernia, pneumothorax or pneumomediastinum may lead to collapse of the lungs as a result of external pressure and may therefore limit gaseous exchanges. Pneumonia contracted after prolonged rupture of the membranes limits the passage of air into the alveoli and exchange of gases.

Failure of the pulmonary circulation except in such conditions as transposition of the great vessels and atresia of the pulmonary artery is a rare case of respiratory failure. It has been suggested that disturbance of the pulmonary circulation at capillary level could be responsible for the respiratory distress syndrome.

Failure of the systemic circulation for any reason is inevitably followed by hypoxia. Newborn infants are often found to be hypotensive with marked peripheral vasoconstriction and it is difficult to know whether this state of shock is due to disorder of the nervous, circulatory or of the respiratory systems.

Interrelationship of systems. It is important to realize that successful adaptation at birth depends on the interrelationship of the central nervous system, the circulatory system and the respiratory system. Although only one of the systems may be under strain initially, depression of the remaining systems frequently follows and gives rise to a state of general depression and a vicious circle is established. Conversely, treatment of one system may break the cycle and lead to general improvement. If, for example, the depression is due to apnoea IPPR will result in an improvement in the circulation, more oxygen will be supplied to the brain which in turn enables the establishment of spontaneous respiration and a lessening of the general depression. Similarly the successful treatment of cardiac failure will improve tissue oxygenation and correct depression of the central nervous system caused by previous hypoxia.

OXYGEN-CONSERVING ADAPTATION

Faced with a gradual reduction in oxygen supply due to such conditions as toxaemia and postmaturity the fetus reacts by means of a compensatory adaptation of its circulation. In this oxygen-conserving adaptation of the fetal circulation, which is regulated by the autonomic nervous system, the blood flow and hence the oxygen supply to a number of less important parts of the body, such as the extremities, abdominal viscera and lungs, are reduced by vaso-constriction. The oxygen saved in this way then becomes available for use by the vitally important brain and heart.

Acidosis. Local tissue hypoxaemia leads to an increase in the formation of lactic acid with a lowering of the pH of the blood as a result of anaerobic glycolysis. Fetal blood sampling allows an estimate of the condition of the fetus before delivery. If acidosis is present it can be corrected at birth by the immediate intravenous injection of 8.4 per cent sodium bicarbonate (Chap. 5).

Fetal heart rate. As the blood supply to the brain and heart are maintained as a result of the oxygen-conserving adaptation of the fetal circulation the degree of change in the heart rate as recorded by the cardiotocograph does not indicate the degree of fetal hypoxia as efficiently as fetal blood sampling.

EFFECTS OF FETAL HYPOXIA

Oxygen-conserving adaptation can be held responsible for many clinical conditions present at birth.

Light-for-dates babies. Reduction of blood flow to the skin leads to cessation of sebum production and the desquamation associated with fetal malnutrition as seen in light-for-dates babies.

Asphyxia pallida. Generalized pallor of the skin as found in 'asphyxia pallida' represents an advanced stage of oxygen-conserving adaptation.

Meconium staining. Reduction of blood flow to the bowel is associated with hyperperistalsis and discharge of meconium, the time-honoured sign of 'fetal distress'.

A fatal massive adrenal haemorrhage may follow the normal delivery of a chronically hypoxic fetus.

Pulmonary vasoconstriction. The respiratory problems which frequently arise in postnatal life following intrauterine hypoxia may be a consequence of oxygen-conserving adaptation. As a result of pulmonary vasoconstriction there is reduced blood flow through the lungs. This may be responsible for the deficiency of surfactant found in the respiratory distress syndrome (Chap. 15).

ACUTE OXYGEN DEPRIVATION

Acute oxygen deprivation is not accompanied by oxygen-conserving adaptation. Sudden obstruction of the respiratory passages from whatever cause results in violent respiratory movements and deep, generalized cyanosis to which the term 'asphyxia livida' was formerly applied.

Clinical Signs of Intracranial Injury

Premonitory factors. Whether they be due to trauma, haemorrhage or hypoxia the signs of intracranial injury are the same. Such signs are to be expected where the birth has been associated with prolonged or premature labour, with operative, high instrumental or precipitate delivery, with breech or face presentation, or with fetal distress or neonatal hypoxia. In these circumstances a newly born baby should be kept under observation in the special care baby unit for at least 48 hours.

CLINICAL EVIDENCE

Clinical evidence of intracranial damage manifests itself in many ways.

Limpness. Frequently but not invariably the infant is severely shocked at birth, lies limply in the cot, and may be pale or ashen-grey in colour. He may be unmistakably quiet or fretful. Respirations can show almost any kind of abnormal variation and are often associated with an excess of mucus secretion which is sometimes noticeably viscid. The child may deteriorate as evidenced by increasing depression of respiratory and other vital functions. Limpness and cyanosis become intensified and life may slowly ebb away, usually within a few hours of birth.

Irritability. On the other hand and in the majority of instances the general condition gradually improves. Clinical signs of irritation may appear some 12 hours after birth. Their first appearance is rarely later than the second or third day of life. From being limp and quiet the infant becomes restless and may be heard to utter a high-pitched shrill or even piercing cry.

The facial expression (Fig. 12.26) is that of an unnaturally wide-awake baby of many weeks and not of one a few days old, and seems to betray alertness and apprehension. The brow is wrinkled

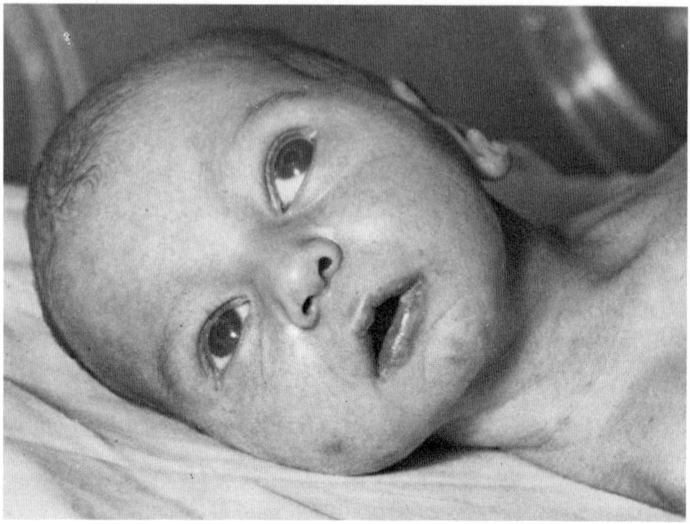

Figure 12.26 The alert expression and wide open eyes of a baby aged 2 days with pronounced signs of intracranial irritation.

and shows an unnatural frown which increases with disturbance or movement. Responses to touch, light and sound are excessive to the point of being violent.

Twitching movements may occur affecting the digits, the extremities, the angles of the mouth or the eyes, and in the most severe cases true convulsions develop.

Stiffness of the limbs is sometimes detectable. It may vary in degree. Occasionally the arms are held rather rigidly in a position of 'surrender', and the fists may be firmly clenched.

Head retraction occurs rarely but there is often some degree of stiffness of the neck in the absence of actual retraction (Fig. 12.27).

The fontanelle if large may be bulging (Fig. 12.28) or feel tense or spongy on palpation. Little information of value can be obtained from examination of a small fontanelle.

Rapid darting protrusive movements of the tongue are characteristic of intracranial irritation.

PROGNOSTIC SIGNS

Prognostically vomiting, convulsions, and sudden phases of intensified cyanosis are especially serious. The temperature may be subnormal, normal or moderately raised. There are no characteristic variations in the rate of the pulse or respirations. Loss of sucking and swallowing reflexes is rare.

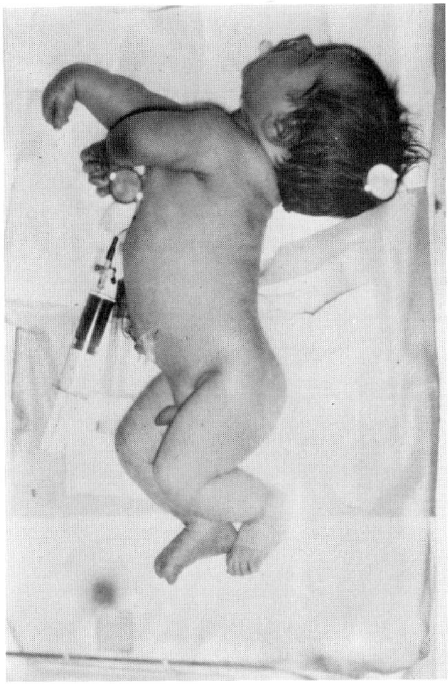

Figure 12.27 Head retraction in baby with severe hypoxic brain damage.

EARLY RECOGNITION

Any of the signs enumerated may appear in a baby with intracranial damage. Rarely are they all present. Realization of this is fundamental. Diagnosis and treatment depend for success upon early recognition. The implied challenge is to anticipate and to observe the individual signs in the absence of the complete clinical picture and to realize their possible significance in relation to the antenatal and natal histories. The midwife has a special responsibility because more often than not she is the first individual to witness signs of intracranial disturbance, which in the early stages are liable to be stimulated by feeding and napkin changing.

SUBDURAL HAEMATOMA

Findings suggestive of a subdural haematoma include failure to thrive, disinclination to feed and a measure of inactivity in an infant more than a week old. There is no constant time in relation to delivery when clinical signs first appear. Even after making allowances for delayed and missed diagnoses, available evidence suggests that clinical signs rarely develop in the first week of life and may not

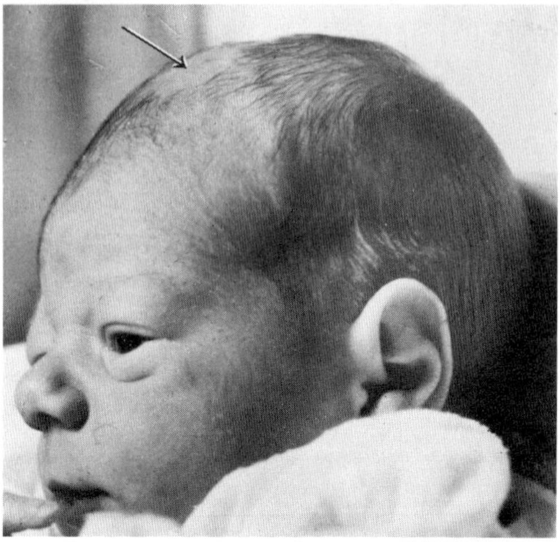

Figure 12.28 Bulging fontanelle in a baby with intracranial trauma.

appear until after the neonatal period. Occasionally vomiting subsequently complicates the picture. Usually after a further interval of a few days isolated convulsions occur. The fontanelle may be moderately full and the head slightly enlarged. A difference in resistance and in the note elicited on gentle percussion of the cranium can sometimes be detected on comparing the two sides but is of little value in locating the site of the effusion. Retinal haemorrhages are almost always present. Paralysis is exceptional at this stage. Confirmation of diagnosis depends upon aspiration of blood or significantly blood-stained cerebrospinal fluid from the subdural space (Chap. 19).

DIFFERENTIAL DIAGNOSIS

Clinically it is rarely possible to differentiate signs due to intracranial haemorrhage from those due to intracranial congestion or oedema. Moreover, signs suggestive of intracranial disturbance are not infrequently found at postmortem examination to have been due to congestion or hypoxia secondary to some other condition such as congenital heart disease. In such circumstances there may be nothing of significance on macroscopic examination of the brain. Fortunately the principles of treatment are the same regardless of the exact nature of the intracranial pathology. Despite the difficulties of arriving at a precise diagnosis lumbar puncture should only be used as a diagnostic aid when the need arises to exclude meningitis.

Management of Intracranial Injury

ANTENATAL

Treatment begins with careful antenatal supervision and obstetrical measures intended to prevent intracranial damage. These consist in avoiding circumstances favouring hypoxia, in the early recognition of situations which may call for episiotomy or instrumental delivery, and in offsetting as far as possible the risks attendant upon preterm delivery, low birth weight, and abnormal presentations.

AFTER DELIVERY

Quietness. The keynotes to care of the newly born infant with suspected intracranial disturbance are continuous, meticulous, careful clinical observation, the exclusion of all potentially disturbing stimuli, and the reduction to a minimum of handling and attention to the baby. Weighing, measuring and bathing are dispensed with temporarily. A room or place in the nursery should be selected for its quietness and warmth.

Apnoea monitor. Attention must be paid to the respiratory pattern, making special note of hypoventilation. An apnoea monitor (Chap. 10) should be used to give audible warning of periods of apnoea.

The air passages must be kept clear of mucus. Provided there is no excess of mucus, the head should be slightly raised.

Feeding. The decision as to whether feeding will be by bottle or tube is determined by the condition of the individual baby. Fluids must be offered in amounts appropriate to the infant's maturity, age and weight and should not be reduced because of the symptoms he is manifesting. The baby is not taken out of his cot for feeding or napkin changing.

Anticonvulsants. For the infant who is extremely irritable or actually convulsing anticonvulsant drugs may be used. It is most important, however, that their use to control signs should not be allowed to hide the necessity for establishing the cause of the convulsions. Hypoglycaemia, hypocalcaemia, hypomagnesaemia and other similar metabolic disturbances may occur in the infant with intracranial injury and require specific treatment.

Where brain injury is the sole cause of fits, treatment with phenobarbitone 5 to 10 mg per kg per day given intramuscularly or orally divided into four to six doses is often effective. More recently diazepam up to 1 mg per kg per dose given intravenously has proved very effective in the immediate control of convulsions. Chloral hydrate in a dose of 30 to 60 mg by mouth continues to be the first line of treatment in some centres.

Dexamethasone has proved its value in the treatment of cerebral oedema in older children and adults, but less is known about its use in the newborn period. Given intramuscularly or intravenously in a dose of 0.5 to 1.0 mg it does appear to relieve some forms of congestion or oedema of the brain.

The treatment of bleeding disorders is considered in more detail in Chapter 17. A special problem arises in the case of low birth-weight babies in whom a low thrombotest assessment is found together with signs of intracranial disturbance. If the baby's condition is not immediately critical, treatment can be limited to vitamin K intramuscularly, the thrombotest being repeated at intervals. Otherwise a transfusion of fresh frozen plasma or fresh blood should be given in an effort to improve the clotting status.

Treatment of encysted subdural haemorrhage is by repeated aspiration or continuous drainage. Open operation is sometimes required.

Prognosis

It is not always easy to give an accurate prognosis of the likely long-term effects of cerebral birth injury when the injury is first diagnosed. In general prolonged ante- or postnatal hypoxia is more likely to have permanent significant effects than an acute but short-lived period of hypoxia, or mechanical injury at birth. It may be weeks, months or years before the full effect of hypoxic brain damage becomes evident.

Increasing knowledge of the normal pattern of neurological behaviour in the newborn period and the first few weeks of life is making it easier for paediatric neurologists to make a more accurate prognosis at an early stage. Expert knowledge and skill is essential for this type of forecasting. Even with that knowledge it is still necessary to follow any infant in whom hypoxia or mechanical brain damage has been suspected at a suitable centre over several years.

MINIMAL BRAIN DAMAGE

Such long-term follow-up into school age has revealed some children with learning and co-ordination problems which are not readily demonstrable on routine neurological examination but which cause sufficient difficulty to the child to result in a sense of frustration. Because of difficulty in fine movements such children may not be able to function in the school setting at the level expected for their level of intelligence. This may lead to emotional problems and add to their schooling difficulties.

Minor impairment of sensory function particularly of the special senses may similarly cause educational problems.

ASSESSMENT CENTRES

Assessment of minor as well as major handicap requires the co-ordinated investigation of a number of specialists. This can best be organized in the form of assessment centres which are now established in many parts of the country. Further development of such centres and a review of their findings will in the future give us a more accurate assessment of the significance of perinatal injury in the production of long-term handicap.

POSTNATAL INJURY

After delivery the infant continues to be exposed to risk of injury either from his own actions or from those of his attendants.

He may scratch his own face (Fig. 12.29) or cause local abrasions

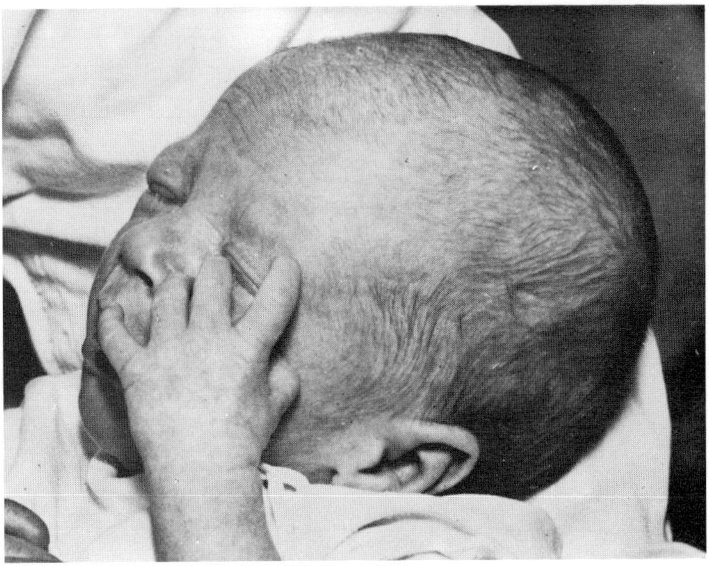

Figure 12.29 Scratching—a possible cause of minor superficial injury.

by rubbing a knee with the heel of the opposite leg (Fig. 12.30). Burns may occur due to lapses in nursing technique in the use of electric blankets. The use of unsuitable napkins or careless attention to napkin changing can give rise to local irritation. Loose threads inside a mitten may occlude the circulation in a finger and lead to gangrene with possible loss of part of a finger (Fig. 12.31, 32). Overzealous attention to the hygiene of the mouth, too vigorous extraction of mucus from the pharynx (especially during resuscitation), and impatient use of the feeding bottle can all injure the

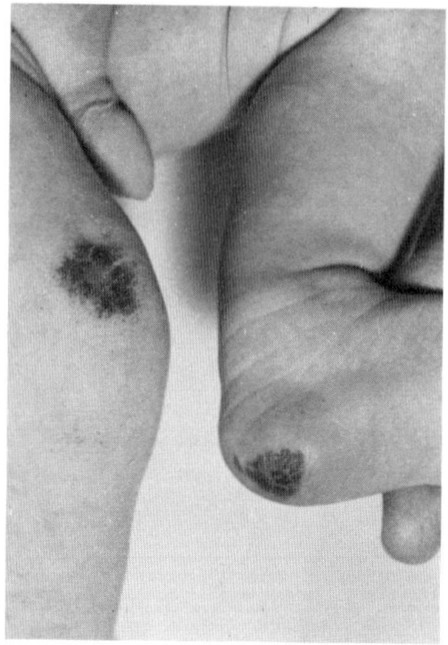

Figure 12.30 Abrasions caused by rubbing.

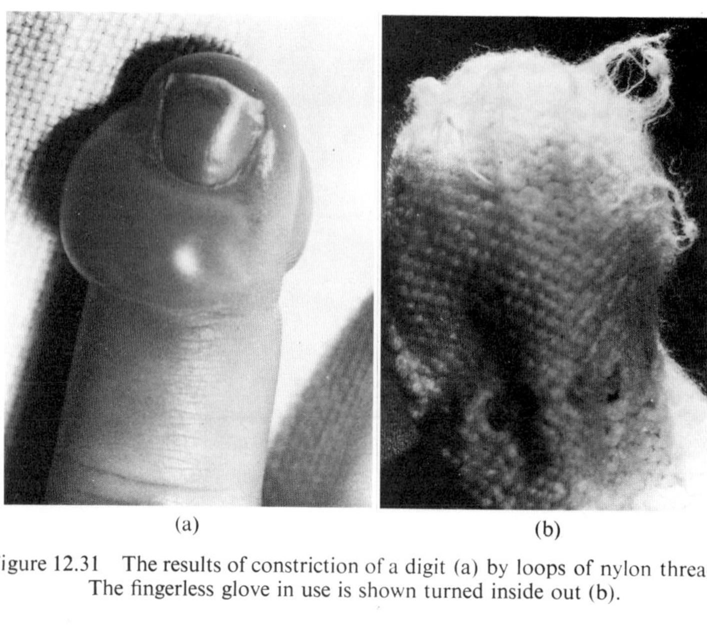

(a) (b)

Figure 12.31 The results of constriction of a digit (a) by loops of nylon thread. The fingerless glove in use is shown turned inside out (b).

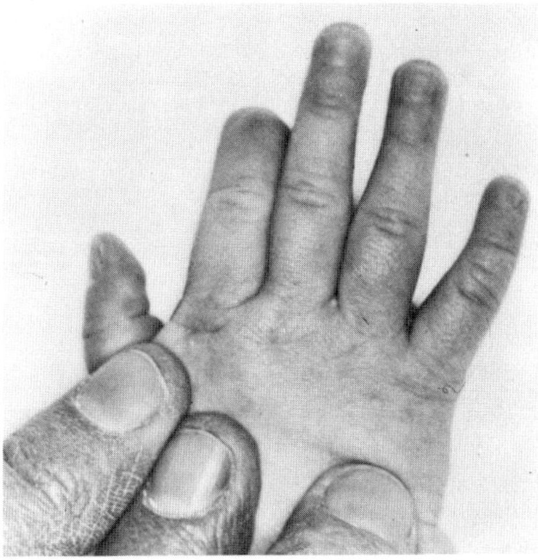

Figure 12.32 Loss of distal phalanx of index finger following constriction by a loose thread in a mitten.

buccopharyngeal mucous membrane. Mismanagement of physiological engorgement of the breasts may lead to tissue destruction and suppurative mastitis. These are instances of avoidable trauma which, if they occur, are a reflection on the standards of nursing care.

FURTHER READING

SALING, E. Z. (1970). Oxygen-conserving adaptation of the fetal circulation. In *Modern Trends in Paediatrics*, vol. 3. Edited by J. Apley. London: Butterworths.

13

Infection

The fetus *in utero* is protected from infection by his isolation from the external environment. This protection is not absolute but the fetus is in a very much safer situation than the newborn infant who is exposed to invasion by the organisms of whatever environment he may enter. Under favourable circumstances this invasion is accomplished without harm to the infant and some benefit may accrue. This is termed colonization as opposed to clinical infection which occurs when the number or virulence of the organisms encountered overwhelms the defence mechanisms of the infant. As many of the factors involved in the colonization of infants are under the control of those caring for the newborn most infections are preventable. Adequate preventive measures depend upon a knowledge of the source and spread of organisms and of the infant's capacity to resist invasion. With this knowledge a logical policy of management can be prepared and kept under review. This chapter will therefore deal with the general principles involved in preventing infection as well as discussing the diagnosis and management of particular infections. As the effect of infection alters as pregnancy progresses, the fetus as well as the newborn infant will be considered.

INTRAUTERINE INFECTION

Transplacental Infection

While the uterine membranes are intact the most probable route by which infection can reach the fetus is via the maternal bloodstream across the placenta into the fetal circulation.

RUBELLA

From extensive studies of pregnant women exposed to the virus of rubella (German measles) it is clear that this virus readily crosses the placenta and affects the fetus.

Abortion. In the very early stages of pregnancy the infected embryo may die and be aborted. During the first eight weeks, when the organs are developing, transplacental rubella infection may cause abnormal development of one or more organs but allow life to continue.

The heart, eyes and ears are the commonest sites of abnormality (Chap. 11). At later stages in pregnancy more disseminated evidence of infection is found in those infants who survive to delivery.

Purpura occurs because of thrombocytopenia, the liver and spleen are enlarged and there may be jaundice.

The long bones on radiological examination often show evidence of areas of translucency and increased density.

Retinal pigmentation is evident on ophthalmoscopy.

Microcephaly may be present at birth or be noted on later examination.

Incidence. When the mother has been infected in the first four months of pregnancy 20 to 25 per cent of the infants will show evidence of intrauterine infection.

PREVENTION

There is no treatment for rubella virus infection. Following exposure protection can be given by the injection of specific antirubella IgG where this is available. There is insufficient evidence to justify the use of standard IgG in the previously recommended doses but larger doses may be more useful.

Immunization. Knowledge of the harmful effect of rubella infection in pregnancy is widespread and causes great anxiety to many mothers. In pregnant women with no natural immunity who have been exposed to infection the question of a therapeutic abortion has to be considered seriously. The development of an effective rubella vaccine gives promise of a more efficient means of eliminating this problem. In many areas school girls who have no immunity from natural infection are immunized with rubella vaccine. It is hoped that this will provide complete protection during later pregnancies. With wider application of prophylactic immunization it should be possible to eliminate rubella as a problem during pregnancy.

OTHER VIRUS INFECTIONS

Rubella has been selected from the virus diseases because it is a common condition and readily recognized. It has therefore been relatively easy to establish a connection between rubella infection in the mother and abnormality in the fetus. Other virus infections cross the placenta and several are known to be associated with an increased incidence of abortion. In infections such as measles, chickenpox, smallpox, vaccinia and herpes simplex the fetus may be infected and if the infection occurs late in pregnancy the infant may be born with the characteristic rash of the infection. Figure 13.1 shows an infant of 2 days with chickenpox. Mother developed her rash one day after the infant.

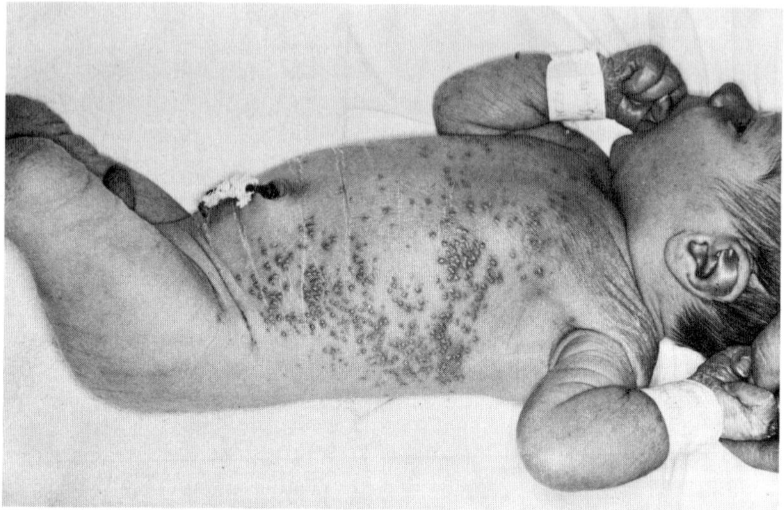

Figure 13.1 Chickenpox on second day of life. Mother developed her rash the following day.

OTHER INTRAUTERINE INFECTIONS

Other intrauterine infections may become evident only after the infant has been delivered as the mothers have shown no evidence of illness during pregnancy. Typical of these is cytomegalovirus (CMV) infection.

Cytomegalovirus infection. As the mother will rarely have symptoms it is not possible to fix the time of infection. Infection is probably transplacental during the period of maternal viraemia. The infant may be stillborn or alive but ill. In those severely infected there is enlargement of the liver and spleen, jaundice, haemorrhage, purpura and choroidoretinitis. There may be evidence of encephalitis with cerebral calcification on X-ray examinations. No treatment is available and it is unusual for infants to survive more than a few hours or days.

Toxoplasmosis. Similar clinical features are found in infants with congenital toxoplasmosis due to transplacental infection with a protozoon, *Toxoplasma gondii.*

Syphilis. Some non-viral maternal infections such as syphilis can be recognized by antenatal serological testing. Where infection is present, appropriate treatment in early pregnancy will prevent infection of the fetus, which does not occur before the fourth month and is more likely to occur later in pregnancy. Affected infants may be stillborn. Those born alive have an enlarged liver and spleen and develop snuffles, a watery and later purulent nasal discharge. A skin rash appears from the second week onward, X-ray of the long bones shows osteochondritis and periostitis in about 90 per cent of affected infants. Treatment with penicillin is highly effective.

Ascending Infection

PREMATURE RUPTURE OF MEMBRANES

Premature rupture of membranes allows organisms present in the maternal vagina to spread to the amniotic cavity and to be inhaled by the fetus.

Intrauterine pneumonia. The resulting infections are generally in the form of a diffuse pneumonia and the organisms isolated include non-haemolytic streptococci, *Escherichia coli* and other Gram-negative bacteria, *Listeria monocytogenes* and Monilia. Death may occur before delivery but in those born alive prompt and appropriate antibiotic therapy may prevent death.

Bacterial swabs taken from the ear in which infected liquor may have been trapped can give early indication of the organisms involved.

Treatment. Opinions differ as to the advisability of giving antibiotic treatment to the mother when membranes have ruptured prematurely, or to the infant following delivery. Controlled trials have not shown that prophylactic antibiotic treatment reduces mortality or morbidity. Careful bacteriological screening of infants suspected of having suffered intrauterine infection is advisable so that the appropriate antibiotic therapy can be started at the first clinical sign of infection.

Intrapartum Infection

The differentiation between infection acquired *in utero* following rupture of the membranes and infection acquired during passage of the fetus down the birth canal is mainly one of timing.

The organisms acquired are similar but the infant infected during delivery will not show clinical evidence of infection for a day or more after birth.

LISTERIA MONOCYTOGENES

Listeria monocytogenes infection acquired before delivery generally presents at birth as aspiration pneumonia. Other infants present later in the first week of life with signs of septicaemia and meningitis. In these infection was probably acquired during delivery. Treatment with ampicillin alone or in combination with penicillin or kanamycin has proved effective if given sufficiently early.

GONORRHOEA

Infants of mothers suffering from gonorrhoea are liable to a severe form of conjunctivitis due to contamination of the conjunctival sac during delivery.

Ophthalmia neonatorum. With the present increase in the incidence of gonorrhoea, gonococcal ophthalmia neonatorum is once again appearing. Diagnosis may be delayed by the use of chloramphenicol eye drops which suppress clinical signs without eradicating the infection in many cases.

Prophylaxis. The use of prophylactic antiseptic eye drops (e.g. 1 per cent silver nitrate) is associated with a chemical conjuctivitis in some infants and is not fully effective in preventing infection.

Prenatal screening of mothers, particularly of those with a vaginal discharge, and appropriate treatment of those shown to be infected is the most effective prophylaxis for the infant. Unfortunately gonococcal infection may be atypical and not suspected clinically. The affected infant should be treated with penicillin given locally and systematically.

OTHER ORGANSIMS

Other organisms including Gram-negative bacilli and Monilia may be acquired in sufficient numbers during delivery to cause subsequent clinical infection of the skin or deeper tissues, particularly where there has been a break in the skin surfaces.

Colonization

The great majority of infants are free of organisms when labour begins and pick up only small numbers during delivery. Swabs taken from skin surfaces after birth produce growths of organisms of the type found in the maternal vagina.

ENVIRONMENT

During the first few days of life these are generally replaced by other organisms acquired from the infant's immediate environment. In the 1950s the predominant organism in most hospital nurseries was the staphylococcus and many studies were made of the pattern of spread of this organism in the progressive colonization of individual infants.

SITES OF COLONIZATION

These studies showed that the infant's nose, throat, umbilicus, axillae and perineum which are normally sterile at birth became colonized within the first few days of life. The umbilicus is the first site to be colonized. Of the skin sites the perineum and axillae tend to become heavily colonized. The spread of organisms from one infant to another may take place by contact with attendants' hands, common surfaces into which more than one infant comes into contact or from the dust suspended in the air. New organisms are introduced by infected attendants or by symptomless carriers.

GRAM-NEGATIVE ORGANISMS

Although much of our knowledge of the spread of organisms in nurseries came from studies of staphylococci these organisms are no longer the dominant organisms in most nurseries and their place has been taken by a variety of Gram-negative organisms including *E. coli*, *Bacillus proteus* and *Pseudomonas pyocyanea*. Less is known about the method of spread of these organisms. As they flourish in a moist environment they are often called the 'water bugs'. They are particularly likely to contaminate incubators, suction apparatus and respirators.

VIRUSES

Our knowledge of viral colonization of the newborn infant is relatively scanty because of the difficulty and expense involved in isolation of viruses. As will be shown later, clinical viral infections occur in the newborn and it is reasonable to suppose that infants can be colonized by viruses without clinical infection when the defence mechanisms are sufficient to contain the number of viruses encountered.

Spread of Organisms

PROPHYLACTIC MEASURES

Several factors have been shown to be involved in the spread of organisms to newborn infants in a nursery environment and, as many of these are controllable, increasing knowledge has led to improved means of reducing the environmental flora to levels at which colonization occurs with minimum risk of infection. Such methods have also reduced the risk of epidemic spread of infection should this be introduced. The overall morbidity and mortality from infection is therefore less of a problem where suitable precautions are taken but there is always a risk that with the success achieved precautions are relaxed and infection can immediately become a major menace.

The prophylactic measures advisable are matters of policy in the design and staffing of nurseries as much as the detailed management of the individual infant.

Adequate space per infant, preventing infants' cots being closely packed together, has in our experience been as important as expensive methods such as air conditioning of nurseries.

Good architectural design of nurseries avoiding dust traps and allowing easy cleaning together with planning which prevents excessive movement of personnel help to reduce the number of air-borne organisms.

Design of equipment should bear in mind the possibility of organisms becoming trapped in inaccessible areas and allow for the effective disinfection of all equipment used. This helps to reduce sources of organisms previously often not suspect.

The use of disposable equipment has greatly improved the situation although at a considerable financial cost.

PROCEDURES

Of equal importance are the detailed planning of medical, nursing and other procedures in areas where infants are being nursed. In general the object is to reduce the contact between the infant, other infants and the staff to an absolute minimum. Such contact may be direct or indirect by objects which touch more than one infant. Apart from the air the most likely shared surfaces are the hands of the infants' attendants.

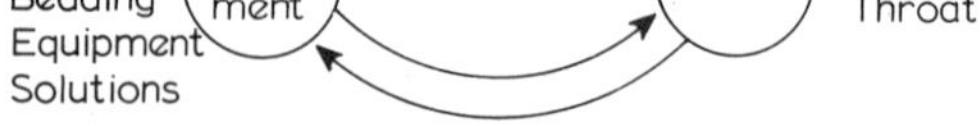

Figure 13.2 Circle of contact whereby infection is transferred.

A circle of contact (Fig. 13.2) can be envisaged and it is essential to break this wherever possible without making life unreasonable for the mother, infant or hospital staff. By using disposable materials such as paper to cover common points of contact like the pan of a weighing machine direct spread of infection can be prevented.

Cot nursing the infant reduces many of the periods of common contact in changing or bathing rooms.

Rooming-in, with the baby nursed alongside the mother, has many advantages where adequate space has been allowed for this.

Cohort nursing, whereby batches of infants born about the same time are nursed together in small nurseries, is aimed at reducing the number of infants with whom an individual infant comes into contact. The small nurseries are emptied as each cohort leaves and thoroughly cleaned before the next cohort is admitted. Such a system is costly in space, equipment and staff and is seldom justifiable under normal circumstances. It is, however, an important means of management when clinical infection such as gastroenteritis has appeared in a nursery.

Resistance to Infection

As was explained earlier, clinical infection will appear in the infant only where the number or virulence of the organisms present is greater than the infant's ability to resist infection.

The balance may be upset by an overwhelming number of invading organisms or by lack of resistance on the part of the host.

DEFENCE MECHANISMS

At all ages the body provides a number of defence mechanisms against infection.

The skin and mucous membranes remain our first and principal line of defence. During delivery the skin may be abraded and any break offers a route of access for organisms. Resuscitative measures are liable to damage the mucous membranes of the nose, mouth, pharynx and larynx.

The inflammatory response is well established before birth but the newborn infant has poor ability to concentrate the response at the site of infection.

IMMUNOGLOBULINS

Maternal immunoglobulins do not cross the placenta with the exception of IgG, which crosses to the fetus in significant amounts. This transfer occurs mainly during the last trimester of pregnancy and maternal IgG gradually disappears from the infant during the first few weeks of life.

Fetal immunoglobulins IgG, IgM and probably IgE are produced in the spleen from about midterm onwards but in the absence of an antigenic stimulus during pregnancy there is no IgA or IgM in the cord blood. Where intrauterine infection has occurred both IgA and IgM may be raised in the cord blood.

Newborn immunoglobulins. IgA appears in secretions after birth before it appears in the serum. Synthesis of IgM is increased from shortly after birth but the process is slower in immature infants. IgG synthesis is slower to develop. As antibodies against Gram-negative bacteria belong mainly to the IgM group the relative lack of IgM in the newborn may explain their susceptibility to Gram-negative infection. Maternal IgG, on the other hand, grants temporary protection to many virus diseases.

IMMUNOLOGICAL COMPETENCE

Contrary to earlier belief it is now clear that the newborn infant is immunologically competent to deal with infection. It would appear, however, that the male is less efficient than the female in resisting infection as is shown by the male preponderance in morbidity and mortality from infective causes. There is evidence to suggest that immunoglobulin synthesis is related to a gene locus on the X chromosomes thus favouring females, who have a greater genetic diversity having inherited one X chromosome from each parent.

CLINICAL INFECTION

GRAM-POSITIVE ORGANISMS

When staphylococci and other Gram-positive organisms such as pyogenic streptococci are the causative organisms the first clinical signs of infection are often superficial and therefore visible with clinical signs of inflammation in the form of redness, swelling and production of pus. Blood spread to the deeper organs such as the lungs and bones may follow.

GRAM-NEGATIVE ORGANISMS

With Gram-negative organisms the reverse is frequently the case and infection presents in a widespread form with bacteraemia, urinary tract infection and meningitis. In such a situation the infant is systematically ill with a variety of clinical signs which are not specific to infection. It is unusual for a local site of inflammation to be obvious.

In this chapter infection has been divided into superficial visible infection and the less obvious deep systemic infection. This division is artificial and there is a considerable overlap between the two types. The distinction is, however, useful clinically and therapeutically. Superficial infections are more likely to contaminate the environment, and whereas they may be less of a risk to the individual affected they may create a greater risk to other infants. Deep infections are a more immediate threat to the infant concerned but, with the exception of gastroenteritis, are less likely to be a risk to other infants. Antibiotic therapy is essential for the management of deep infection but may not be called for in superficial infection.

Superficial Infection

Although the nose, throat, umbilicus and groins are the first sites to be colonized by organisms the commonest sites of superficial infection are the conjunctiva and the skin.

STICKY EYE

Sticky eye occurring in the first day of life is only rarely associated with bacterial infection and cleansing with saline is the only treatment required provided that swabs have been taken for culture.

CONJUNCTIVITIS

Conjunctivitis occurring after the first day or two of life may be due to a variety of organisms including viruses (Fig. 13.3). Treatment

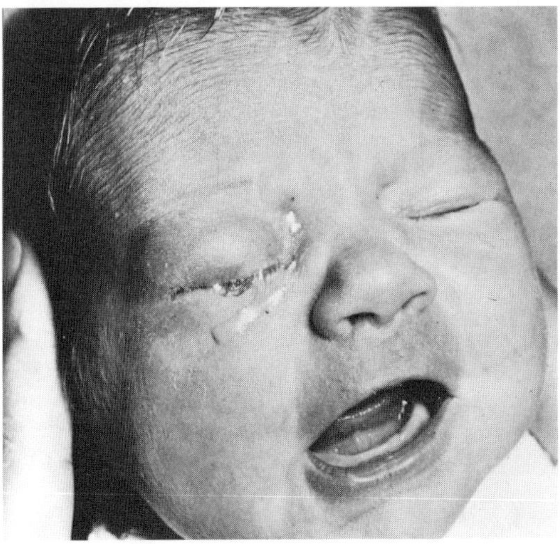

Figure 13.3 Purulent conjunctivitis.

should not be started until adequate specimens have been taken for bacteriological examination. The infant should be isolated and all swabs used for wiping the eyes kept in a disposable bag and burned. The mother should be asked about any vaginal discharge before delivery: bacteriological reports may be available to help in the choice of treatment. Chloramphenicol eye drops (0.25 per cent) are a suitable initial therapy remembering that the irrigant effect may be as important as the antibiotic effect. If the response is not satisfactory increase in frequency of treatment is more important than increase in number of drops per instillation. The risk of masking gonococcal infection has already been noted earlier. Should the initial smear or culture suggest the presence of gonococci treatment should be changed to a combination of local and systemic penicillin.

SKIN INFECTION

Skin infection with staphylococci has practically disappeared since the introduction of hexachlorophane washes for the skin of infants. The unconfirmed risk associated with this form of management has reduced the popularity of this preparation and skin sepsis is reappearing.

Pustules are the commonest presentation and present (Fig. 13.4)

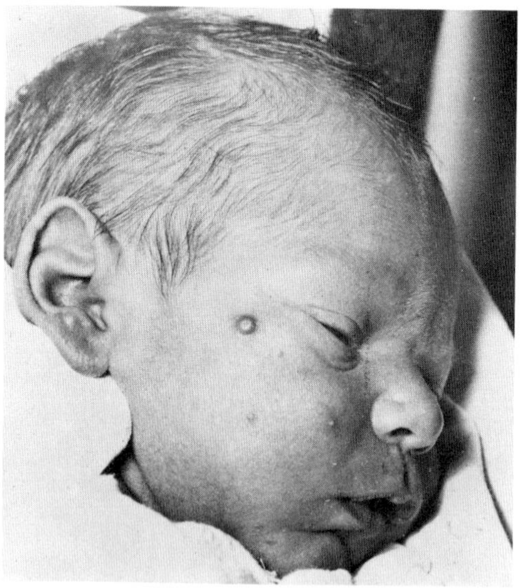

Figure 13.4 Skin pustules.

as small 1 to 2 mm vesicular projections containing pus and surrounded by an area of erythema. The yellow colour of the pustule distinguishes it from papular urticaria (Chap. 6). Rupture of the pustule leaves an ulcerated area and discharges highly infective material.

Pemphigus. Larger vesicles, particularly over the buttocks and trunk, may occur with staphylococcal or streptococcal infection and are termed *impetigo* or, in their most severe forms, *pemphigus.*

Ritter's disease. A more severe but fortunately rare form of skin infection produces exfoliation of large areas of skin (Fig. 13.5) and is called Ritter's disease or exfoliative dermatitis.

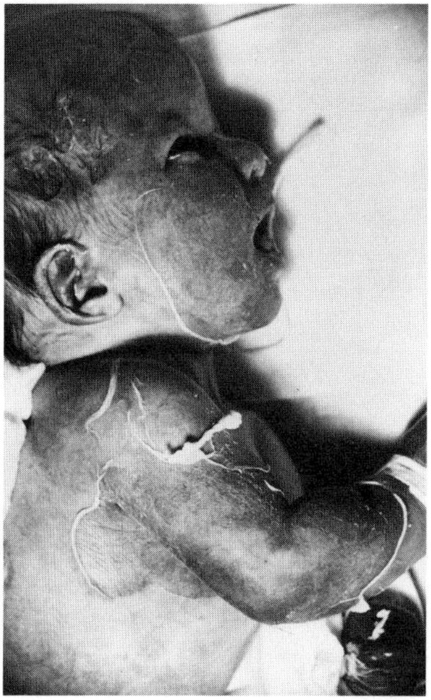

Figure 13.5 Exfoliative dermatitis (Ritter's disease).

Prevention. The most important aspect of treatment is prevention of contamination of the skin by the methods described above.

Isolation and barrier nursing are necessary for the child with skin infection.

Antiseptics, antibiotics. In the milder cases with skin pustules local antiseptic washes with pHisoHex solution or a similar preparation are often sufficient but in more severe cases of pemphigus and exfoliative dermatitis a systemic antibiotic is necessary. Penicillinase-resistant penicillins such as cloxacillin are generally the most suitable choice.

Flexures. Skin infection particularly in the flexures such as the axillae and groins may be due to Gram-positive and Gram-negative organisms. Between the buttocks and occasionally around the neck and behind the ears Monilia may be responsible. These sites are normally moist and poorly ventilated. Exposure and drying aid in treatment. Local antiseptic preparations such as surgical spirit or 1 per cent gentian violet in spirit may also be necessary.

PARONYCHIA

Paronychia is infection occurring in the nail folds of the skin. It is an added risk to the infant because of the ease with which he can infect other parts of his body by scratching. Because of the tightness of the skin around the nails the oedema of inflammation produces a rapid rise in pressure and infection may spread to proximal and deeper tissues (Fig. 13.6). In addition to the general treatment of skin

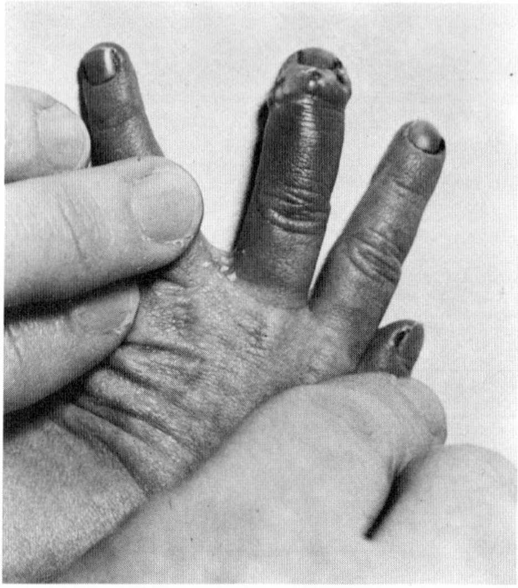

Figure 13.6 Paronychia.

infection the infant's limb should be immobilized and mitts applied so that he cannot scratch himself or his mother's breast with the infected finger.

ABSCESSES

The scalp, ears and face may be injured during delivery and local infection follow. Infection of the subcutaneous tissues gives rise to abscess formation. This may be seen in the infant's breast particularly if it is engorged. Laceration of the skin also allows access for organisms to deeper tissues and abscesses may be formed. A subcutaneous haemangioma is an ideal culture site for invading organisms.

OMPHALITIS

The umbilical stump is colonized early and occasionally clinical infection, omphalitis, occurs with spread to the surrounding skin. Further spread of infection may occur along the umbilical vein to the liver where abscess formation may occur.

STUFFY NOSE

Stuffy nose is the commonest manifestation of infection of mucous membranes and varies from a slight mucoid nasal discharge to a profuse mucopurulent discharge which seriously hampers breathing during feeding and therefore causes the infant distress. Viruses or a combination of virus and bacteria are generally responsible. Decongestant nose drops such as $\frac{1}{2}$ per cent ephedrine in saline relieve symptoms and the condition generally clears without further treatment. Should the infection pass down the respiratory tract a more serious situation develops.

THRUSH

The mouth is a relatively common site of infection particularly with *Candida albicans* producing thrush. This generally presents as a white coating of the tongue (Fig. 13.7) which cannot be removed with

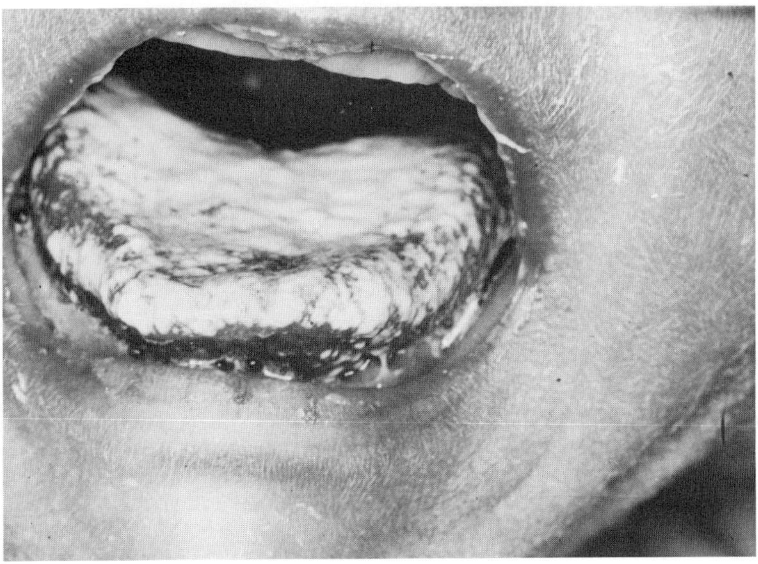

Figure 13.7 Extensive thrush on the tongue.

a spatula as can milk curds. Spread to the mucous membranes of the gums, cheeks and soft palate produces a deeper form of infection which is more difficult to eradicate. It is important therefore to recognize monilial infection as early as possible, when treatment with 1 per cent aqueous solution of gentian violet applied locally is likely to be effective. This is a messy form of treatment but cheaper than the alternative of nystatin 100000 units q.i.d. given by dropper into the mouth. Spread of thrush downwards into the gastrointestinal tract can produce a severe form of infection which in debilitated infants may prove fatal. This is a particular risk where wide-spectrum antibiotic therapy has been given for other forms of infection.

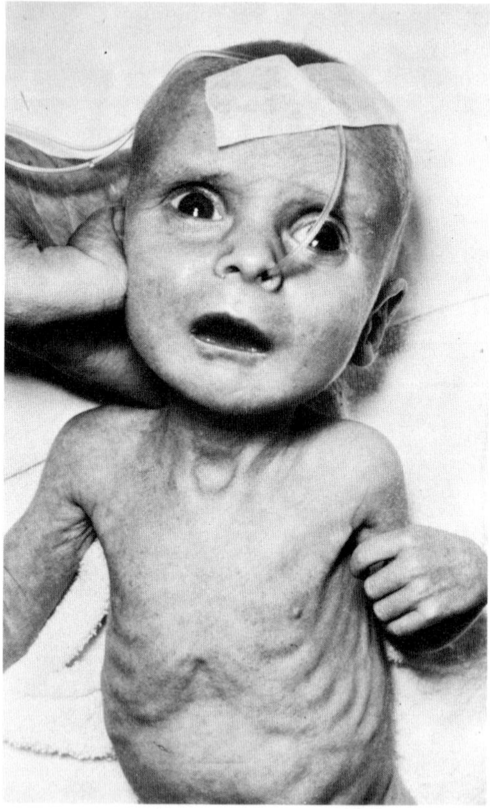

Figure 13.8 Seriously ill infant with Gram-negative bacteraemia and meningitis.

Deep Infections

As has been mentioned earlier, the signs of infection in the organs and deeper tissues are non-specific and this applies particularly to infection with Gram-negative organisms (Fig. 13.8) when there is rarely any superficial sign of inflammation as often occurs with Gram-positive infections.

BACTERAEMIA

Many deep infections are accompanied by bacteraemia and infection may occur simultaneously in several parts of the body. Infants dying of such infection may show at postmortem examination that there has been pyelonephritis, meningitis, pneumonia, osteomyelitis, arthritis or pericarditis (Fig. 13.9). The liver and spleen are

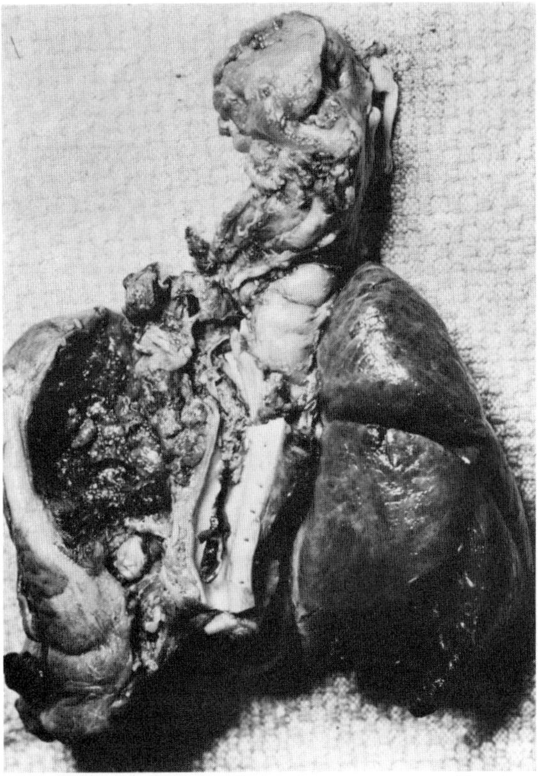

Figure 13.9 Postmortem specimen of infant who had widespread staphylococca infection with pyopneumothorax, mycotic aneurysm of the aorta and thrombosis.

frequently enlarged and abnormal as the result of circulating toxins. Widespread haemorrhage often occurs and death follows bleeding into the adrenal glands, lungs or brain. Microscopical examination in such cases often shows evidence of disseminated intravascular coagulation (Chap. 17).

CLINICAL PRESENTATION

Clinically such infants present with inactivity, feeding difficulty, weight loss, and these progress to circulatory collapse with a greyish pallor, episodes of cyanosis and rapid, shallow breathing and poor pulse. The abdomen becomes distended, the liver and spleen are large, jaundice and haemorrhages may develop. With renal infection the kidneys may be palpable and tender. The fontanelles become tense in meningitis. Joint swelling and bone tenderness may be noted. Vomiting and diarrhoea can develop whether or not infection is present in the gastrointestinal tract. The loss of fluid and electrolytes causes a further rapid deterioration in the infant's general condition and metabolic acidosis develops rapidly.

GASTROENTERITIS

Gastroenteritis in the newborn without systemic spread of infection produces a similar clinical picture of dehydration and collapse which cannot be distinguished clinically from parenteral infection. In both enteral and parenteral infection the downward course tends to be rapid and early recognition and treatment are essential. A rise in temperature is not always due to infection and in severe infection the temperature often falls to subnormal levels. The volume of the pulse is as important as the pulse rate. Above all it is the change in an infant's general activity and well-being which must be noted as a possible sign of infection.

INVESTIGATIONS OF DEEP INFECTIONS

Although physical examination may indicate the main site of infection it is essential that adequate specimens be obtained to check the possibility of infection at other sites before treatment is started. The bacteriological investigations suggested are shown in Table 13.1.

Table 13.1 Specimens to be taken for bacteriological examination in suspected deep infections

Swabs from
Nose
Throat
Ear
Umbilicus
Groin
Blood culture
Urine (preferably by suprapubic aspiration)
Stool
Cerebrospinal fluid

Our experience shows that urine culture is the investigation most likely to be omitted unless its importance is appreciated. Techniques for obtaining urine including suprapubic aspiration of the bladder are described in Chapter 19.

ANTIBIOTICS

Once the bacteriological specimens have been obtained antibiotic treatment should be started. The choice of individual antibiotic depends on knowledge of the antibiotic sensitivity of the likely invading organism or of the environmental flora (see below).

Intravenous fluids are generally required both to restore the circulation and to correct coexistent metabolic disorders. Where bleeding is occurring the cause must be defined and appropriate treatment given (Chap. 17).

Intensive therapy. Severely infected infants require intensive therapy and where suitable facilities do not exist early transfer to a suitably equipped centre is advisable before the infant deteriorates to a state which would make a journey unjustifiable. This implies close observation and recognition of the earliest signs of infection.

Source of Infection

Outbreaks of infection in nurseries indicate a break in the preventive measures employed. With low birth-weight infants nursed in incubators the problem is often a local one involving that one infant only. When several large well babies become infected, however, a source of infection with access to many infants has to be sought. This may be a member of staff or a mother who has a clinical infection or who is a carrier.

Spread may occur by direct contact or indirectly by common objects handled. The maximum risk occurs if an infected person is involved in preparing feeds. The common types of organisms to be introduced into nurseries by adults are streptococci, staphylococci, shigellae and salmonellae.

EPIDEMICS

Epidemics of skin and umbilical infection have been virtually eliminated by skin antisepsis. Gastroenteritis remains the main epidemic infection in nurseries. A number of organisms may be involved but the most frequent belong to the group of typeable *E. coli* such as O–26, O–55, O–86, O–111, O–125 and O–126.

Epidemic diarrhoea of the newborn is a serious threat to nurseries and should an outbreak occur treatment of the individual infant must be accompanied by control of the epidemic. This involves barrier nursing of affected infants and cohort nursing of clean babies for whom separate clean accommodation and staff must be available. Should such measures fail the unit may have to be closed to further admissions until the outbreak has been controlled. Consultation between all members of the nursing, medical, laboratory and administrative staff is essential to make sure that each understands the other's position. Rapid planning will frequently curtail an outbreak before it is established.

Transferable drug resistance. The ability of organisms to transfer drug resistance to previously sensitive organisms can cause major problems in treatment if antibiotics are used unnecessarily. Co-ordination and planning are again essential.

Antibiotic Policies

Antibiotic policies are frequently talked about, less frequently put into effect. Nurseries for the newborn are suitable situations in which to formulate and test antibiotic policies. Our own experience has convinced us of the advantage of a firm policy for the use of antibiotics which limits the primary choice to a single antibiotic or antibiotic combination, the choice of which is based on knowledge of the environmental flora. The antibiotic chosen was originally changed at intervals of six months but this has now been extended to 12 months.

PROPHYLACTIC ANTIBIOTICS

Opinions differ as to the advisability of using antibiotics prophylactically. We have progressively reduced the use of antibiotics in the absence of suspected clinical infection without evidence of increase in infection. An antibiotic policy must be based on local information and no single policy is universally applicable.

REASSESSMENT

Any change in the environmental flora should lead to a reassessment of the antibiotic being used.

Throughout this chapter stress has been laid on the importance of policy decisions in the prevention and control of infection in hospital nurseries. Advance in the understanding of sources and spread of organisms have provided a basis on which sound policies can be based. The responsibility for carrying out such policies rests with the staff of the unit concerned. Education of new members of staff is essential, and regular reviews of results and reassessment of policy decision are necessary to maintain a high standard of vigilance and efficiency. Without these, infection continues to be a potential hazard to all infants in newborn nurseries.

FURTHER READING

Davies, P. A. (1971). Bacterial infection in the fetus and newborn. *Archives of Disease in Childhood*, **46**, 1–27.

Edelmann, C. M., Ogwo, J. E., Fine, B. P. & Martinez, A. B. (1973). The prevalence of bacteriuria in full-term and premature newborn infants. *Journal of Pediatrics*, **82**, 125–132.

Scopes, J. (1971). Problems of the newborn: vomiting, diarrhoea and infection. *British Medical Journal*, iv, 739–741.

Lancet (1971). Proteus in the nursery. i, 640.

14

Jaundice

Jaundice is the commonest abnormal physical sign in the newborn period, so much so that jaundice is described as being 'physiological' in the majority of affected infants. As jaundice may be associated with cerebral dysfunction and death it is clearly not always physiological and must be considered as a potentially serious condition. To understand the investigation and management of a jaundiced infant it is useful to have some knowledge of the metabolism of the pigment bilirubin which is the cause of the yellow discoloration of the tissues known clinically as jaundice.

Physiology

Bilirubin is one of the breakdown products of haemoglobin which the body excretes by two main forms of metabolism, hepatic conjugation and photodecomposition.

HEPATIC CONJUGATION

Conjugation of bilirubin with glucuronic acid changes fat-soluble bilirubin to water-soluble bilirubin diglucuronide which can then be excreted in the bile. The laboratory will report fat-soluble bilirubin as indirect-acting bilirubin and water-soluble bilirubin diglucuronide as direct-acting bilirubin. This process takes place in liver cells and is catalysed by the enzyme glucuronyl transferase which is not present in sufficient quantity in the first few days of life to deal with all the bilirubin presented to the liver. The level of bilirubin in the blood rises causing jaundice. In term babies enzyme activity is generally sufficient to deal with the bilirubin load by the third or fourth day of life, but in preterm babies it may not be present in the quantities required until the sixth or seventh day. Jaundice is therefore likely to be more marked in preterm infants. Jaundice from this cause is due to immaturity of liver function.

HEPATIC EXCRETION

Excretion of conjugated bilirubin into the bile canaliculi is an active process.

Obstructive jaundice occurs when the liver is unable to excrete conjugated bilirubin into the gastrointestinal tract by the bile duct system. The problem may occur in the liver cell, the intrahepatic biliary system or in the extrahepatic bile ducts. Particularly when the liver cell is involved both direct- and indirect-acting bilirubin may be abnormally raised in the blood and tissues.

Enterohepatic recirculation of bile occurs as some of the conjugated bilirubin passed into the bowel is deconjugated and reabsorbed.

PHOTODECOMPOSITION

Photodecomposition of bilirubin to water-soluble dipyrroles takes place in the skin under the stimulus of blue light and is not dependent on enzyme action. The dipyrroles are excreted in the urine. How much bilirubin is decomposed depends on the area of skin exposed to light and the length of exposure. In a clothed infant under normal lighting conditions the amount is probably small and special conditions have to be created to make this method of disposal of bilirubin of clinical importance. This is described later in this chapter as phototherapy.

Pathology

BILIRUBIN ENCEPHALOPATHY

If neither of these pathways is sufficient to dispose of the bilirubin formed the level of bilirubin in the serum rises progressively and the infant becomes increasingly jaundiced as bilirubin passes from blood into the skin and other tissues such as the brain which accept fat-soluble substances. Brain cells do not tolerate the presence of bilirubin, and cell death may occur. The clinical effect of this is called bilirubin encephalopathy, which is evident clinically as lethargy, disinclination to feed, drowsiness and eventually coma. A sunsetting appearance of the eyes may be obvious (Fig. 14.1). As brain damage increases, twitching, convulsions and episodes of cyanosis occur. Recovery is possible in all but the most severely affected infants but there are frequently permanent residual signs in the form of high tone nerve deafness and cerebral palsy of the athetoid type.

KERNICTERUS

Where death results from bilirubin encephalopathy examination of the brain shows areas of yellow discoloration in the basal nuclei and other parts of the brain and spinal cord (Fig. 14.2). These are due to deposition of bilirubin and cell death. The condition is termed kernicterus. Treatment of kernicterus is not possible and management must aim at forestalling the passage of bilirubin into brain cells. This can best be done by recognizing those infants in which bilirubin encephalopathy is liable to occur, watching their progress carefully and applying treatment at a stage when the risk of brain

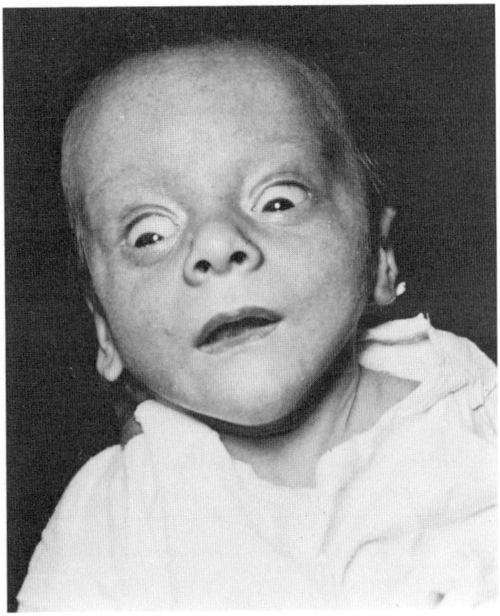

Figure 14.1 Sunsetting appearance of eyes in infant with kernicterus.

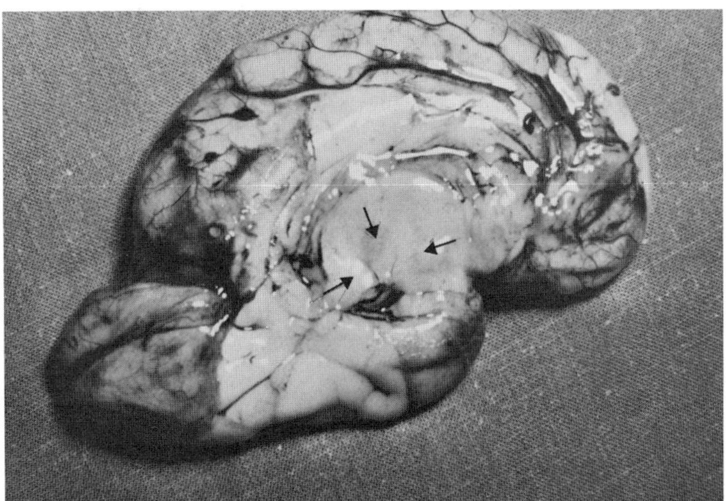

Figure 14.2 Brain of infant of 28 weeks gestation who died from kernicterus. The arrows indicate where yellow staining was evident.

damage exceeds the risk of the treatment proposed. It is therefore necessary to be able to assess the chances of brain damage occurring in any jaundiced infant and to know the relative dangers of possible therapeutic regimes.

CONTRIBUTORY FACTORS

Hyperbilirubinaemia. The risk to the infant increases with progressive rise of serum indirect-acting bilirubin but the level of bilirubin at which encephalopathy occurs varies from infant to infant.

Acidosis, *hypoglycaemia*, *hypoxia* and presence in the blood of substances such as free fatty acids which compete with bilirubin for albumin-binding sites are other factors involved. We have seen kernicterus in severely acidotic immature infants in whom the serum bilirubin did not exceed 13 mg per 100 ml. Healthy mature infants have had bilirubin levels of 25 mg per 100 ml or more and shown no evidence of bilirubin encephalopathy. The serum bilirubin level remains, however, the best means available at present of assessing the risk of brain damage in jaundiced infants.

Albumin-binding capacity. When the molar concentration of the bilirubin/albumin ratio exceeds 1/1 the albumin-binding capacity is likely to be exceeded and the infant is in danger. This ratio corresponds to a serum bilirubin level of 20 mg per 100 ml at an albumin concentration of approximately 3 g per 100 ml. It must be stressed, however, that immature acidotic infants may be at risk at bilirubin levels well below 20 mg per 100 ml.

CLINICAL CAUSES

Our chief concern in the management of the jaundiced infant is the prevention of bilirubin encephalopathy. As bilirubin is no longer toxic once it has been made water soluble it is important to differentiate those causes of non-obstructive jaundice which are associated with high levels of indirect-acting bilirubin from those causing obstructive jaundice in which direct-acting, water-soluble, bilirubin is a major cause of jaundice. As the risk of bilirubin encephalopathy is highest in non-obstructive jaundice, and as this is much more common than the obstructive type, it will be dealt with first and at greater length.

Non-obstructive Jaundice

The commoner factors likely to increase the serum indirect-acting bilirubin and to produce a non-obstructive jaundice are shown in Table 14.1.

Immaturity of Liver Function

Adequate liver function is essential for the conjugation of bilirubin and its excretion into the biliary tract. In some term infants and in the majority of preterm infants liver function is temporarily inadequate. The more mature the infant the more rapidly does liver function mature to cope with the load of bilirubin presented. The longer the delay until such maturity of function occurs the greater the risk of bilirubin rising in the serum to levels which may produce bilirubin encephalopathy.

Table 14.1 Causes of non-obstructive jaundice

IMMATURITY OF LIVER FUNCTION
Physiological jaundice
jaundice of immaturity
INHIBITION OF LIVER FUNCTION
Breast milk jaundice
HAEMOLYTIC ANAEMIAS
ABO incompatibility
Rh incompatibility
Glucose-6-phosphate-dehydrogenase (G6PDH) deficiency
Spherocytosis
Haemoglobinopathies
Severe infections
Drug sensitivity
Extravasated blood
Other rare causes
Hypothyroidism
Crigler-Najjar syndrome
Congenital pyloric stenosis
Malrotation of the intestine
Cystic fibrosis

TIME SCALE

Time is therefore of great importance in the assessment of jaundice. The earlier the jaundice appears and the longer it persists the greater is the risk to the infant. In term healthy infants physiological jaundice, which is due to a relatively minor degree of hepatic immaturity, appears on the second or third day of life and clears in two or three days as liver function improves. In preterm infants the onset is also on the second or third day but persists for longer and may not reach its maximum until the end of the first week of life.

Jaundice in the first 24 hours. Jaundice appearing on the first day of life must never be accepted as physiological and is highly suggestive of a haemolytic anaemia or of severe liver dysfunction as may occur in infection.

Persistence of jaundice. Similarly, any jaundice which persists for more than 10 to 14 days after birth must always be investigated thoroughly with particular reference to signs of obstructive jaundice. If there is no evidence of biliary obstruction the possibility of hypothyroidism has to be considered, as persistent jaundice in the neonatal period may be the first clinical evidence of this condition.

Haemolytic Anaemias

The incidence of haemolytic anaemia varies according to the racial background of the infant. In European countries Rh incompatability was until recently the most frequent cause of severe haemolytic anaemia. As shown below, preventive treatment may soon make this problem a rarity. Throughout the world incompatibility of the fetus and mother for the ABO blood groups is the most frequent potential cause of haemolytic anaemia but fortunately it seldom results in severe degrees of jaundice. In some Mediterranean races, in Negroes and Far Eastern races deficiency of the enzyme glucose-6-phosphate dehydrogenase (G6PDH) is a much commoner cause of haemolytic anaemia than Rh incompatibility. Abnormalities of red cell membrane in such conditions as thalassaemia and elliptocytosis are associated with unusual haemoglobins and are a cause of haemolysis in certain races.

Blood Group Incompatibility

Blood group incompatibility occurs when the fetus has inherited from its father a blood group such as the Rh factor which is not present in the mother. Should fetal red blood cells pass across the placenta into the mother in sufficient numbers she may become sensitized to these foreign red cells and produce an antibody (immunoglobulin) which promotes the destruction of the foreign cells. Should such an immunoglobulin pass back to the fetus across the placenta it will cause haemolysis of the fetal cells, haemoglobin will be released and break down, with resulting anaemia and the production of bilirubin. *In utero* this bilirubin is excreted via the placenta into the maternal circulation and dealt with by the mother. If the placenta has not been able to excrete all the bilirubin presented the infant at birth may be slightly jaundiced and jaundice is likely to increase rapidly. The infant may also be anaemic and have a large liver and spleen due to increased intrauterine haemopoiesis. Where haemolysis has been very marked *in utero* the degree of anaemia can be sufficient to cause cardiac failure with the accumulation of oedema which, when severe, is called *hydrops fetalis* (Fig. 14.3). In severe cases haemorrhage may occur into the skin or deeper tissues. The infant may be stillborn.

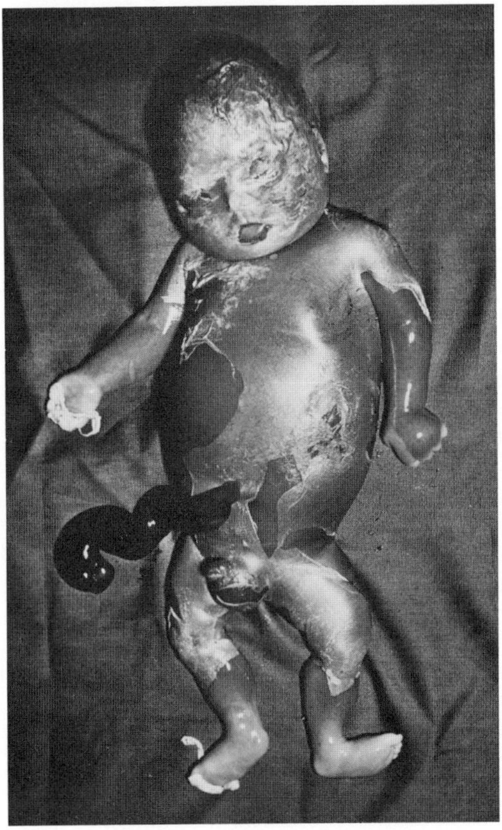

Figure 14.3 Hydrops fetalis.

ABO INCOMPATIBILITY

Incompatibility of the ABO blood groups occurs in the situations shown in Table 14.2. Fortunately even where incompatible fetal cells enter mother's circulation and immunoglobulin reaches the fetus the resulting haemolytic anaemia is generally relatively mild and rarely causes jaundice of a severity likely to require treatment.

Table 14.2 ABO incompatibility

Mother's group	Fetus group Compatible	Fetus group Incompatible
O	O	A, B, AB
A	O, A	B, AB
B	O, B	A, AB
AB	O, A, B, AB	

Where both ABO and Rh incompatibility occur in the same pregnancy the ABO incompatibility frequently protects mother from being sensitized by Rh-positive fetal cells.

Rh Incompatibility

PREVENTION

Rhesus (Rh) incompatibility occurs where mother is Rh-negative and father and fetus Rh-positive. Among European races approximately 15 per cent of the population is Rh-negative. It is now possible to prevent almost all Rh-negative women from being sensitized by Rh-positive cells from the fetus. The passage of cells from the fetus to mother is likely to occur late in pregnancy most frequently during labour, particularly where there are such complications as toxaemia of pregnancy, caesarean section and breech delivery. Fetal red cells can be recognized in mother's blood by the acid elution technique. Injection of an immune anti-D (Rh) globulin into mother destroys the fetal red cells before sensitization takes place. Where Rh-negative mothers are adequately supervised throughout all pregnancies it should therefore be possible to eliminate Rh incompatibility as a cause of jaundice in infants.

SENSITIZATION

Women may be sensitized to the Rh and other factors which they do not themselves possess by means other than pregnancy. These generally involve the injection of blood or blood products containing the antigen. This is now fortunately an unusual ocurrence but in spite of the widespread use of preventive measures the possibility of blood group sensitization must always be kept in mind as a cause of jaundice in the newborn.

ANTENATAL RECOGNITION

Some blood group incompatibilities can be recognized antenatally by examination of maternal serum and liquor amnii as discussed in Chapter 4. Such examination may indicate that a fetus is severely affected and in danger of dying within a few days. In such situations the obstetrician and paediatrician have to consult together to decide whether it is safer to induce labour and accept the risk of delivering the infant prematurely, or to transfuse the infant *in utero* in an attempt to prolong fetal life until the risk of the haemolytic anaemia outweighs the risk associated with that period of gestation.

Intrauterine transfusion. In general intrauterine transfusion is preferable to induction of labour before 32 weeks gestation but the advantage lies with delivery after 32 weeks. Decisions of this nature should only be made at centres used to dealing with such problems.

With the decreasing incidence of Rh incompatibility it is important that sensitized mothers be referred for advice as to management to a limited number of regional centres who can maintain the high standard of judgment based on experience necessary to produce a successful outcome.

OTHER CAUSES OF HAEMOLYTIC ANAEMIAS

In spite of the likely continuing decline in the incidence of Rh incompatibility, jaundice in infants will remain a major problem for those managing nurseries for the newborn because of the other factors involved in the production of jaundice. With the increase in movement of families between countries there is need for awareness of causes of jaundice which were previously rare in this country. These include deficiency of the enzyme G6PDH, which results in increased liability to haemolysis as does the presence of an abnormal haemoglobin within the cell. Infections, particularly with Gram-negative organisms, must always be looked for where jaundice is otherwise not satisfactorily explained. Drugs such as Synkavit, the synthetic analogue of vitamin K, in doses of 15 mg or more per day is associated with an increase in haemolysis. Extravasated blood as in a large bruise or cephalhaematoma increases the load of bilirubin and may be a significant contributing cause of jaundice.

INHIBITION OF LIVER FUNCTION

Breast milk jaundice. Substances which may impair liver function include some steroids. The increased incidence of jaundice in breast-fed infants may be related to a steroid contained in the milk of some mothers giving rise to 'breast milk jaundice'. Infants of mothers who have been taking the 'pill' shortly before conception occurred are reported to have higher levels of bilirubin than infants of mothers who were not on the 'pill'. Novobiocin is believed to inhibit the activity of glucuronyl transferase.

RARER CAUSES OF JAUNDICE

The persisting jaundice associated with hypothyroidism is due to depression of enzyme activity whereas in families with the Crigler-Najjar syndrome there is inherited deficiency of glucuronyl transferase. In infants with obstruction of the pylorus or small intestine, jaundice may, at least in part, be non-obstructive and clears with correction of the obstruction to the bowel.

Obstructive Jaundice

Obstructive jaundice has a greenish tinge which may be distinguishable clinically from the purer yellow of jaundice associated with raised levels of indirect-acting bilirubin. Observation of the stool and urine is important in any infant with jaundice. Where the jaundice is of obstructive type the urine will be dark brown in colour due to the excess of bile pigments (but not of urobilinogen) and the stools are very pale in colour and will be white in the early stage of complete obstructive jaundice. Blood examination will show raised levels of direct-acting bilirubin which will fall if the obstruction is relieved.

Obstructive jaundice can be due to hepatitis or to abnormality of the bile duct system.

HEPATITIS

Hepatitis may be due to infection or to the toxic effect of certain chemical substances.

Infective hepatitis evident at or shortly after birth would have been acquired antenatally by the passage of organisms across the placenta. Syphilis, cytomegalic inclusion body disease and toxoplasmosis are acquired by this method. During delivery viruses such as *Herpes simplex* or bacteria such as *Listeria monocytogenes* may be acquired and cause hepatitis within a few days of birth. Infection may be introduced into the umbilical vein following umbilical sepsis, particularly if a catheter has been introduced through the infected area. Further spread of infection to the liver occurs by the portal venous system, and multiple liver abscesses or a more generalized hepatitis follows. All of these conditions will be associated with jaundice and enlargement of the liver. In addition there are often enlargement of the spleen and signs of more generalized infection (Chap. 13).

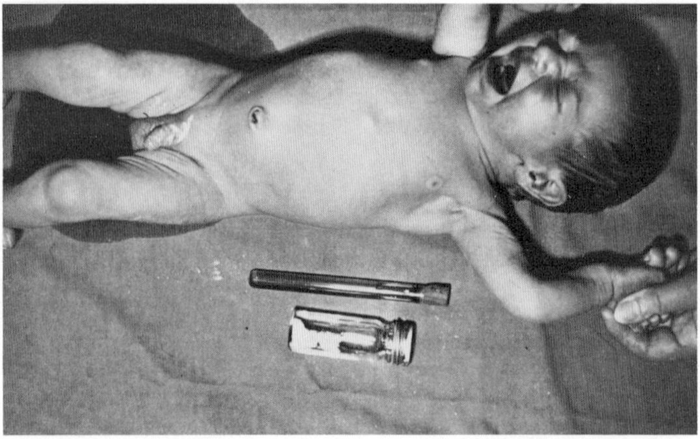

Figure 14.4 Obstructive jaundice showing dark urine and pale stool.

Chemical hepatitis. More rarely hepatitis may also occur in the first week of life because of the deposition of toxic chemical substances in liver cells. Jaundice due to such hepatitis may be the presenting sign of galactosaemia (Chap. 11).

ABNORMALITIES OF THE BILE DUCTS

Congenital obliteration of the bile ducts may occur within the liver or in the extrahepatic system and cause the clinical signs of obstructive jaundice (Fig. 14.4). A cyst of the bile duct (choledochal cyst) may result in intermittent or permanent obstruction of the biliary system. The differential diagnosis between hepatitis and mechanical obstruction of the bile ducts is difficult during the first month of life. In the infant who is not acutely ill and in whom treatable causes of hepatitis have been excluded there appears to be no advantage in carrying out a diagnostic laparotomy until the third or fourth month of life.

Assessment of the Jaundiced Infant

Clinical assessment must bear in mind significant information obtained from the mother's antenatal history which may clearly suggest Rh incompatibility or other cause of haemolytic anaemia.

TIME OF ONSET

Infants who are active and feeding well and in whom the onset of jaundice occurred after 24 hours of age require less urgent investigation than the sick infant who has become jaundiced on the first day of life. In such an infant urgent investigation is necessary to establish the cause of jaundice and to apply appropriate treatment in the hope of preventing the onset of bilirubin encephalopathy and kernicterus.

HISTORY AND EXAMINATION

The following aspects of the history and clinical examination require particular attention:

- Maternal and family history
- Time of onset of jaundice: N.B. first 24 hours
- Rate of increase in depth of jaundice
- General state of the infant including gestational age, activity, ability to feed
- Size of liver and spleen
- Pallor
- Signs of haemorrhage
- Colour of urine and stool.

The laboratory investigations required will vary with the history and clinical findings but in all significantly jaundiced infants the following investigations are necessary to determine the need for further investigation or treatment:

Infant and mother
- ABO and Rh blood groups
- Coomb's test

Infant
- Serum bilirubin—direct- and indirect-acting
- Haemoglobin or packed cell volume.

DIFFERENTIAL DIAGNOSIS

On the basis of the history, the clinical examination and the investigations listed it should then be possible to decide if the jaundice is due to a haemolytic anaemia or to some form of hepatitis. In the absence of indications of either of these conditions it is probable that the jaundice is due to immaturity of hepatic function. Further investigation of the cause of unexplained haemolytic anaemia will involve more detailed examination of the racial and family history and is likely to require some or all of the following investigations:

- Blood film
- Reticulocyte and platelet count
- Red cell fragility
- Red cell enzymes
- Haemoglobin electrophoresis
- Blood culture
- Urine culture.

Where the preliminary findings indicate the probability of hepatitis the following additional investigations are indicated:

- Blood culture
- Urine—microscopic examination, chemical tests for reducing substances, glucose, bile, urobilinogen, culture for bacteria and viruses
- Liver function tests.

When the preliminary investigations do not establish a diagnosis and if the infant's condition is deteriorating referral to a regional centre for more detailed investigation will be indicated.

TREATMENT

The treatment of the jaundiced infant must include both the correction of the underlying condition causing the jaundice where this is possible and the protection of the infant from the potentially harmful effects of bilirubin. Investigation to establish the cause of the jaundice is therefore an essential part of the management of the jaundiced infant. Similarly it is necessary to assess the urgency of the need for treatment. The majority of jaundiced infants suffer no ill effect from their short period of mild jaundice and require no treatment other than that of close observation.

ASSESSMENT OF URGENCY

Prophylactic treatment by prevention of preterm delivery, prevention of acidosis by early feeding, stimulation of photo-decomposition by exposure to phototherapy, enzyme induction by phenobarbitone will all reduce the need for more active treatment and are most important factors in the management of the jaundiced infant. These methods are, however, insufficient to deal with more severe degrees of jaundice and more active and immediate treatment is required for the infant in whom the jaundice is deepening rapidly, particularly if there are early signs of bilirubin encephalopathy. Other signs indicating urgency are profound anaemia, signs of haemorrhage and marked enlargement of the liver and spleen.

PROPHYLAXIS

Reduction of the incidence of preterm delivery and the early institution of feeding have already been discussed in Chapters 4, 8 and 9.

PHOTOTHERAPY

Phototherapy, which aims at increasing the decomposition of bilirubin in the skin to non-toxic water-soluble dipyrroles can be achieved by exposing the infant to a potent source of blue light. This is most readily carried out in an incubator with the infant fully exposed apart from the eyes which should be covered by a mask made from non-irritant material (Fig. 14.5). In Britain natural daylight varies so considerably in intensity that it cannot be relied upon to provide an adequate source of blue light for a long enough period each day.

Artificial light sources are therefore required and are most readily available in the forms of fluorescent tubes which emit more blue light than tungsten filament bulbs. The fluorescent tubes can be mounted with reflectors in frames which are mobile and can be placed over an incubator (Fig. 14.6). Such phototherapy units deliver about 200 foot candles of light at the level of the infant.

Indications. As phototherapy is more effective in preventing a rise in serum bilirubin than in reducing a high level of bilirubin, treatment

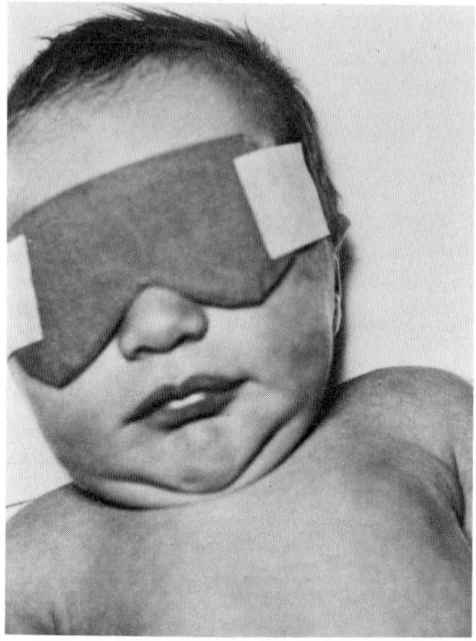

Figure 14.5 Mask for protecting eyes during phototherapy.

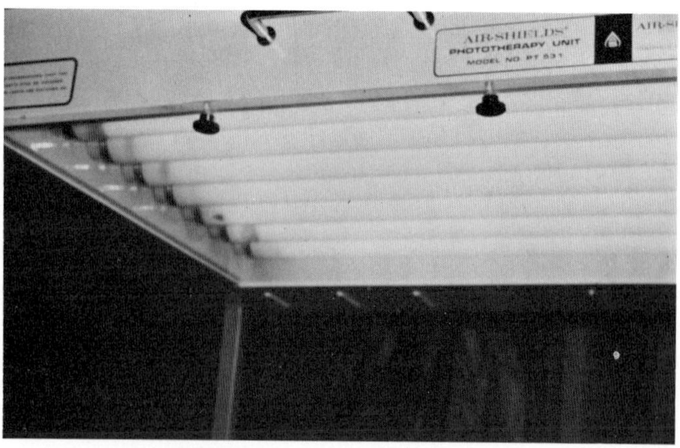

Figure 14.6 Phototherapy unit.

should be given to jaundiced infants as soon as their serum bilirubin reaches 10 mg/100 ml. Some paediatricians prefer to expose the infant to phototherapy intermittently for limited periods of say four hours with an interval of four hours. This appears to be almost as effective as continuous exposure and allows other infants to share the use of the light source. With certain incubators it is possible for two incubators to be placed under one phototherapy unit.

Length of treatment. As skin colour is no longer a useful indication of depth of jaundice in infants under treatment with phototherapy it is necessary to take blood for serum bilirubin estimations to decide on the length of treatment required. This is likely to vary with the gestational age of the infant being longest in the most immature infants. Phototherapy is most suitable for the treatment of jaundice due to immaturity of liver function but may also be used prophylactically in infants with haemolytic anaemias. In such cases a particularly careful watch must be kept on the serum bilirubin as photodecomposition may not be sufficient to deal with all the bilirubin being released. It has, of course, no effect on the associated anaemia.

Side effects of phototherapy have not yet been fully evaluated. As there has been a suggestion that brain growth may be disturbed caution must be observed in its use until more is known about possible side effects. Infants being treated by phototherapy often have loose stools.

ENZYME INDUCTION

Reference was made in Chapter 4 to the induction of enzyme activity in the fetus by giving phenobarbitone to the mother antenatally. At birth the infant is therefore better prepared to deal with the load of bilirubin presented to the liver. Giving phenobarbitone to the infant from birth has a similar but delayed effect and is therefore less valuable. There is no point in giving phenobarbitone to an infant who is already jaundiced. As it is not possible to recognize antenatally all mothers who will deliver their infants before term or to recognize at birth all infants who will become jaundiced, treatment with phenobarbitone would have to be given unnecessarily to large numbers of mothers and infants to make sure that all infants who were due to become jaundiced had been treated in time. This raises ethical problems. As there is no evidence that treatment with phenobarbitone has any advantage over phototherapy the authors prefer the latter.

Early feeding helps to reduce the danger of high bilirubin levels by reducing the risk of acidosis and preventing the rise of free fatty acids which compete with bilirubin for albumin binding sites.

CORRECTION OF ACIDOSIS

Correction of acidosis by intravenous alkali will restore the capacity of albumin to bind bilirubin.

ALBUMIN INFUSION

The place of infusions of salt-free albumin to boost albumin binding capacity has not been settled. Given through the umbilical vein in a maximum dose of 1 per g per kg body weight as a replacement for an equal volume of blood this method has proved safe in very small infants (below 1 kg) and may prevent the need for exchange transfusion in infants seriously ill for other reasons.

Exchange Transfusion

The object of an exchange transfusion is to remove blood containing harmful substances such as bilirubin from a patient and to replace it by healthy donor blood. Similarly, blood of low packed cell volume (PCV) can be replaced by blood of normal PCV so that severe anaemia can be corrected without overloading the circulation. In Rh incompatibility Rh positive cells can be replaced by Rh-negative cells. The procedure is generally carried out through a catheter in the umbilical vein. Various techniques can be employed and some of these are discussed in Chapter 19.

RISKS

In all procedures there is a risk to the infant which depends upon a number of factors such as the skill and experience of the operators, the type of donor blood used and the technique involved. 'Unexplained death' during exchange transfusion is in well ordered centres now very much rarer than previously but the complex physical and chemical changes which take place during exchange transfusion still constitute a risk for infants. The decision as to when this method of treatment should be employed depends upon knowledge of the risk to the infant of the condition being treated, the availability of other safer methods of treatment and the risk of exchange transfusion in the unit concerned. Only when the risk of exchange transfusion is less than the risk of the infant developing bilirubin encephalopathy should exchange transfusion be the treatment of choice.

Expertise. Because of reassessment of the situation along the lines indicated above many centres carried out fewer exchange transfusions in the 1960s than they did in the 1950s. This in turn led to some loss of expertise and possibly to a greater risk to the infant. Because of reduced numbers there may be long periods without serious mishap and it becomes difficult to assess the risk involved.

Complications. Even with experienced staff, however, the risk of exchange transfusion itself is probably not lower than a mortality rate of 1 in 100 transfusions. Non-fatal complications such as portal vein thrombosis, hepatitis, peritonitis following perforation of the bowel also have to be borne in mind.

INDICATIONS

It therefore follows that knowledge of the risk to the infant of the degree of anaemia or jaundice present is equally important when considering the indications for exchange transfusion. In each infant more than one factor is likely to be involved and the ultimate decision is therefore a clinical one and should not be made entirely on laboratory evidence. As clinical impressions are difficult to quantify some laboratory guide-lines are useful.

Laboratory criteria. We recommend that exchange transfusion be carried out in patients with proven blood group incompatibility for the following indications: at birth and in the first 72 hours of life, a cord or venous haemoglobin of 10 g per 100 ml or less: at any age jaundice with early signs of bilirubin encephalopathy or a serum indirect-acting bilirubin of 20 mg per 100 ml or more.

In infants with no cause other than immaturity for jaundice the indications for exchange transfusion are early signs of bilirubin encephalopathy or a serum indirect-acting bilirubin of 25 mg per 100 ml or more.

In infants with Rh or other cause for haemolytic anaemia we have not found that the bilirubin level in cord blood is a useful indication of the need for immediate exchange transfusion. Early exchange transfusion in such infants does little to prevent the need for subsequent exchange transfusion and may increase the total number of transfusions required.

The urgency of treatment must always be assessed. Where the prenatal findings in an Rh-sensitized mother suggest a severely affected infant arrangements must be made in good time before delivery so that an immediate exchange transfusion can be carried out at birth. This will be required in severely anaemic and oedematous infants (hydrops fetalis)—(Fig. 14.3) from whom peritoneal and pleural fluid may have to be aspirated to allow respiration to continue. Jaundiced infants are not such urgent problems provided that frequent assessment of their clinical state has been made and that the rate of rise of serum bilirubin is known. Estimations at four-hourly intervals of serum bilirubin allow a useful graph to be plotted, and the pattern of further development can be estimated with a surprising degree of accuracy. A rapid rise to 15 mg per 100 ml followed by a slower rise may indicate that dangerous levels of bilirubin will not be reached. If an exchange transfusion is carried out in such an infant who is well at a level of say 17 mg per 100 ml serum bilirubin, the bilirubin may fall but rise again with the entry of bilirubin from the tissues into the blood stream. A second transfusion may then be required. If the first transfusion had been delayed the second transfusion might not have proved necessary.

DONOR BLOOD

Blood for exchange transfusions must be fresh (less than 48 hours old) accurately tested for compatibility and restored to the infant's true packed cell volume by withdrawal of plasma (e.g. 100 ml). Rh-negative blood of appropriate ABO group is used for Rh-sensitized infants. The blood must be slowly warmed to body temperature. Where citrated donor blood is used injections of calcium gluconate are commonly given at regular intervals. These are not indicated in all infants and others prefer to give 1 ml of 10 per cent calcium gluconate slowly intravenously only when the infant shows evidence of overexcitability.

PROCEDURE

Monitoring. Observation of the infant during exchange transfusion is of first importance to detect the earliest changes in general condition, body temperature, pulse rate and volume and irritability. Many centres use recording apparatus for this purpose but where this is not available good clinical observation can be as effective provided that there is no relaxation of concentration.

Temperature control. Maintenance of a stable body temperature

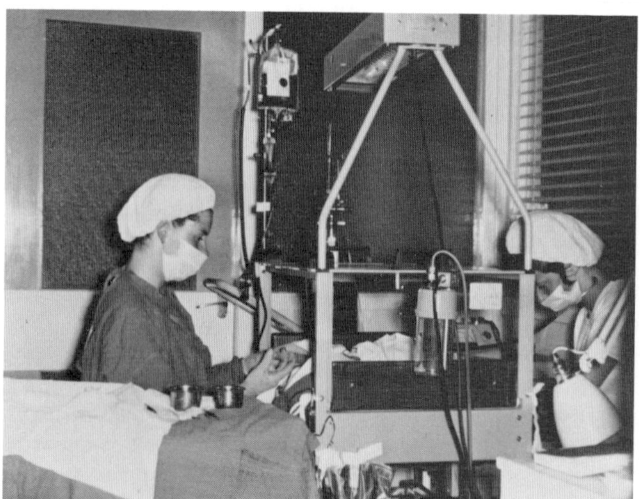

Figure 14.7 Exchange transfusion being carried out in a controlled environment.

may require special arrangements for heat control. This may be an incubator, overhead heating panel or heating pad below the infant (Fig. 14.7). Frequent recording of the infant's central temperature is indicated. An oesophageal thermocouple and temperature recorder is an advantage.

Volume control. Careful control of the volumes of blood removed and transfused is essential to prevent changes in the infant's blood volume. Where mechanical control is not available the importance of careful recordings of the volumes used in each cycle cannot be overstressed.

Access for resuscitation Particularly where several leads from recording instruments are involved it is important to ensure that free access to the infant's head is always available in case of vomiting or the need for resuscitative procedures.

Prevention of infection. As the umbilical vein is a ready source of entry for pathogenic organisms antiseptic and aseptic precautions must be rigidly enforced. It is useful to take a bacteriological swab from the umbilicus before cannulation and after the transfusion to send the distal end of the catheter for bacteriological examination. Most centres prefer to give prophylactic antibiotic cover following an exchange transfusion.

EFFECTIVENESS

Exchange of red cells. A mathematical study of the effectiveness of exchange transfusion in removing an infant's red cells shows a decrease in efficiency, as the exchange proceeds, as more and more of the blood being removed is donor blood.

Removal of bilirubin. When the indication is jaundice a different pattern emerges. As the serum level of bilirubin falls a gradient is established and bilirubin passes from the tissues into the blood. This movement is encouraged by the provision of 'clean' albumin in the donor blood. Thus more bilirubin can be removed from the body than was in the blood at the beginning of the transfusion. This advantage can be further improved by priming the infant with albumin 1 g per kg body weight at least 30 minutes before the exchange, and the priming can be repeated during the procedure. Whether the advantage gained is justified is debatable. Even without priming with albumin the mass of bilirubin removed may be as much as 150 per cent of the bilirubin in the infant's plasma before exchange transfusion. The speed of transfusion is of some importance and there are advantages from increased safety and increased bilirubin output in not exceeding a rate of exchange of 2 ml per kg body weight per minute.

The total volume exchanged may be limited by the number of units of blood available but a suitable objective is 200 ml per kg body weight. At the rate quoted this would mean that the transfusion would extend over 100 minutes.

Cord stump. Following withdrawal of the umbilical vein catheter bleeding should be controlled by pressure and the umbilical cord stump sealed with a suitable agent (e.g. Nobecutane). If bleeding persists a ligature should be inserted to control the bleeding but this is not often required. It is advisable to leave the stump exposed so that any secondary bleeding can be observed quickly.

PREVENTION

The prevention of maternal Rh sensitization, the recognition and early treatment of affected infants together with contraceptive advice or sterilization of mothers liable to have further seriously affected infants should progressively reduce the problem of Rh incompatibility. It is less easy to forecast further development in relation to jaundice of immaturity which is now the most frequent cause of possible bilirubin encephalopathy. Better understanding of the metabolic processes involved has already reduced the frequency of the most severe forms of this condition, and as safer forms of therapy are introduced it can be hoped that this cause of jaundice will be less of a problem in the future.

Treatment of Obstructive Jaundice

Urgency. The treatment of obstructive jaundice is less urgent unless the cause is infective, in which case rapid identification of the causative organisms and appropriate antibiotic or other treatment is indicated.

INFECTIVE

It is unfortunately only in the case of bacillary infections and syphilis that satisfactory therapy exists. Toxoplasmosis may respond to pyrimethamine (Daraprim) but in infants infected before birth and showing evidence of hepatitis at delivery the outlook is poor. In other forms of hepatitis due to virus infection no treatment other than supportive is available but the prognosis is not necessarily poor. Evidence of spontaneous recovery may not be evident for several weeks.

SURGICAL TREATMENT

Surgical treatment of obstructive jaundice should not be undertaken until hepatitis has been excluded as a cause of the obstructive jaundice. Premature surgical interference decreases the chance of recovery in infants with hepatitis and there is no evidence that early surgical treatment is necessary in the management of the rare cases of operable extrahepatic biliary obstruction.

The treatment of galactosaemia is withdrawal of lactose-containing foods from the diet.

FURTHER READING

BERGSMA, D., HSIA, D. Y. Y., & JACKSON, C. (Eds.) (1970). *Bilirubin Metabolism in the Newborn.* Baltimore: Williams & Wilkins.

BRITISH MEDICAL JOURNAL (1971). Prevention of Rh haemolytic disease: final results of the 'high risk' clinical trial. A combined study from centres in England and Baltimore, ii, 607–609.

BRITISH MEDICAL JOURNAL (1972). Phototherapy in neonatal jaundice, ii, 62–63.

CLARKE, C. A. (1972). Practical effects of blood group incompatability between mother and fetus. *British Medical Journal*, ii, 90–95.

LUCEY, J. F. (1972a). Neonatal jaundice and phototherapy. *Pediatric Clinics of North America*, **19,** 827–839.

LUCEY, J. F. (1972b). The unsolved problem of kernicterus in the susceptible low birth-weight infant. *Pediatrics*, **49,** 646–647.

MAURER, H. M., SHUMWAY, C. N., DRAPER, D. A. & HOSSAINI, A. A. (1973). Controlled trial comparing agar, intermittent phototherapy, and continuous phototherapy for reducing neonatal hyperbilirubinaemia. *Journal of Pediatrics*, **82,** 73–76.

TABB, P. A., INGLIS, J., SAVAGE, D. C. L. & WALKER, C. H. M. (1972). Controlled trial of phototherapy of limited duration in the treatment of physiological hyperbilirubinaemia in low birth weight infants. *Lancet*, ii, 1211–1213.

15

Dyspnoea and Cyanosis

The healthy baby generally breathes within a few seconds of birth. Once established, respirations assume a rhythmic, although not precisely regular, pattern. Inspiration and expiration through the nose follow each other in uninterrupted succession with preterm babies breathing at a rate of about 55 per minute and mature babies 45 per minute. Normally breathing is diaphragmatic, rather than thoracic, with indrawing of the lower ribs and intercostal spaces on inspiration.

DYSPNOEA

The terms dyspnoea and respiratory distress are applied to breathing which is difficult, distressed, laboured or rapid. Dyspnoea usually assumes the form of rapid shallow breathing which is often accompanied by more pronounced costal recession (Fig. 15.1). In any condition in which there is obstruction of the upper airways or decreased lung compliance (lack of elastic recoil) as in some forms of congenital heart disease with a left to right shunt, costal recession becomes very much greater. With increasing dyspnoea breathing takes place through the mouth. Inspiration is accompanied by backward movement of the head and expiration by a characteristic grunt.

SILVERMAN SCORE

In an effort to evaluate the degree of severity of dyspnoea Silverman introduced a scoring system based on five objective signs (Table 15.1). Each sign is given a score and the total score can range from 0 to 10. Silverman scoring is of particular value in assessing

Table 15.1 Silverman assessment of dyspnoea

Sign	Score 1	Score 2
Respiratory rate	Over 60	Over 80
Chest recession	Slight	Marked
Grunt	Heard with stethoscope	Heard without stethoscope
Nostril dilation	Slight	Marked
Cyanosis	Slight	Marked

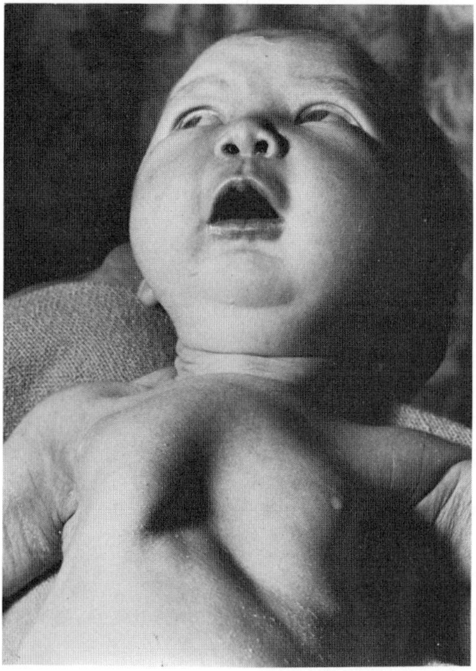

Figure 15.1 Costal recession in dyspnoeic infant.

improvement or deterioration rather than as an indication for treatment. The authors use a score of 6 on more than two occasions, or over 6 on one occasion, as an indication for arranging for blood gas analysis.

Causes of Dyspnoea

A great variety of disorders cause dyspnoea (Table 15.2). In preterm babies the commonest causes of dyspnoea are the respiratory distress syndrome and pulmonary haemorrhage, whilst in term infants massive aspiration and pneumonia head the list.

OBSTRUCTION OF THE UPPER AIRWAY

Nasal obstruction. Obstruction of the nasal passages in the newborn is a frequent finding. It varies considerably in degree. Complete obstruction may result from bilateral choanal atresia (Chap. 11). Obstruction by nasal secretions is recognized by the noise (snuffles) in the nose accompanying inspiration and expiration. A discharge from the nose is rarely seen in the newborn, although on occasion dried particles of mucus can be detected adherent to the nostrils.

Table 15.2 Causes of dyspnoea

OBSTRUCTION OF THE UPPER AIRWAY
Nasal obstruction
Choanal atresia
Laryngeal obstruction
Tracheal compression
LUNG PARENCHYMAL DISEASE
Primary atelectasis
Secondary atelectasis
Respiratory distress syndrome
Pulmonary haemorrhage
Pneumonia
Emphysema
Pneumothorax
Wilson-Mikity syndrome
Transient neonatal tachypnoea
INTRATHORACIC DISORDERS
Developmental defects of the lung
Pulmonary agenesis
Pulmonary cysts
Pulmonary sequestration
Disorders of the diaphragm
Hernia
Paralysis
Oesophageal atresia
Intrathoracic tumours and cysts
Pleural effusion
MISCELLANEOUS DISORDERS
Heart failure
Intracranial lesions
Severe anaemia
Febrile conditions
Metabolic acidosis

Discharge, when present, tends to drain posteriorly into the nasopharynx.

Stuffy nose syndrome. Not all nasal secretion is due to infection. The nasal mucous membranes of the newborn infant are notably susceptible to changes in temperature and humidity of the atmosphere, and react quickly to foggy conditions. Nasal swabs taken from babies born in hospital often give growths of staphylococci on culture but these organisms may not belong to pathogenic strains. A combination of staphylococci and an adenovirus appear to be the cause of what is called the stuffy nose syndrome, which is descriptive. Neither organism on its own produces the same effect. Even when the result of infection, nasal catarrh is not accompanied by symptoms of general systemic disturbance unless spread to the pharynx, trachea or bronchi takes place. Signs and symptoms if present are essentially local and take the form of mild to moderate dyspnoea and of difficulty in feeding. Unable to breathe effectively through the nose, the infant has periodically to release his grasp of the areola or teat in order to breathe through his mouth.

Snuffles, an early sign of congenital syphilis, is now rarely seen in this country.

Treatment of nasal catarrh is only necessary where feeding difficulties arise.

Decongestant nasal drops such as 0.5 per cent ephedrine in saline serve to relieve the vascular congestion of the mucous membranes. One drop is instilled into each nostril before feeds as required. If the discharge is purulent a close watch should be kept for early signs of descent of infection as bronchitis in the newborn can rapidly assume serious proportions.

LARYNGEAL OBSTRUCTION

Laryngeal obstruction giving rise to congenital laryngeal stridor may be first noticed at birth or at any time during the first two weeks of life. If the obstruction is severe it gives rise to marked inspiratory stridor which becomes worse in the presence of a respiratory infection.

Laryngomalacia. The condition has been variously ascribed to an unusually soft larynx which collapses on inspiration (laryngomalacia), an epiglottis of abnormal shape and size, and redundant aryepiglottic folds. Phonation is unimpaired but stridor is present.

Laryngeal web. Stridor is present and phonation may be abnormal in the presence of a laryngeal web.

Laryngeal stenosis. Stridor present in both inspiration and expiration can result from laryngeal stenosis.

Oedema of the larynx and epiglottis may follow tracheal intubation at birth when stridor will also be present both in inspiration and expiration. Placing the baby in the prone position improves the airway and relieves the stridor.

TRACHEAL COMPRESSION

Tracheal compression from a vascular ring (Fig. 15.2) or from a mediastinal tumour is rare.

A vascular ring is in effect a double aortic arch which encircles and compresses both the trachea and oesophagus. The condition should be suspected in the presence of dyspnoea and swallowing difficulty. In order to improve the airway the baby holds his head in extension. Forcible flexion of the head may completely occlude the airway. The diagnosis is confirmed by barium swallow examination and surgical removal of the accessory arch relieves all symptoms.

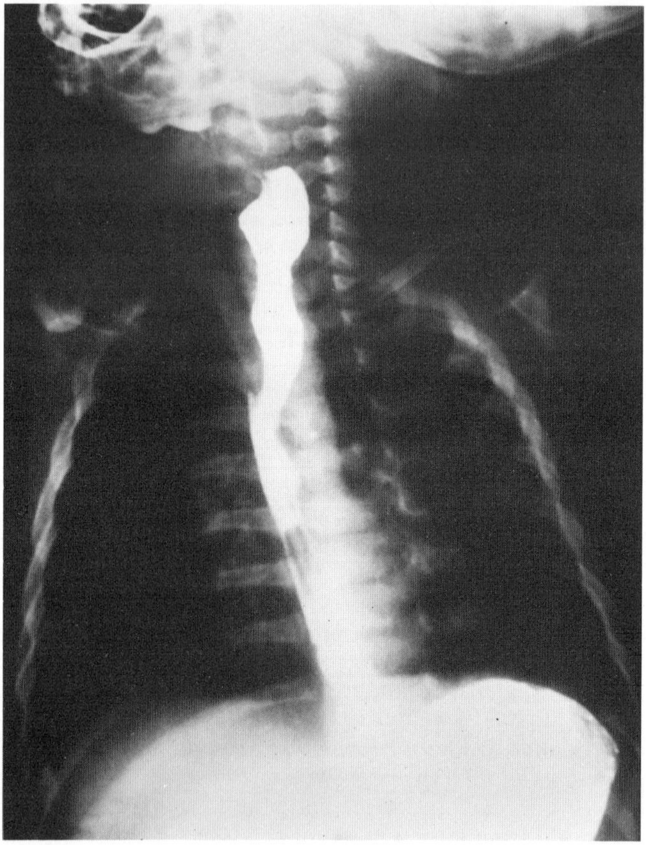

Figure 15.2 Vascular ring compressing the oesophagus and trachea.

Lung Parenchymal Disease

PRIMARY ATELECTASIS

During fetal life the lungs are not required for ventilation and are filled with fluid. With the first breaths after delivery air fills the bronchial tree and the alveoli are progressively expanded and fill with air. Areas of the lung, however, may not expand and in these areas there is primary atelectasis. If the total area of primary atelectasis is small the clinical effect is minimal, but if larger areas fail to expand, there is dyspnoea and cyanosis.

If a major bronchus remains filled with fluid a whole lung or lobe of a lung may fail to expand. Treatment consists of laryngoscopy and aspiration of the trachea and major bronchi by a suction catheter passed through the larynx. When the obstruction is relieved expansion of the alveoli follows.

SECONDARY ATELECTASIS

Aspiration syndromes. A baby may aspirate fluid into the lungs before, during or after birth, the mortality being high in those who aspirate meconium.

Meconium aspiration is most frequently seen where there has been prenatal hypoxia with onset of respiration before delivery.

If inspiration takes place after premature separation of the placenta the lungs may be filled with maternal blood.

Aspiration pneumonia. Aspiration of infected amniotic fluid or vaginal secretions is a common cause of postnatal pneumonia. It is generally agreed that conditions tending to produce fetal hypoxia cause the fetus to gasp in the uterus or birth canal. When aspiration has occurred *in utero* it often follows fetal distress marked by the presence of meconium staining of the amniotic fluid.

Postnatal aspiration of gastric contents may be found in depressed infants who are tube fed.

The aspiration of foreign material leads to severe irritation of the lungs with congestion, oedema and haemorrhage resulting in patchy and emphysema, atelectasis and secondary collapse.

Physical signs. The baby may be severely hypoxic at birth requiring immediate intubation and intermittent positive pressure respiration. On examination of the chest there will be found tachypnoea, costal recession, dullness on percussion and crepitations on auscultation. The baby continuously produces mucus which is stained with meconium or blood.

X-ray examination of the chest shows coarse, irregular densities together with focal areas of emphysema and collapse. The domes of the diaphragm are usually flattened.

Treatment. Thorough clearing of the airway at birth should be followed by aspiration of the stomach aimed at preventing further vomiting and aspiration. The baby is nursed in an incubator with extra oxygen as necessary. Antibiotics are given to prevent *E. coli* pneumonia, which commonly complicates meconium aspiration. It may be necessary to correct metabolic acidosis (Chap. 12).

Prognosis. Babies who aspirate amniotic or vaginal contents generally do well and recover within two or three days. Deaths are common following massive aspiration associated with intrauterine hypoxia. Some develop pneumomediastinum and/or pneumothorax as a result of progressive emphysema. This usually absorbs spontaneously. Others develop pneumonia as a result of aspirating infected liquor, maternal secretions or meconium.

RESPIRATORY DISTRESS SYNDROME

The respiratory distress syndrome (RDS) occurs most commonly in preterm babies. Other predisposing factors, such as caesarean delivery, maternal diabetes and fetal distress due to antepartum haemorrhage, have been thought to be of importance in the past but their significance is now less clear.

INCIDENCE

As there are no universally accepted criteria on which to base the clinical diagnosis the incidence and mortality rate of the respiratory distress syndrome are impossible to assess accurately. However, it probably occurs in 10 to 15 per cent of preterm babies and the mortality varies from 25 to 40 per cent.

AETIOLOGY

Pulmonary immaturity. RDS is more common in preterm infants but may occur in some term infants. The immaturity of such infants' lungs is related to inability to produce sufficient amounts of surfactant which acts as a surface tension reducing agent.

Surfactant is a phospholipid normally produced by certain cells lining the alveoli. It reduces the surface tension within the alveoli and allows the lungs to expand normally at birth. Lack of surfactant probably causes diminished lung compliance making it even more difficult to expand the lungs and as a consequence there is also increased pulmonary vascular resistance and right to left shunting of blood through the foramen ovale, ductus arteriosus and atelectatic portions of the lungs. These are all characteristic signs of respiratory distress syndrome and it is clear that lack of surfactant is of major importance in the aetiology of this condition. The lack of surfactant is not due to immaturity alone as surfactant can be found in fetal lung as early as 24 weeks gestation. Deficiency is presumably a failure of adequate production. A possible explanation of this failure in production was given in Chapter 12. It will be recalled that one of the consequences of oxygen-conserving adaptation accompanying intrauterine hypoxia was persistent pulmonary vasoconstriction after birth with marked increase in the right to left shunting of blood through the ductus arteriosus. Many authors believe that this reduced pulmonary blood flow is responsible for deficiency or absence of surfactant.

PATHOLOGY

At postmortem examination the lungs are found to be atelectatic with a typical eosinophilic hyaline membrane (Fig. 15.3) lining the

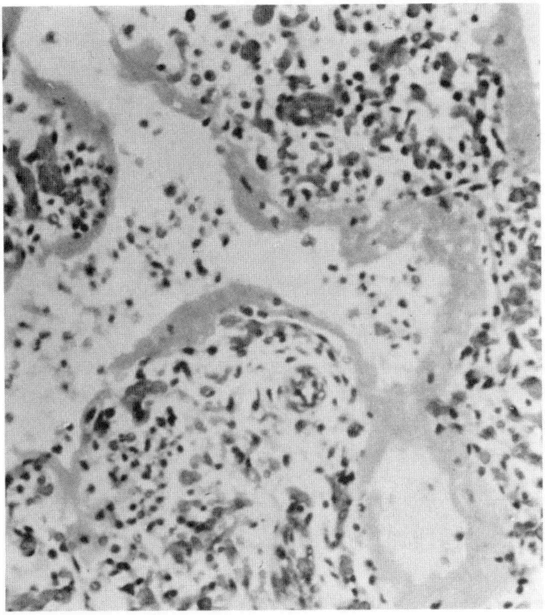

Figure 15.3 Microscopic appearance of lung with hyaline membrane.

alveoli and terminal bronchioles. The origin of the membrane is doubtful but it is probably formed as a result of exudation from pulmonary capillaries.

Pulmonary hyaline membrane disease is to be regarded as a pathological and not a clinical diagnosis.

Intraventricular haemorrhage is not an uncommon finding at postmortem examination.

CLINICAL SIGNS

The diagnostic signs of the respiratory distress syndrome are costal and sternal recession, increased respiratory and heart rate, expiratory grunting and decreased air entry on auscultation, present during and persisting beyond the first three hours of life in the absence of co-existing disease.

The respiratory rate steadily increases after birth to a peak of about 75 per minute at 24 hours of age.

The heart rate increases to 130 to 170 per minute.

The temperature often falls.

Central cyanosis is common. There may be pitting oedema of the hands and feet.

Crepitations may be heard in the lungs.

In addition to the tachycardia other cardiovascular signs include liver enlargement, hypotension and a ductus arteriosus murmur. Because of difficulty in feeding excessive weight loss may occur. Cerebral irritation as a result of hypoxaemia may confuse the diagnosis.

X-ray. Typically the chest X-ray shows a fine ground-glass mottling throughout both lung fields, and the contrast between this mottling and air in the bronchi accounts for the air bronchogram. Chest X-ray is of more importance in excluding other conditions such as aspiration syndrome, congenital unilobar emphysema, diaphragmatic hernia and pneumothorax, than of confirming the clinical diagnosis of respiratory distress syndrome.

Assessment. As mentioned earlier in this chapter repeated observation using the Silverman score gives an objective measure of change in condition and an indication as to when blood gas analysis should be undertaken.

BIOCHEMICAL CHANGES

Acidosis. The pH falls and may be as low as 7.0 or in very severe cases even lower. This fall in pH is due to a mixture of respiratory and metabolic acidosis. Estimations are commonly carried out on the Astrup apparatus calculating the results from the Siggaard-Andersen nomogram.

Respiratory acidosis results from retention of carbon dioxide, and $P\text{CO}_2$ may reach 80 to 100 mmHg.

Metabolic acidosis develops because of the excessive respiratory muscle activity, low oxygen tension and the accumulation of lactic acid. The negative base excess may be 20 mEq per litre or more.

Oxygen tension in arterial blood falls progressively to below 60 mmHg because of poor ventilatory exchange and right to left shunting of blood.

MANAGEMENT

Prevention. As preterm delivery is the most important single factor in the aetiology of respiratory distress syndrome, measures which reduce the incidence of preterm delivery are of major importance in the management of the respiratory distress syndrome.

Delivery at a time when the lungs are capable of producing an adequate amount of surfactant is the most direct method of preventing RDS. It has recently been suggested that the respiratory distress syndrome can be prevented in infants of under 32 weeks gestation if labour can be delayed for 24 hours during which time the mother is given betamethazone. The glucocorticoid appears to act by accelerating lung maturation in the fetus.

Observation. The diagnosis of RDS is primarily clinical and requires close observation of all newborn infants, particularly of those of low birth weight during the first few hours of life. Should there be any sign of respiratory distress frequent or constant observation of colour, activity, grunting, use of accessory respiratory muscles, respiratory rate, heart rate and temperature should be made.

Incubator. Such observations can most readily be made with the infant exposed in an incubator, preferably with constant recording of skin temperature.

A Silverman score should be recorded at least every quarter of an hour.

X-ray. In order to exclude other causes of respiratory difficulty a chest X-ray should be arranged. In infants with RDS there is a characteristic ground-glass appearance of the lung fields with an air bronchogram.

Arterial blood gases. If the infant's condition is showing signs of deterioration, with a Silverman score of 6 or more, arterial blood gases should be measured (Chap. 19).

Oxygen. The environmental oxygen concentration should be raised sufficiently to maintain the infant's arterial blood Po_2 between 60 and 90 mmHg. Regular estimation of the oxygen concentration within the incubator should be made using an oxygen analyser.

In the absence of facilities for arterial Po_2 measurement the lowest oxygen concentration which allows the baby to remain a good colour should be used. Because of the risk of retrolental fibroplasia following the use of unnecessarily high concentrations of oxygen it is most important that the oxygen concentration within the incubator be limited and carefully controlled. If this cannot be done the infant should be transferred to a unit where suitable facilities are available.

Correction of acidosis. Metabolic acidosis can be corrected by giving alkali. This is most readily done by the intravenous injection of 8.4 per cent sodium bicarbonate, which provides 1 mEq per ml. The volume to be given is calculated from the formula:

negative base excess × weight in kg × 0.3 ml = 8.4 per cent bicarbonate solution.

This dose should be given slowly intravenously, but in mild cases where an intravenous line is not already established, it may be given by tube into the stomach. Correction of acidosis must be confirmed by further biochemical estimation of base excess or of bicarbonate in the blood.

Respiratory acidosis is indicated by a raised Pco_2. This can only be reduced by increasing the efficiency of ventilation. With the natural improvement which takes place in many infants with RDS this can occur without further treatment than that already outlined. If the infant shows signs of progressive deterioration of respiratory function with fall in Po_2 and rise in Pco_2 further treatment will be required.

Ventilator care. This will involve intermittent positive pressure respiration (IPPR) controlled manually or by a ventilator. For further information with regard to ventilator care reference should be made to more specialized publications on the intensive care of the newborn. In general it is preferable that infants likely to require respirator management should be transferred to an intensive therapy nursery for such treatment as necessary.

Continuous positive pressure respiration. More recently interest in the management of RDS has centred on a variety of methods of maintaining continuous positive pressure respiration (CPPR). The object of CPPR is to prevent the collapse of alveoli on expiration by

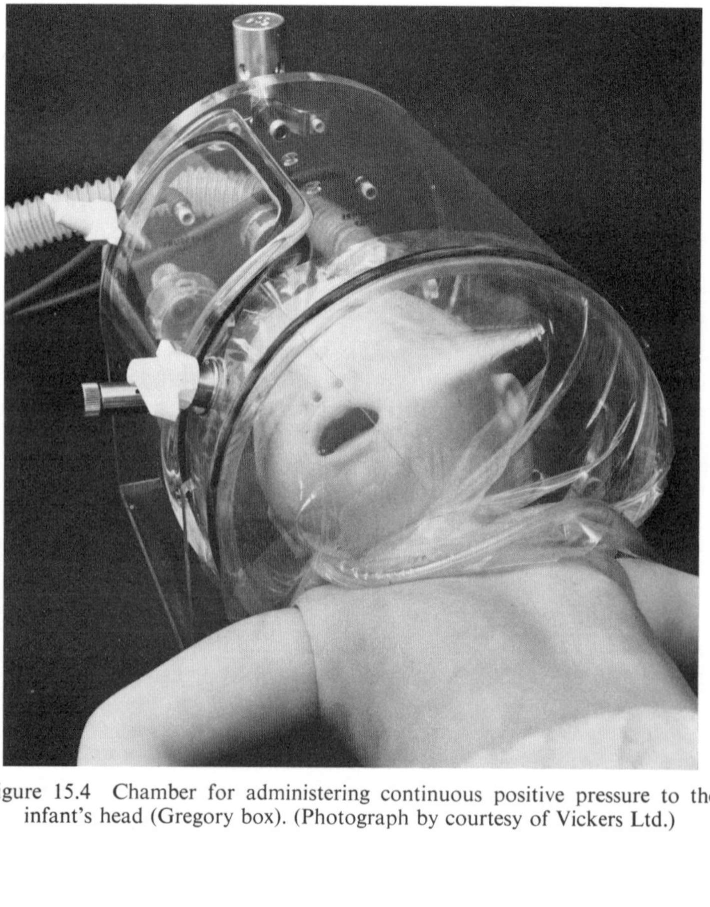

Figure 15.4 Chamber for administering continuous positive pressure to the infant's head (Gregory box). (Photograph by courtesy of Vickers Ltd.)

maintaining a positive pressure in the airways throughout the respiratory cycle. This can be achieved by a variety of methods which maintain a raised pressure around the infant's head in a box or bag (Fig. 15.4) or, if an endotracheal tube is in place, by arranging a positive end expiratory pressure. It has been suggested that a similar effect can be obtained by using bilateral nasal catheters with a continuous gas flow. Other methods have applied continuous negative pressure to the chest with the infant's trunk in a negative pressure chamber leaving the infant's head free (Fig. 15.5).

The value of CPPR in the management of RDS has yet to be established and the relative merits of the various methods employed will have to be assessed carefully before this type of treatment becomes standard. Early reports are promising but it must be remembered that overenthusiastic reports on other forms of treatment of RDS have led to subsequent disappointment after more extensive evaluation.

COMPLICATIONS

Include apnoeic episodes, pneumothorax, pulmonary haemorrhage, intracerebral haemorrhage. Where IPPR has been used through an endotracheal tube there is a risk of pulmonary infection which increases with the length of time for which IPPR is required.

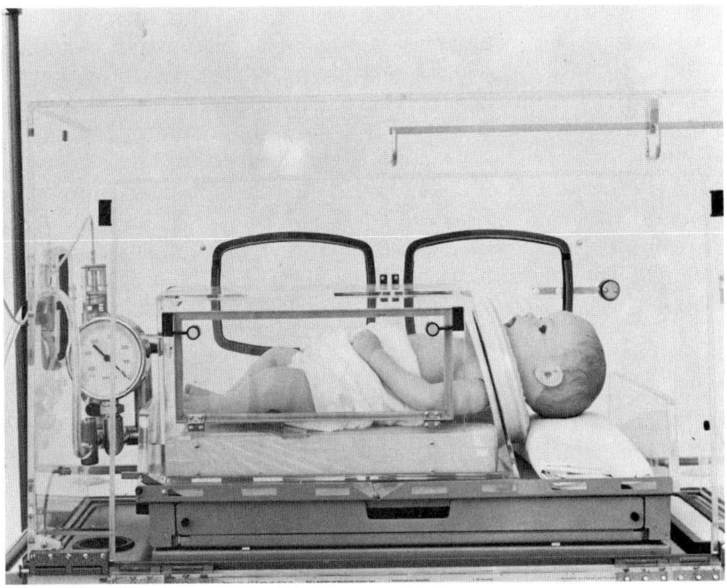

Figure 15.5 Chamber for administering continuous negative pressure to the infant's trunk. (Photograph by courtesy of Draeger Ltd.)

Prognosis. RDS is unfortunately a condition for which we cannot guarantee a cure. Many infants who are mildly affected will survive without specialized treatment. In the most severely affected death may occur in spite of the most sophisticated treatment. With intensification of supportive management the mortality rate is steadily falling and in the best hands is as low as 25 per cent but in other centres may still be 40 per cent.

In individual infants the response of the arterial Po_2 to increase in the concentration of inspired oxygen gives some indication of prognosis, the poorer the response the poorer the prognosis. Acidosis which is not readily correctable by the methods outlined similarly carries a poor prognosis. Conversely an infant with a minor degree of acidosis and a Po_2 which is easily kept within the normal range has a good prognosis.

Recovery. Most infants who survive for three days without major disturbance of their pH or Po_2 will show progressive improvement in respiratory function and general activity. Recovery is complete and not associated with long-term respiratory problems.

PULMONARY HAEMORRHAGE

Dyspnoea associated with the coughing up of blood-stained secretion or the aspiration of blood-stained material from the trachea is highly suggestive of pulmonary haemorrhage. This diagnosis can, however, only be proved at postmortem examination and may then be found without any clinical evidence of its presence during life.

Pulmonary haemorrhage is often a terminal event after fulminating infection or severe RDS. It occurs most commonly in low birth-weight infants, particularly in those who are light for dates. It is one of the manifestations of disseminated intravascular coagulation and is found in severe hypothermia.

Treatment is symptomatic and supportive by giving extra oxygen when required, by antibiotic if infection is present and by correction of hypothermia.

PNEUMONIA

Pneumonia is found at postmortem examination more often than any other infective disease. About 10 per cent of perinatal deaths are due to congenital pneumonia following the inhalation of liquor amnii in association with fetal hypoxia. The source of infection in early, as distinct from strictly congenital, pneumonia may be material aspirated before, during or after birth. Alternatively, the infection may be air-borne or part of a bacteraemia of antenatal or postnatal origin. The use of prophylactic antibiotics in cases of known maternal infection or prolonged rupture of the membranes is of doubtful value.

The newborn baby is particularly susceptible to staphylococcal pneumonia but infection by streptococci, pneumococci, *E. coli* and *Pseudomonas aeruginosa* are not uncommon. Staphylococcal pneumonia is particularly dangerous by reason of the tendency to form lung abscesses which rupture into the pleural cavity, with resultant pyopneumothorax (Fig. 15.6).

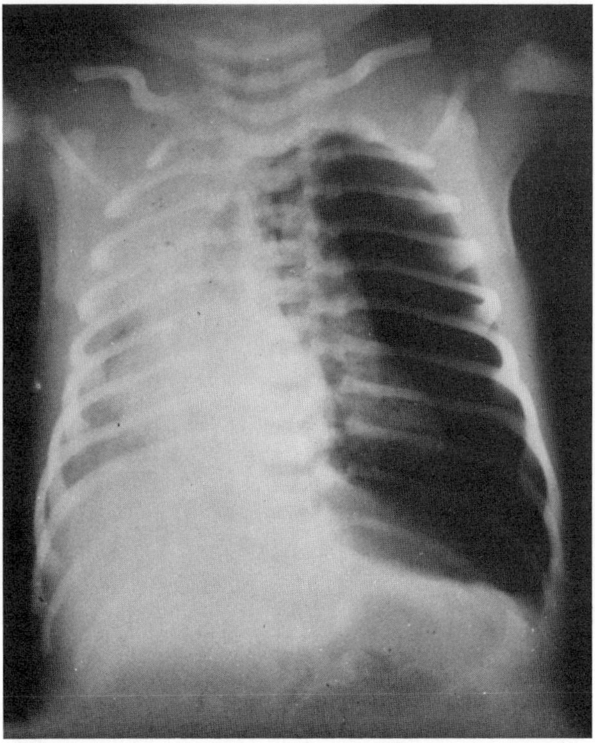

Figure 15.6 Staphylococcal pneumonia complicated by left pneumothorax.

Clinical evidence of pneumonia is frequently absent. The presence of an acute infection is suggested by anorexia, drowsiness, vomiting, pallor, irregular temperature, dyspnoea and cyanosis. Chest signs are limited to generalized crepitations, the other signs of pneumonia being rarely found. Chest X-ray (Fig. 15.7) is frequently helpful in arriving at a diagnosis.

Humidified oxygen in sufficient concentration is given to relieve cyanosis. Before starting antibiotic treatment blood culture should be arranged and swabs should be taken from the nose, throat, ears and umbilicus. The antibiotics chosen should have a sufficiently broad spectrum to cover all likely infections. Suitable combinations are penicillin and kanamycin or ampicillin and cloxacillin. These should be given intramuscularly or intravenously.

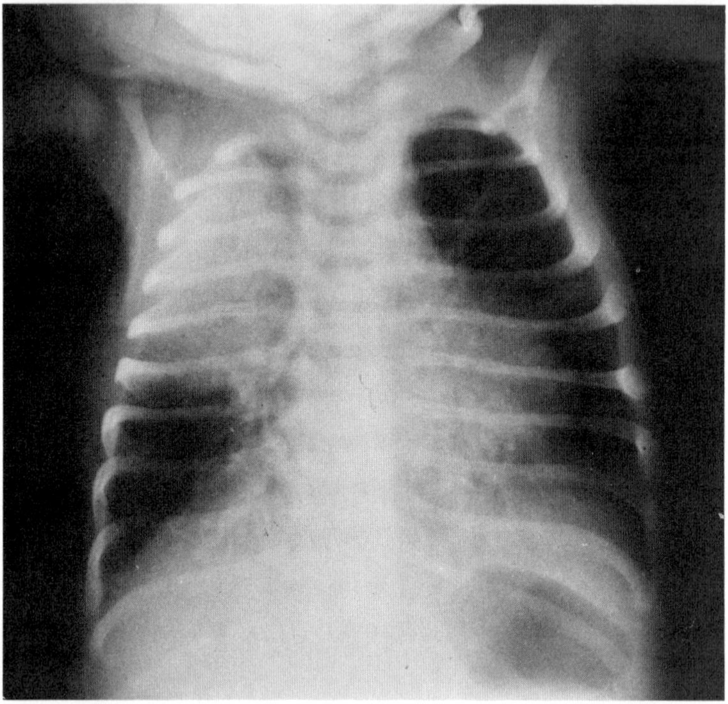

Figure 15.7 Pneumonia right upper lobe (age 6 days).

Feeds should be given in small quantities frequently. If bottle feeding proves exhausting then tube feeding should be instituted. Severely ill infants should be given intravenous fluids.

EMPHYSEMA

Compensatory emphysema occurs in healthy lung tissue as a result of negative intrathoracic pressure attributable to persisting atelectasis elsewhere.

Obstructive emphysema. Massive inhalation of foreign material can give rise to impaired expulsion from, but continued air entry into, alveoli with resultant obstructive emphysema.

Interstitial emphysema. Necrosis of parenchymatous lung tissue in staphylococcal pneumonia sometimes enables air to escape from the lungs along the perivascular spaces producing interstitial emphy-

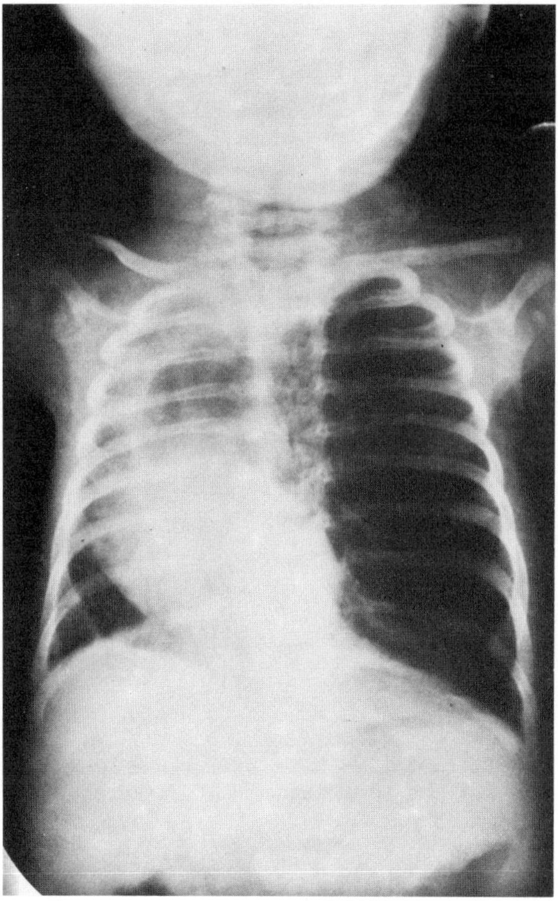

Figure 15.8 Unilobar emphysema.

sema. Rupture of alveoli with extensive emphysema can readily follow resuscitative methods employing excessive pressures. This danger is decreased in any system in which the pressure is restricted, by a blow-off valve which limits the pressure to 30 cm of water (Chap. 5).

Unilobar emphysema can give rise to signs and symptoms resembling those in pneumothorax. There are cyanosis and dyspnoea of increasing severity, hyperresonance over the affected lobe and mediastinal displacement. X-ray findings (Fig. 15.8) are characteristic. Lobectomy (Fig. 15.9) provides prompt and permanent relief and is associated with low mortality risk.

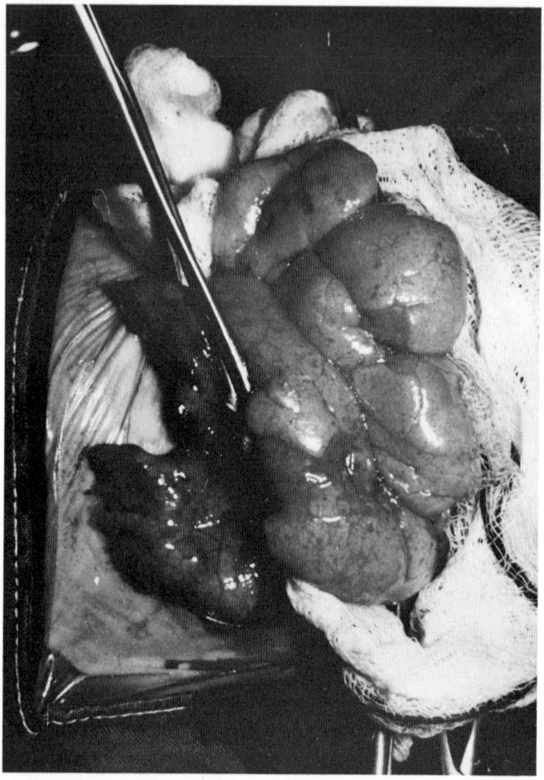

Figure 15.9 Unilobar emphysema. Exposure of affected lobe prior to operative removal. (By courtesy of Mr D. A. Watson, F.R.C.S.)

PNEUMOTHORAX

Rupture of emphysematous areas of the lungs releases air into the pleural cavities causing a pneumothorax. The commonest causes are overvigorous initial resuscitation or the use of excessive pressure during subsequent ventilation. Spontaneous rupture of an emphysematous lobe may occur. Pneumothorax may also be a complication of RDS.

Symptoms and signs will depend on the volume and pressure of air in the pleural cavity. Small pneumothoraces under low pressure may only be discovered on X-ray examination and require no treatment.

Pressure pneumothorax will occur if there is a valve effect at the site of the alveolar rupture which only allows air to pass outward into the pleural cavity. As the pressure rises the lung collapses and the infant shows increasing evidence of dyspnoea. The heart and mediastinum will become displaced away from the side of the pneumothorax and the contralateral lung may be compressed. As the infant finds breathing progressively more difficult cyanosis develops and the infant will die unless treated quickly.

Drainage of the pneumothorax may be carried out surgically with a catheter from the pleural cavity leading to an underwater seal. Where immediate surgery is not available life can be saved by passing a needle into the chest and connecting this to a Heimlitz valve (Chap. 19).

WILSON-MIKITY SYNDROME

This condition, of unknown aetiology, is restricted to immature babies of less than 36 weeks gestation. Affected babies are usually dyspnoeic at birth and present a clinical picture not unlike that seen in the respiratory distress syndrome. Improvement takes place within one to two weeks to be followed by the insidious onset of cyanosis and costal recession which may then persist for several months. During this period the baby requires extra oxygen to prevent cyanosis. Rhonchi are to be heard in the lungs. Other babies have no respiratory symptoms at birth, receive no added oxygen, yet some weeks later develop the symptoms described above. The condition is associated with fracture of the ribs but this association has yet to be explained unless it be due to overvigorous external cardiac massage.

X-ray of the chest is normal during the first weeks of life but later bilateral, coarse infiltration and cystic changes are seen. Complete clearing of these lung changes takes place any time up to two years. Abnormalities of pulmonary function including carbon dioxide retention, substantial right to left shunts, reduction of lung compliance and increased airways resistance have been reported.

Treatment consists of supportive measures and sufficient oxygen to relieve cyanosis.

TRANSIENT NEONATAL TACHYPNOEA

It has been suggested that a condition termed transient neonatal tachypnoea is due to delayed absorption of alveolar fluid, and possibly of inhaled amniotic fluid. The delay is due to damage to capillaries caused by hypoxia. This condition occurs in term babies following a period of prenatal hypoxia. Within a few hours of birth the respiratory rate increases to between 80 and 120 per minute and remains high for two to five days. No signs are heard in the chest but X-ray examination may show signs of emphysema and possibly an enlarged heart. The radiological signs return to normal within about five days.

Intrathoracic Disorders

DEVELOPMENTAL DEFECTS OF THE LUNGS

Developmental defects of the lung, including pulmonary agenesis, pulmonary cysts and sequestered lobes, are very rare causes of dyspnoea in the newly born infant.

Pulmonary agenesis. Failure of development of the primitive lung bud may lead to all gradations of underdevelopment of the lung ranging from hypoplasia of one segment or lobe to complete absence of both lungs. Affected babies experience great difficulty from birth with dyspnoea and cyanosis. Those who survive are prone to repeated respiratory infections.

Pulmonary cyst. Dyspnoea is usually the first recognizable sign of the presence of a pulmonary cyst (Fig. 15.10) whether of congenital or acquired origin. Signs may appear suddenly or gradually and at any time in the neonatal period, dependent upon the rate

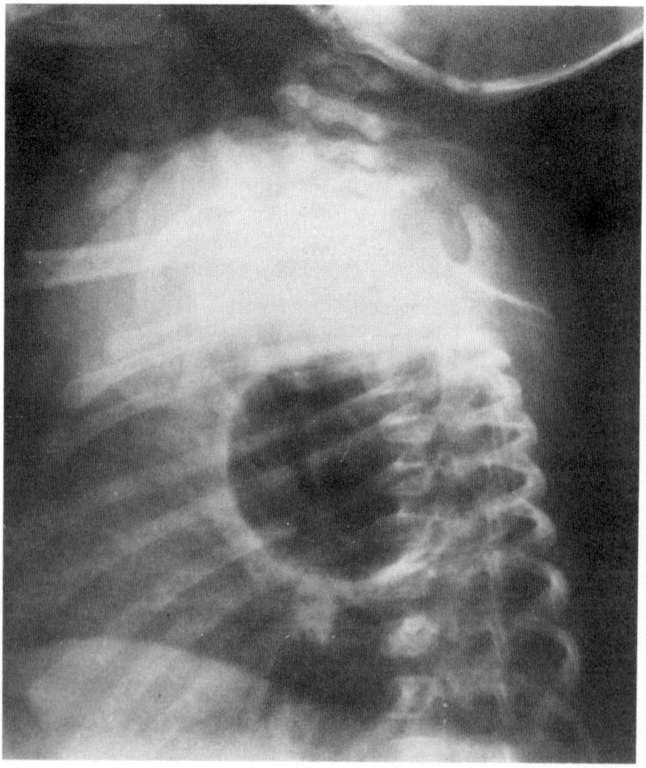

Figure 15.10 Pulmonary cyst.

of distension by air of the cyst. Cystic lesions of the lung may be single or multiple (Fig. 15.11) and are sometimes asymptomatic being discovered accidentally in the course of X-ray examination. Immediate operative intervention is an urgent necessity where tension in a cyst is increasing, and is indicated when the cyst contains pus.

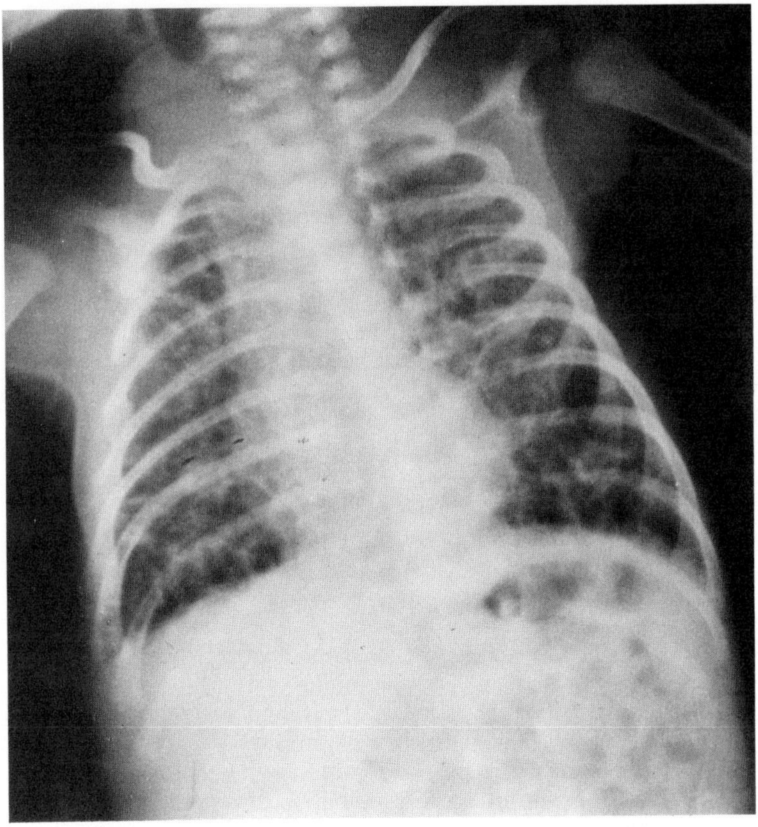

Figure 15.11 Congenital multiple cystic disease of the lungs.

Sequestered lobe. Sequestered lobes, which mainly affect the left lower lobe, rarely give rise to symptoms in the newborn period. They are usually detected on chest X-rays taken for other reasons. Sequestered lobes are the site of repeated infection so they should always be resected.

DISORDERS OF THE DIAPHRAGM

Diaphragmatic hernia sometimes gives rise to clinical signs including dyspnoea closely resembling those of extensive atelectasis.

Abdominal contents protrude into the thorax through a defect in the diaphragm. Dyspnoea and cyanosis may be present from birth. To limit inflation of the gut oxygen should not be given by mask but endotracheal intubation should be carried out. As pointed out in Chapter 11 early operation is essential. Suspected dextrocardia on first examination is an indication for a chest X-ray, as the heart may be displaced to the right by a diaphragmatic hernia.

Diaphragmatic paralysis is an occasional complication of Erb's palsy (Chap. 12) when nerve roots C5 and 6 are damaged during delivery. Dyspnoea in such circumstances should be investigated by X-ray screening.

Elevated diaphragm. Abdominal distension due to intestinal obstruction causes dyspnoea due to pressure on the diaphragm.

OESOPHAGEAL ATRESIA

Excessive secretion in the buccopharynx of a newly born baby, or secretion which tends to 'drool' more or less continuously should immediately raise the question of oesophageal atresia. Likewise an obstetric history of hydramnios should always raise the suspicion of oesophageal atresia. Any fluid given overflows from the blind upper portion of the oesophagus into the respiratory tract. Pneumonia results and is only too liable to be followed by death after, or even before, operation. If the infant is unfortunate enough to be given a feed the milk overflows into the larynx when he will cough, his face will become blue, some of the milk will be aspirated and he will become very dyspnoeic.

Investigation. Immediate investigation is indicated. The tip of a firm radio-opaque catheter will be arrested some 10 cm beyond the alveolar margin, and on X-ray screening is found to be on a level with the fourth thoracic vertebra. The blind ending of the upper portion of the oesophagus may be outlined by injecting contrast medium down the catheter. The contrast medium should always be removed on completion of the examination to prevent an aspiration pneumonia.

Management. Once the diagnosis has been made the infant should be maintained in a sitting position to prevent acidic stomach contents passing through the lower oesophageal segment to the lungs and should have the contents of the upper oesophageal segment aspirated at 15 minute intervals pending operation. Details of operative procedure vary according to the exact nature of the defect. In general it can be said that the operation consists of end to end anastomosis of the two segments of the oesophagus with closure of any accompanying tracheo-oesophageal or broncho-oesophageal fistula.

INTRATHORACIC TUMOURS AND CYSTS

These cause dyspnoea by compressing the lungs and airways. A large variety of solid tumours and fluid-filled cysts have been found in the chests of newly born infants. Malignant tumours occur less frequently than cysts of gastrointestinal origin, dermoid cysts and teratomatous tumours. Lesions may arise in the posterior (neuroblastoma, duplications of the gut, bronchogenic cysts), middle (vascular tumours) and anterior (enlarged thymus, teratomas) mediastinal spaces. Fibrosarcomas and hamartomas may be found in the lung substance itself.

These tumours and cysts give rise to increasing dyspnoea and frequently become infected and come to light on X-ray examination of the chest. Treatment consists of excision followed by irradiation when indicated.

PLEURAL EFFUSION

A massive effusion into the pleural cavity will cause dyspnoea and cyanosis with dullness on percussion and diminished breath sounds. Pleural effusions were found in babies severely affected by rhesus incompatibility. A rare cause is chylothorax which usually occurs for no obvious reason but cases have been reported in babies born with the umbilical cord tightly around the neck when the thoracic duct has been torn.

If the chylothorax persists despite repeated aspiration then surgical intervention is indicated.

HEART FAILURE

Dyspnoea due to congenital disease of the heart is not usually severe but increases in the presence of cardiac failure. Dyspnoea of cardiac origin is liable to be aggravated by crying and disturbance, and in the more severe cases is associated with restlessness. An infant suffering from extreme respiratory distress due to intrathoracic infection or to terminal cardiac failure frequently lies with his neck retracted, suggestive of intracranial disease. At the same time he lies panting desperately, his fixed gaze conveying the impression of extreme apprehension. The treatment of cardiac failure was dealt with in Chapter 11.

Extrathoracic Causes of Dyspnoea

CEREBRAL

Cerebral birth trauma may cause apnoeic attacks going on to generalized cyanosis and convulsions. Following an apnoeic attack respirations are often slow and gasping or periodic in nature when the breaths are of increasing and decreasing depth. These symptoms, which are due to raised intracranial pressure, are also found in hypoxaemia, hypoglycaemia and meningitis. When the anterior fontanelle tension is raised, and lumbar puncture has excluded meningitis, then bilateral subdural taps should be carried out to exclude an encysted haematoma (Chap. 12).

SEVERE ANAEMIA

Dyspnoea is seen in the presence of severe anaemia secondary to haemorrhage. Severe anaemia at birth and within the first few days of life may be due to fetal haemorrhage into the maternal circulation or into the circulation of a twin, bleeding from a placental tear, accidental incision during caesarean delivery, accidental haemorrhage from the umbilical cord or due to severe haemorrhagic disease, bleeding into a massive cephalhaematoma or under the aponeurosis of the scalp, and rupture of the liver, spleen or adrenals. Severe anaemia is also a feature of haemolytic disease. A strikingly pale and dyspnoeic infant at birth must have a haemoglobin estimation carried out immediately and must be given blood when indicated. Severe anaemia may cause death within a few hours of delivery as a result of shock and cortical necrosis of the kidneys.

FEBRILE CONDITIONS

Dyspnoea may be seen in conditions accompanied by pyrexia, e.g. urinary tract infection, acute respiratory infections and septicaemia.

METABOLIC ACIDOSIS

Dyspnoea is a feature of metabolic acidosis. In severe cases respirations are both deep and rapid.

Due to increased catabolism of body tissue acidosis is commonly found in small immature babies for the first few days of life. This is best corrected by early feeding—especially with breast milk.

Metabolic acidosis is a feature of the respiratory distress syndrome and also accompanies fetal hypoxia. As described earlier fetal hypoxia results in anaerobic glycolysis with the accumulation of lactic acid in the blood. In both situations the acidosis is corrected by the administration of sodium bicarbonate.

NURSING OBSERVATIONS

Observations made by the midwife concerning dyspnoea are of importance in recognizing the presence of disease and in assessing clinical progress. Thus changes in the rate, rhythm and depth of respiration are of great significance in the first 48 hours of life in evaluating the trend of clinical events in a baby who has been born hypoxic or prematurely. An increase in the rate of respirations may be the first sign of disease or the spread of infection from pharynx to the trachea, bronchi or lungs. The sudden onset of dyspnoea should always suggest an emergency which may have its explanation in a pneumothorax, a fulminating infection or massive haemorrhage.

CYANOSIS

Cyanosis is a blue colour of the skin or mucous membranes which is usually due to the presence of an excessive amount of reduced haemoglobin in the small blood vessels of the tissues. Very occasionally it is due to the presence of methaemoglobin or sulphaemoglobin. There must be at least 5 g of reduced haemoglobin per 100 ml blood before cyanosis occurs, consequently cyanosis does not occur in presence of severe anaemia.

Cyanosis can be either peripheral or central. In central cyanosis the arterial blood is unsaturated whereas in peripheral cyanosis the arterial blood is normally saturated but the extraction of oxygen from the blood in the tissues is excessive. The distinction is best made by examining the buccal mucous membranes where blood flow is always good. If these are blue the cyanosis is of the central type. In cases of doubt the baby should be compared with a healthy infant. The various causes of cyanosis are detailed in Table 15.3.

Table 15.3 Causes of cyanosis in the newborn

PERIPHERAL CYANOSIS
Poor peripheral circulation
Traumatic cyanosis
CENTRAL CYANOSIS
Transitory
Primary apnoea
Secondary apnoea
Airway obstruction
RDS
Intrathoracic
Infective
Persistent
Congenital heart disease
Polycythaemia
Methaemoglobinaemia

Peripheral Cyanosis

Peripheral cyanosis occurs when the flow of blood through the superficial skin and mucous membranes is unusually slow with the result that most of the oxygen in the normally oxygenated blood passes into the surrounding tissues. This form of cyanosis is present in the hands and feet (and sometimes the face) of a large proportion of babies during the early hours of life, and in the lips and extremities of newly born babies of any age who have become chilled. In lethargic infants or in infants whose circulation has become temporarily slow (as in sleep) circumoral cyanosis may develop but disappears with a return of normal activity.

TRAUMATIC 'CYANOSIS'

Traumatic cyanosis, which results from venous compression followed by extravasation of blood, is limited to the head and neck and follows when the cord has been wrapped tightly around the neck or when the head has been on the perineum for some considerable time. In addition to the cyanosis, which contrasts with the normal pink of the trunk and extremities, close inspection will reveal the presence of tiny petechiae in the scalp and skin of the head and neck. Subconjunctival haemorrhages may also be present. In the absence of a serious complicating condition traumatic cyanosis need not cause concern and does not interfere with normal progress.

In traumatic cyanosis petechiae are limited to the head and neck but where petechiae are distributed over the whole body the possibilities of congenital rubella, toxoplasmosis, cytomegalovirus infection and congenital thrombocytopenic purpura must be entertained.

Central Cyanosis

Reduction of the oxygen content of all the blood is evident as central cyanosis. The hypoxaemia may be due to lack of oxygen in the inspired air, failure to absorb oxygen in the lungs or to mixture of venous and arterial blood within the heart or great vessels.

Central cyanosis is always significant and requires immediate investigation and treatment. The causes of transitory cyanosis are in general different from those of persistent cyanosis.

TRANSITORY CYANOSIS

Primary apnoea. At birth the infant will be cyanosed until respiration is satisfactorily established.

Secondary apnoea. Any cause of secondary apnoea will also result in cyanosis. This may occur in low birth-weight infants, in infants with RDS and in those who are hypoglycaemic. It will also occur during convulsions or as a separate manifestation of cerebral birth injury.

Airway obstruction. Aspiration of milk or secretions, blockage of the airway by the tongue in Pierre-Robin syndrome or any other form of obstruction of the airway will produce cyanosis.

The serious significance of severe hypoxaemia and cyanosis in RDS has already been discussed earlier in this chapter.

Intrathoracic causes include diaphragmatic hernia, pulmonary agenesis, emphysema, pneumothorax and lung cysts which have already been discussed.

Infections, whether in the lungs or in other parts of the body, may cause cyanosis.

PERSISTENT CYANOSIS

Congenital heart disease. Persistent central cyanosis is the presenting sign of certain congenital heart lesions involving a right to left shunt of deoxygenated blood. Lesions include transposition of the great vessels, pulmonary atresia, tricuspid atresia and total anomalous pulmonary venous drainage. Central cyanosis of later onset is associated with Fallot's tetralogy.

Polycythaemia. Cyanosis due to polycythaemia may be detected at or shortly after birth. This may be the result of antenatal transplacental maternofetal bleeding or, in a twin pregnancy, of an arteriovenous shunt from the placenta of one to that of the other twin. Infants born to diabetic mothers have a naturally high colour which may lead to suspicions of cyanosis more especially when they are crying.

Methaemoglobinaemia. Central cyanosis is an early sign in congenital methaemoglobinaemia in which a deficiency of the methaemoglobin reductase system in the red cells leads to an accumulation of methaemoglobin. The absence of signs of illness in the presence of deep cyanosis is diagnostic. The baby is not dyspnoeic and the cyanosis is not increased by crying or diminished by the administration of oxygen. Blood examination shows no evidence of either anaemia or polycythaemia, and methaemoglobin bands are seen on spectroscopic examination. Reducing agents in the form of ascorbic acid (200 to 500 mg daily) and methylene blue (4 mg per kg daily by mouth in three divided doses) have been used in treatment for many years without ill effects. There is risk in the use of benzocaine and related anaesthetics and of long-acting sulphonamides in these babies.

NURSING OBSERVATIONS

Cyanosis of sudden onset requires immediate investigation and treatment. Baby's air passages must be cleared of any obstruction and the effect on respiration noted. Increased respiratory movement suggests continuing obstruction and tracheal intubation and aspiration may be required.

16

Convulsions and Other Abnormal Behaviour

In this chapter consideration will be given to convulsions, hyperactivity, hypertonia, hypotonia, drowsiness and abnormal posture.

CONVULSIONS

Convulsions are repetitive jerky movements which may be accompanied by apnoea, rigidity and loss of consciousness (Fig. 16.1). They vary considerably in form and in degree.

Tonic. A tonic phase may be followed by clonic movements and

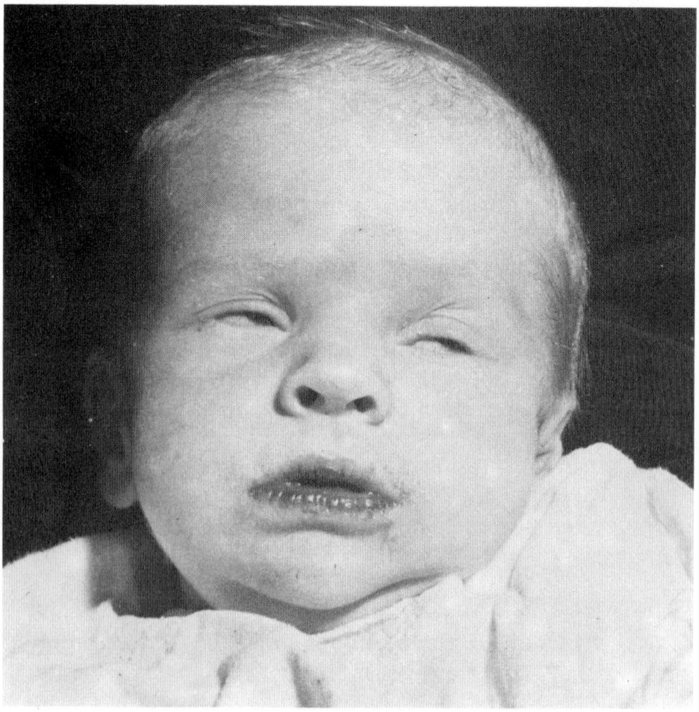

Figure 16.1 The facies and deviation of the eyes during a convulsion. At the time this photograph was taken baby was momentarily unconscious and there were clonic movements of the extremities.

unconsciousness; there may be only isolated but prolonged tonic incidents; or there may be brief clonic phases without associated tonicity or unconsciousness. A grunt or cry may precede a convulsion but is usually absent.

Clonic. Generalized clonic convulsions may occur in infants who have sustained an intraventricular cerebral haemorrhage. Cyanosis, neck rigidity and opisthotonus are occasionally present. Convulsions in the small preterm infant may be evident as rhythmic movements involving the fingers, the toes, the angles of the mouth or the eyes.

Jitteriness. Convulsions should not be confused with neuromuscular hyperexcitability, an exaggerated form of the Moro reflex, sometimes referred to as the 'dithers' or the 'jitters'.

The clinical conditions in which convulsions occur are listed in Table 16.1 and the more common conditions with time of onset are listed in Table 16.2.

Table 16.1 Clinical conditions associated with convulsions

Cerebral disorders
Hypoxia, haemorrhage and trauma
Maldevelopment
Hypoglycaemia
Hypocalcaemia and hypomagnesaemia
Infection
Meningitis
Tetanus
Overhydration
Morphine withdrawal
Metabolic disturbances
Pyridoxine dependency
Maple syrup urine disease
Hypophosphatasia
Hyperprolinaemia
Glycogen storage disease

Table 16.2 Common causes of convulsions with typical time of onset

First Day	Intracranial injury
Second Day	Hypoglycaemia
Fourth to Sixth Days	Hypocalcaemia
End of First Week	Meningitis
Prolonged Convulsions	Cerebral maldevelopment

Cerebral Disorders

INTRACRANIAL INJURY

This is the commonest cause of convulsions in the newly born infant.

Hypoxia. As pointed out in Chapter 12 hypoxia is the single most important factor.

Intracranial haemorrhage is less common and is usually associated with the rapid delivery of a preterm infant.

Time onset. Convulsions due to cerebral birth trauma commonly occur within the first 24 hours of life, being preceded by irritability, a high-pitched cry, an anxious expression and twitching of the limbs, and followed later in the more severe cases by neck stiffness and a bulging fontanelle. In such cases convulsions in association with vomiting and cyanotic attacks signify a poor prognosis and in those who survive there is a high probability of neurological handicap.

CEREBRAL MALDEVELOPMENT

Convulsions which start within a day or two of birth and which prove resistant to anticonvulsant therapy are suggestive of gross cerebral abnormality with underdevelopment of one or both cerebral hemispheres.

Hypoglycaemia

Whenever a previously healthy newborn infant suddenly has a convulsion or apnoeic episode hypoglycaemia should be suspected. A low Dextrostix reading should be checked immediately in the laboratory by glucose measurements on a whole blood sample to confirm the diagnosis.

Blood sugar. In babies who weigh less than 2 kg at birth the mean blood glucose level on the third day of life is 35 mg per 100 ml. After the third day there is a steady rise to the normal range which is achieved by the tenth day. Hypoglycaemia causing convulsions occurs particularly during the first 72 hours of life when the blood glucose falls below 20 mg per 100 ml.

AETIOLOGY

In Chapter 9 it was suggested that hypoglycaemia is a direct consequence of insufficient stores of energy-producing glycogen with the possible additional factor of temporary adrenocortical hypofunction.

Predisposing factors are fetal malnutrition (light-for-dates infants), hypothermia, respiratory distress syndrome and cerebral damage.

Rare causes of hypoglycaemia, occurring after the first week or so of life, are glycogen storage disease, pancreatic islet cell tumour and leucine sensitivity.

CLINICAL SIGNS

The early signs of hypoglycaemia include apnoeic attacks, semiconsciousness and absence of the Moro reflex despite the fact that the infant is irritable when handled. The later signs are severe apnoeic attacks, convulsions and deep coma. These may mistakenly be attributed to cerebral or adrenal haemorrhage.

TREATMENT

In the presence of symptoms a blood sugar level of less than 20 mg per 100 ml is an indication for immediate treatment to prevent brain damage.

PREVENTION

Early and adequate feeding of low birth-weight infants will prevent the onset of hypoglycaemia in most infants.

Intravenous glucose. In the presence of severe symptoms, such as apnoeic attacks or convulsions, the blood glucose must be elevated quickly by the intravenous injection of 10 to 15 ml of 20 per cent dextrose solution. Treatment is continued with 10 per cent dextrose solution at the rate of 5 ml per kg per hour. Oral feeding is resumed when symptoms have settled and the blood glucose has returned to normal. The intravenous fluids are progressively reduced and then withdrawn.

Steroids. If there is difficulty in maintaining a normal blood glucose steroids should be given as prednisolone 0.5 mg per kg two to four times daily, or as ACTH gel 5 units by injection daily for three days.

Oral treatment. If the only symptom has been jitteriness (dithers) and the blood glucose is above 20 mg per 100 ml oral treatment should be given a trial. Extra feeds of 10 per cent dextrose should be given and extra carbohydrate added to normal feeds.

PROGNOSIS

Infants who have shown evidence of hypoglycaemia in the new-born period should be considered 'at risk' and should be reviewed in a follow-up clinic with particular reference to neurological function.

Severe type. The prognosis for infants with severe and prolonged hypoglycaemia is poor and the majority will prove to have severe cerebral dysfunction.

Mild type. It is more difficult to assess the outlook for infants with slight symptoms but in general it is good. Careful assessment at school age may however show that some of these infants have learning difficulties and other forms of handicap which were not evident at an earlier stage.

Hypocalcaemia

Neonatal tetany is evident as irritability followed by twitching and sometimes repeated convulsions which may be focal in nature. It commonly occurs when the serum calcium falls below 3.5 mEq per litre. External stimulation such as lightly tapping the sternum provokes coarse waving movements of the limbs in association with fine agitation of the fingers.

Early onset. There is a significant difference in the prognosis of infants who develop hypocalcaemia in the first few days of life and in those who develop it later in the first week. Hypocalcaemia occurring in the first three days of life is fairly common in low birth-weight babies, in babies born to diabetic mothers and in babies who have suffered cerebral birth trauma. These infants often have a poor prognosis.

Late onset. Hypocalcaemia occurring toward the end of the first week of life is usually associated with artificial feeding, the low blood calcium level being secondary to hyperphosphataemia, which arises since the immature kidney is unable to deal with the high phosphate content of cow's milk. Late onset hypocalcaemia has a good prognosis.

Hyperphosphataemia. It has been suggested that this condition represents parathyroid insufficiency and should be called 'transient congenital idiopathic hypoparathyroidism', tetany being triggered off by the high phosphate and relatively low calcium intake associated with artificial feeding. The modern trend for early feeding of large volumes of cow's milk preparations provokes clinical manifestations of transient congenital hypoparathyroidism which would otherwise remain unrecognized.

Maternal hyperparathyroidism. Hypocalcaemia may occur in transient congenital hypoparathyroidism associated with maternal hyperparathyroidism. The mother's blood calcium should be checked if her baby develops persisting tetany.

TREATMENT

Treatment of tetany consists of correction of the mineral deficiency and in avoiding unnecessary disturbance.

A low phosphate milk such as breast milk or S.M.A. is advisable.

Extra calcium can be given orally as supplements of 5 to 10 ml of a 5 per cent solution of calcium chloride with feeds. Although calcium chloride may cause intestinal haemorrhage it appears to be more effective in raising the blood calcium level than other oral preparations.

Intravenous calcium. Where oral treatment fails or is not feasible 2 ml of a 10 per cent calcium gluconate solution should be given slowly intravenously. Vitamin D and parathormone are required when supplements of calcium are insufficient to correct the serum calcium.

PROGNOSIS

As far as is known babies who have suffered from transient hypocalcaemia develop normally without any neurological sequelae although dental caries is a recognized complication.

Hypomagnesaemia

Primary hypomagnesaemia may occur with hypocalcaemia and should be suspected whenever an infant with hypocalcaemia does not stop convulsing when the serum calcium returns to normal. The symptoms are identical to those of hypocalcaemia and respond dramatically to treatment with magnesium sulphate given parenterally.

Meningitis

Meningitis is described in Chapter 13. The illness is part of a septicaemia with the infection localizing in the meninges. Persistent lethargy or drowsiness and a 'distant' expression, more rarely slight stiffness of the neck, and occasionally associated convulsions would suggest meningitis. There is sometimes a further hint in the presence of slight exophthalmos. The diagnosis is confirmed by lumbar puncture. Treatment with antibiotics and anticonvulsants is instituted immediately.

Gram-negative bacilli. It is highly probable that the causal organism is *E. coli* or one of the related Gram-negative bacilli, so choice of antibiotics would be from kanamycin, ampicillin, gentamycin, colistin and chloramphenicol.

Listeria monocytogenes. To cover this and other possible infections it is probably wise to start treatment with ampicillin and cloxacillin, adjusting treatment when the results of culture and sensitivity are known.

Initially treatment should be given intravenously.

PROGNOSIS

The chances of complete recovery, even with early diagnosis and treatment, are probably less than 40 per cent. Where diagnosis has been late and treatment delayed, the mortality is high and survivors are likely to be permanently cerebrally damaged.

Tetanus Neonatorum

Convulsions also occur in tetanus. There is spasm of the muscles of the jaw, face, trunk and limbs. The condition is rarely if ever seen in the United Kingdom. In areas where the standard of hygiene is low a sickle blade or dirty knife may be used to cut the cord with the danger that tetanus spores may be introduced. Treatment is by antibiotics, sedation with diazepam, antitetanic serum and general supportive measures. The prognosis is poor in very young infants. Giving the mother tetanus toxoid during pregnancy greatly reduces the risk to her infant.

Rare Causes of Convulsions

OVERHYDRATION

Usually due to excessive intravenous infusion of an electrolyte-free solution, overhydration may cause convulsions. It is unwise to give dextrose infusions for more than 24 hours. Dextrose and saline mixtures rather than dextrose should be used.

Morphine withdrawal. Convulsion may precede coma in babies of mothers addicted to morphine. Treatment consists of sedation with phenobarbitone or diazepam for a few days or weeks as necessary.

METABOLIC DISORDERS

Severe convulsions in the newborn may be a feature of such rare metabolic disorders as maple syrup urine disease, hypophosphatasia, hyperprolinaemia, glycogen storage disease and pyridoxine dependency.

Maple syrup urine disease is a rare condition which can give rise to a clinical picture within a week of birth simulating meningitis or intracranial haemorrhage. Failure to thrive is typical, and the excretion of urine with an odour of maple syrup (or burnt sugar) may suggest the diagnosis. Chromatography reveals multiple aminoaciduria (valine, leucine and isoleucine) with a characteristically abnormal pattern. Slow decline preceded by the onset of spasticity and coma is customary, but trial has recently been given to a special diet with moderately encouraging results.

Congenital hypophosphatasia. Absence of the enzyme alkaline phosphatase explains the occasional finding of congenital hypophosphatasia. Signs can appear in the early days, behaviour being characterized by poverty of movement, and apathy short of extreme drowsiness, disinclination for feeds and unsatisfactory weight progress. There may be convulsions which may or may not synchronize with the development of fullness and tension of the fontanelle. Patchy calcification of the metaphyses and widening of the epiphyseal lines are seen in the radiographs (Fig. 16.2). The condition is usually fatal.

Glycogen storage disease. Rarely Cori's type I glycogen storage disease (von Gierke's disease) may become manifest in the neonatal period. Symptoms usually become manifest some time after birth with abdominal distension due to liver enlargement, loss of appetite, vomiting and convulsions due to hypoglycaemia. The prognosis is grave and affected babies fail to thrive and die of hypoglycaemia and acidosis within the first few years of life. Treatment consists in giving a high protein, low carbohydrate diet. Initially feeds should be

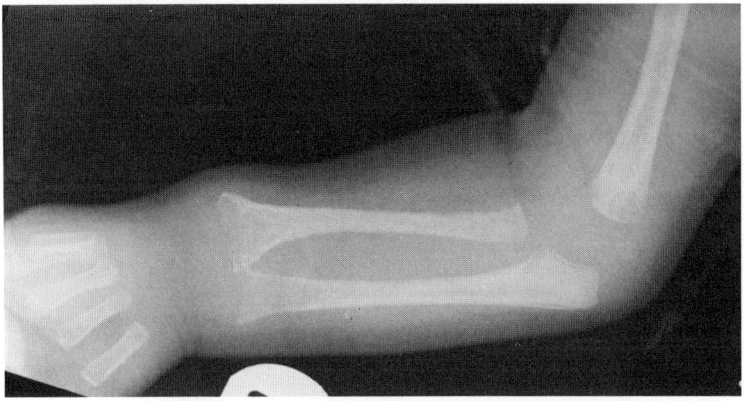

Figure 16.2 Congenital hypophosphatasia. Widening of the distal ends of radius and ulna with defective mineralisation.

given at three or four hourly intervals day and night, and the carbohydrate content of the diet should be in the form of glucose. Hypoglycaemic episodes should be treated vigorously with intravenous dextrose solution.

Hyperprolinaemia. Newly born babies with hyperprolinaemia present a similar clinical picture to that of congenital hypophosphatasia, maple syrup urine disease and glycogen storage disease. The picture is one of sustained cerebral depression continuing in the second, third and fourth weeks of life. Significant features of the picture are an expressionless facies (Fig. 16.3), unresponsiveness to approach and normal stimuli, abnormal quietness, poverty of movement and total disinclination for feeds. It is essential that any baby in whom pronounced signs of disturbed cerebral function persist into the second week should, regardless of the obstetrical background and birth history, be screened for abnormal amino acid and carbohydrate metabolism. This is the more important in view of the known facts that the brain is peculiarly susceptible to damage in disease of inborn errors of metabolism, and that, depending upon the size of the molecule involved, the traumatic process may be initiated *in utero* or in any event shortly after birth.

Pyridoxine dependency is another metabolic disorder in which convulsions are rapidly controlled by the intramuscular administration of 100 mg pyridoxine.

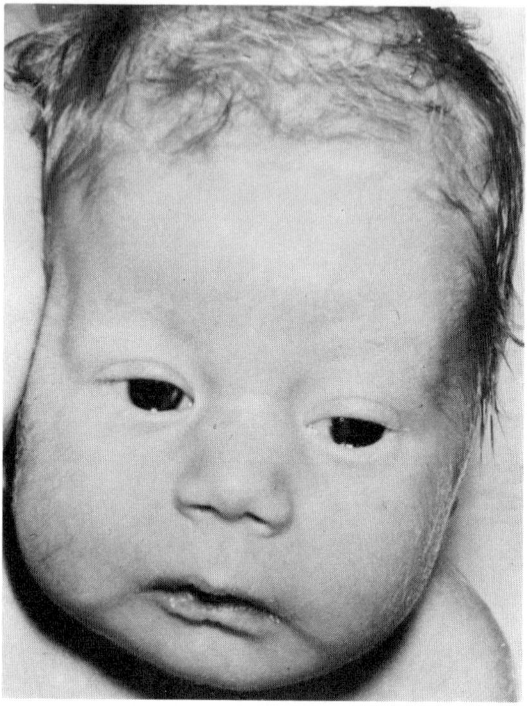

Figure 16.3 Expressionless facies in hyperprolinaemia.

HYPERACTIVITY

Low birth-weight babies are constantly on the move even when asleep. Their abdominal muscles are constantly moving and every now and again a limb will flex and relax in a perfectly natural manner. Occasionally the most immature preterm baby shows remarkable activity during the first day or two of life after which his behaviour resembles that of other preterm babies.

Congenital thyrotoxicosis (Fig. 16.4 and 5) is sometimes seen for a limited period after birth following delivery of a mother with hyperthyroidism, with a history of previous thyroidectomy or with a history of thyroid medication. Symptoms and signs of congenital thyrotoxicosis include tachycardia—sometimes with heart failure, hyperactivity amounting to agitation, abnormal eagerness for feeds, enlargement of the thyroid and exophthalmos. Their onset may be delayed for about a week as a result of prenatal therapy given to the mother. Treatment of the baby is by antithyroid drugs and such

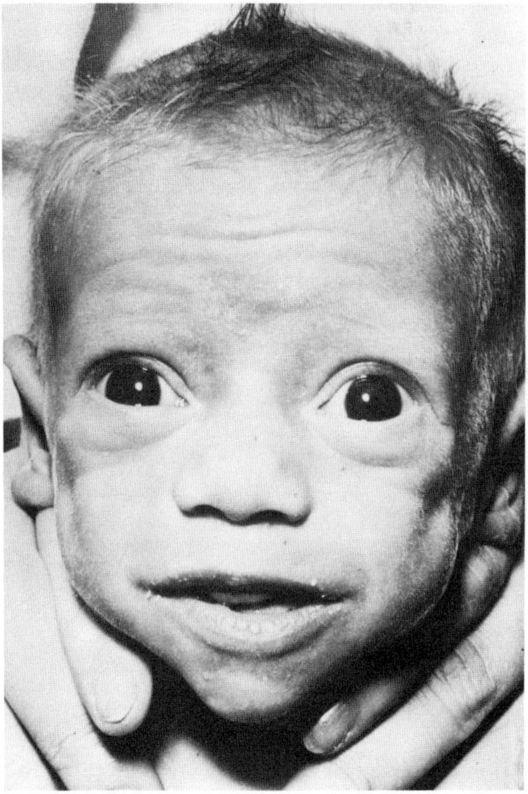

Figure 16.4 Congenital thyrotoxicosis. (By courtesy of Professor A. G. Watkins.)

supportive digoxin therapy as may be indicated by signs of heart failure.

It is now known that the condition is due to the passage of long-acting thyroid stimulator (LATS) across the placenta from a mother with thyrotoxicosis. Like idiopathic thrombocytopenic purpura, myasthesia gravis and possibly congenital diabetes mellitus, congenital thyrotoxicosis has come to be regarded as a possible example of an autoimmune disease. In all these conditions the signs are transient and they disappear with the first six weeks of life with the elimination of maternal immunoglobulins from the infant's circulation.

Stimulants. Apnoeic infants who have been treated with stimulants such as nikethamide (Coramine) or vanillic acid diethylamide

(Vandid) administered to them occasionally show signs of increased neuromuscular excitability, sometimes aptly described as 'Coramine dance'. These signs are more liable to develop in a preterm baby and are evidence of excessive dosage. It is now felt that other methods

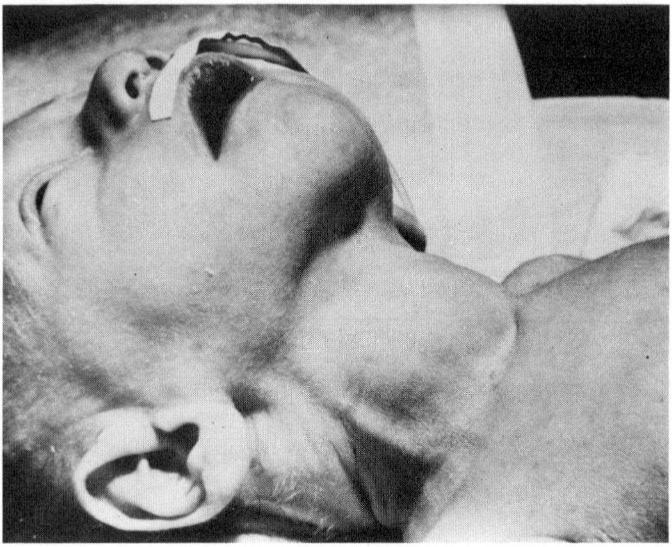

Figure 16.5 Enlargement of thyroid in congenital thyrotoxicosis.

of resuscitation discussed in Chapter 5 are preferable to the use of stimulant drugs.

HYPERTONIA

As in older children and adults convulsions in the newly born infant usually have a tonic component. The tonic phase may be short-lived or prolonged.

HYPOXIA

Babies who have suffered cerebral damage as a result of perinatal hypoxia are hypertonic during the first hours or days after delivery. In this event the hypertonia occurs in association with undue lethargy, feeding difficulty, overexcitability, jitteriness and convulsions. Later the signs of cerebral palsy may become evident.

Increased muscle tone must be differentiated from stiffness due to lack of joint movement as in arthrogryposis (Fig. 16.6) or due to sclerema associated with neonatal cold injury (Fig. 16.7).

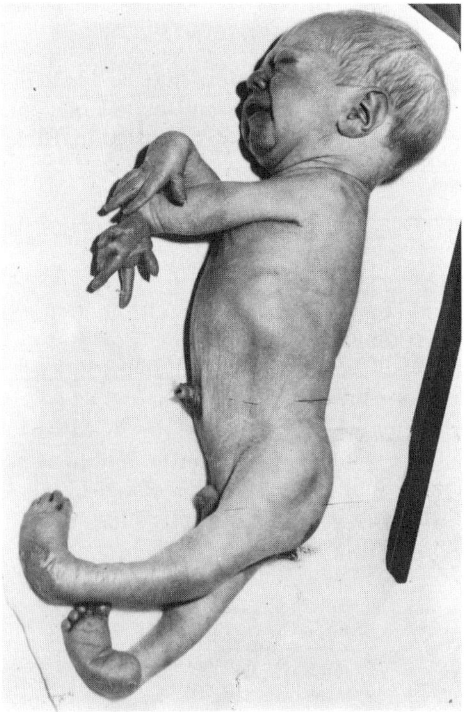

Figure 16.6 Arthrogryposis.

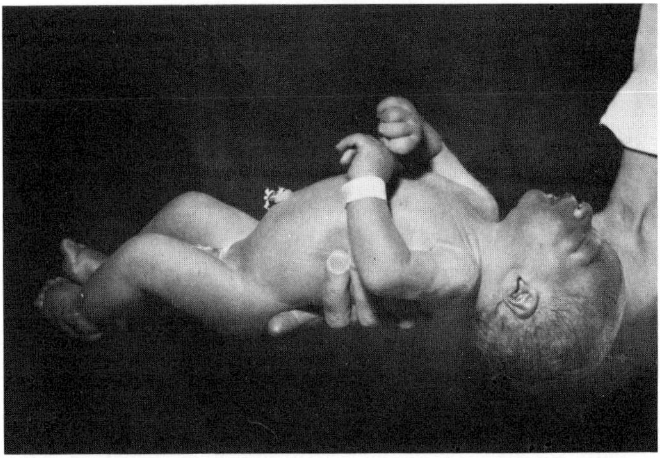

Figure 16.7 Severe hypothermia with generalized rigidity.

HYPOTONIA

Hypotonia in the newly born infant may be due to disorders of the brain, spinal cord, muscles, peripheral nerves or connective tissue. The causes, both common and rare, are listed in Table 16.3.

Cerebral Causes

Hypotonicity is a feature of major dysfunction of the central nervous system.

Birth injury. Extensive injury to the brain whether from hypoxia, mechanical injury or haemorrhage results in hypotonia once the initial phase of irritability has passed.

Maldevelopment of the brain, particularly hypoplasia, is frequently associated with poor muscle tone.

Mental retardation. Abnormality of brain function which later becomes evident as mental retardation may present in the neonatal period as hypotonia and difficulty with feeding. This is seen in infants with Down's syndrome and other chromosomal abnormalities associated with mental retardation.

Table 16.3 Causes of hypotonia in the newborn

Cerebral causes
Birth trauma
Maldevelopment
Mental retardation
Hypoxia
Low birth weight
Rarer causes
Metabolic disturbances
Maple syrup urine disease
Hypophosphatasia
Hyperprolinaemia
Glycogen storage disease
Myasthenia gravis
Werdnig-Hoffmann disease
Muscular disorders
Prader-Willi syndrome
Familial dysautonomia

Severe Hypoxia

In previous chapters repeated reference has been made to the association of hypotonicity with hypoxia and low birth weight. The profound hypotonia of severe hypoxia may be followed by death or, if the baby survives, permanent neurological handicap in the form of cerebral palsy. Less severe degrees of perinatal hypoxia are followed by a stage of hypotonicity of indeterminate length but fortunately, in the majority of cases, without any permanent cerebral damage.

Low Birth Weight

Low birth weight infants, particularly those born well before term, have poorer muscle tone than more mature infants. This hypotonia is the basis for several of the tests discussed in Chapter 9, which are used for the clinical assessment of maturity. Hypotonia is not inconsistent with the periods of hyperactivity seen in low birth-weight infants. Improvement in muscle tone is a sign of normal healthy progress.

Other Rare Causes

Persistent hypotonia in the newly born infant should bring to mind the rarer diagnoses listed in Table 16.3.

METABOLIC DISTURBANCES

As described earlier in this chapter, certain metabolic disturbances including maple syrup urine disease, hypophosphatasia, hyperprolinaemia and the cardiomuscular form of glycogen storage disease all present a similar clinical picture not unlike that presented by the infant who survives perinatal severe hypoxia. In addition to hypotonia these babies exhibit expressionless facies, unresponsiveness to approach and normal stimuli, abnormal quietness and total disinclination for feeds. The baby with glycogen storage disease will have a large heart and tongue.

MYASTHENIA GRAVIS

There are two forms of myasthenia gravis in the newborn.

Juvenile. In the so-called 'juvenile' form signs in the baby persist throughout life, but it is altogether exceptional for them to appear in the first week of life. In these cases the mother has no signs of myasthenia.

Neonatal. The other form is called neonatal myasthenia gravis. The mother is suffering from myasthenia but the signs which are present in the baby at or shortly after birth disappear within a few hours or days, although occasionally they last as long as six to eight weeks. It has been estimated that about 20 per cent of babies of severely myasthenic mothers are affected. Slight delay in the initial appearance of signs in the baby could be explained by therapy given to the mother. Generalized muscular hypotonia dominates the clinical picture, there being symmetrical involvement of face, trunk and limbs. In the severe case there is lack of facial expression, difficulty in sucking and swallowing and poverty of movement. If, as is unlikely with a knowledge of the mother's condition, there is doubt concerning diagnosis, confirmation is obtained by the injection of edrophonium chloride (Tensilon) 0.05 to 0.10 ml or neostigmine methyl sulphate (Prostigmin) 0.01 mg per kg body weight subcutaneously or intramuscularly which will rapidly restore normal muscle tone. Progress is good with the reservation that exceptionally death follows respiratory failure.

Any apparently healthy baby born to a mother with myasthenia gravis should be kept under continuous skilled observation for some two to four days because of the risk of the delayed appearance of myasthenic signs.

WERDNIG-HOFFMANN DISEASE

Werdnig-Hoffmann disease, or spinal muscular atrophy, is an autosomal recessive condition which is characterized by hypotonia and wasting of the skeletal muscles resulting from degeneration of the anterior horn cells of the spinal cord. Fetal movements are feeble or absent, and at birth the baby is limp, flaccid and areflexic. Characteristically the baby lies in a froglike position and there is fibrillation of the tongue. Muscle biopsy shows diagnostic changes and death usually occurs within the first year of life.

MUSCULAR DISORDERS

There are a number of such disorders which may present with hypotonia in the newborn period.

Benign congenital hypotonia improves spontaneously as the infant grows.

Muscular dystrophies usually become apparent well after the neonatal period but affected babies are occasionally noted to be hypotonic at birth.

PRADER-WILLI SYNDROME

Infants with this syndrome are particularly hypotonic and may be unable to cry or suck. In the male child the scrotum is hypoplastic and the testes undescended. As they grow older they become obese.

FAMILIAL DYSAUTONOMIA

Familial dysautonomia, or the Riley-Day syndrome, is an autosomal recessive condition almost exclusively confined to the Jewish race. The condition is transmitted as an autosomal recessive trait and is thought to be a disorder of the autonomic nervous system. Affected infants are hypotonic and areflexic, have difficulty in feeding and swallowing and suffer repeated respiratory infections. In addition there is defective or absent lacrimation, loss of corneal sensation leading to ulcer formation, impaired temperature control, and eventual physical and mental retardation. Treatment is symptomatic and some infants reach adult life.

The Floppy Infant

The differential diagnosis of the hypotonic infant must include consideration of the causes described above. It is often difficult to reach a firm diagnosis in the early stages. The urgency to establish a diagnosis depends upon the severity of the hypotonia and the risk which this implies to the infant's well-being.

Close observation is required and rapid resuscitative measures will be required if a hypotonic infant aspirates mucus or milk. An assessment of change in muscle tone is a most important observation as the final diagnosis may well depend on the recognition of signs of improvement which will eventually appear in a condition such as benign muscular hypotonia.

Investigation. Nerve conduction studies, electromyography, serum enzyme studies and muscle biopsy may be necessary before a final diagnosis and prognosis can be made.

Genetic advice. Accuracy in diagnosis is essential before genetic advice is given.

DROWSINESS

Drowsiness is an indication of poor cerebral function which may occur in small preterm infants, after cerebral injury, with raised intracranial pressure and following sedation. It may also occur with infections, severe hypothermia and in some metabolic disorders.

Cerebral Dysfunction

Preterm infants. The smallest preterm infants, although showing episodes of hyperactivity, periodically tend to be drowsy and inactive particularly after feeds.

Cerebral injury, whether due to mechanical trauma, hypoxia or haemorrhage, may cause profound drowsiness and inactivity.

Raised intracranial pressure. Infants with hydrocephalus or subdural haematoma become increasingly drowsy as the intracranial pressure rises.

Oversedation. Infants whose mothers have been treated with sedatives or hypnotics shortly before delivery may be very drowsy and difficult to resuscitate at birth. If one of the morphine group of drugs has been used an injection of nalorphine should be given. Infants who have been sedated following convulsion will also become drowsy.

INFECTION

Persistent drowsiness and lethargy in association with a 'distant' expression suggests the possibility of widespread infection probably involving the meninges. Lumbar puncture, blood and urine cultures should be arranged and antibiotic treatment given.

NEONATAL COLD INJURY

Severe hypothermia with fall in central temperature is associated with progressive drowsiness as well as the other features already described in Chapter 9.

METABOLIC DISORDERS

Earlier in this chapter mention was made of the drowsiness which forms part of the clinical picture of some metabolic disorders such as maple syrup urine disease and hyperprolinaemia.

ABNORMAL POSTURE

The normal posture at birth is one of generalized flexion which involves both the spine and the limbs. In the course of normal development the primary flexion curve of the spine is modified by secondary extension curves in the cervical and lumbar regions as the baby first acquires head control and later sits, stands erect and walks. Immediately following birth flexion of the limbs is of such a degree that it is frequently impossible to fully extend the limbs. This inability to straighten the legs makes accurate measurement of length at birth both difficult and unreliable.

Abnormal postures result from peripheral nerve palsies, abnormal fetal positions and fractures (Chap. 12).

PERIPHERAL NERVE PALSIES

Dropped wrist is a feature of radial nerve and Klumpke's palsy. In Erb's palsy the arm is rotated internally and hangs limply from the shoulder, the elbow is extended, and the hand is partially closed with the palm directed outwards and posteriorly in the typical 'waiter's tip' position. Obturator nerve palsy results in full external rotation and abduction of the leg with flexion of the knee. Sciatic nerve palsy resulting from unskilled intramuscular injection or mistaken injection into the umbilical artery causes weakness of the leg with a dropped foot.

FRACTURES

Fracture of limb bones causes deformity and possibly pseudoparalysis.

Epiphyseal injuries, usually of the upper epiphyses of the femur and humerus, produce swelling of the part with immobility.

ABNORMAL FETAL POSITIONS

Fetal positions responsible for abnormal postures at birth were described in Chapter 11.

Genu recurvatum is a deformity consisting of abnormal hyper-extension of the knee joint. It may involve one or both limbs and is sometimes complicated by posterior dislocation of the knee. Spontaneous improvement is usual and splinting for a limited period is necessary only in severe cases.

Arthrogryposis. The congenital stiffness of one or more joints together with hypoplasia of related muscles as seen in arthrogryposis congenita multiplex has already been mentioned earlier in this chapter (Fig. 16.6).

Breech delivery. Where the baby has presented at the breech with extended legs the abnormal posture of the legs is maintained for some days after birth. From the clinical point of view it is wise to remember that such an abnormal presentation favours congenital dislocation of the hip.

Talipes. Flexion deformities of the wrist and talipes calcaneo-valgus are not infrequently associated with oligohydramnios. These abnormal postures usually disappear spontaneously within the neonatal period.

Hyperextension of the neck, or opisthotonus, is a worrying sign in the neonate. Possible causes, all of which have already been fully described, include face presentation, meningitis, tetanus, vascular ring and kernicterus.

17

Pallor, Haemorrhage and Purpura

Pallor, haemorrhage and purpura are conveniently considered in one chapter as they often occur together.

PALLOR

The skin of a healthy newborn European infant is sufficiently 'pink' for pallor to be readily recognizable as an abnormal physical sign. Similar lack of coloration from capillary blood can be seen in pigmented races. In any infant pallor must be considered as a serious sign and the cause sought out and treated urgently.

PALLOR OF RECENT ONSET

This is likely to have arisen from one or more of the following: peripheral vasoconstriction, anaemia following haemolysis, anaemia following haemorrhage.

Each of these may occur independently but are often interrelated.

Blood loss may cause immediate peripheral vasoconstriction and be followed by the pallor of anaemia as plasma volume is restored.

Haemolysis, purpura and circulatory collapse may occur together or in quick succession in infants with severe infection.

Several causes of pallor have already been dealt with in previous chapters. The circulatory collapse associated with injury to the brain in Chapter 12, the pallor of severe infection in Chapter 13, the anaemia of haemolytic disease in Chapter 14.

Physiological Anaemia

MARROW INACTIVITY

Pallor of slow onset occurs most frequently in preterm infants and is due to a progressive fall in haemoglobin associated with relative inactivity of the bone marrow (Chap. 5). The resulting 'physiological anaemia' is less marked in more mature infants and does not require treatment. The fall in very small infants is such that by 8 to 9 weeks of age the haemoglobin may have fallen to 7 g per 100 ml, and in addition to pallor the infant may have tachycardia with difficulty in feeding.

Marrow activity improves slowly during the first two to three months, and provided sufficient haemopoietic factors including iron, folic acid, vitamin C, thyroxine and trace elements such as copper and cobalt are available the haemoglobin rises. If there is deficiency of any of the necessary dietary factors anaemia may persist for many months.

HAEMOPOIETIC FACTORS

Recognition of any deficiency of haemopoietic factors is essential to the planning of appropriate therapy.

Iron and vitamin C. In practice iron and vitamin C are the factors most commonly involved, and it is generally considered advisable to give preterm weight infants supplements of these factors from the second month of life. Some feeds are fortified with iron, but where these feeds are not being used a preparation such as ferrous sulphate mixture for infants N.F. 5 ml a day should be given together with ascorbic acid 25 mg a day.

Folate deficiency is difficult to recognize clinically, and measurement of blood folate is necessary to establish the diagnosis. It has been demonstrated that folate deficiency is commoner in preterm infants as a cause of continuing anaemia than was previously realized. Deficiency is particularly likely to occur following infection. The routine prophylactic administration of folate to preterm infants is not generally accepted but the need for treatment of incipient or established deficiency is clear. A therapeutic dose of folic acid in the newborn period would be 0.5 mg per day.

Blood Loss

Infants may lose blood for one or more of the causes shown in Table 17.1.

Table 17.1 Blood loss in newborn infants

BEFORE OR DURING DELIVERY
Fetomaternal transfusion
Feto–fetal transfusion in twins
Rupture of placental vessels
Placenta praevia
Surgical incision
Rupture of cord vessels
Precipitate delivery
FOLLOWING DELIVERY
External blood loss
Cord stump
Gastrointestinal tract
Menstruation in females
From skin injury
From nose
Internal blood loss
Brain, lung, adrenals—often fatal
Liver and spleen
Kidney and muscles

ANTENATAL

Blood loss from the fetus before labour begins is difficult to detect and may only be suspected because of a change in fetal activity or heart rate. Occasionally mothers may experience a mild shivering attack and episode of discomfort if a considerable fetomaternal haemorrhage occurs.

Recognition. Fetal blood can be recognized in the maternal circulation by the acid elution technique of Kleihauer and an estimate made of the volume of blood lost by the fetus.

Twin pregnancies. Bleeding from one twin to another only occurs in homozygous twins with a communicating vessel between the placentae. If this is from the artery of one twin to the vein of the other blood transfer will occur, the one twin becoming progressively more anaemic until intrauterine death may occur. The other twin will be plethoric and is generally the larger of the two at birth. Figure 17.1 shows a fetus papyraceus alongside the placenta of the healthy

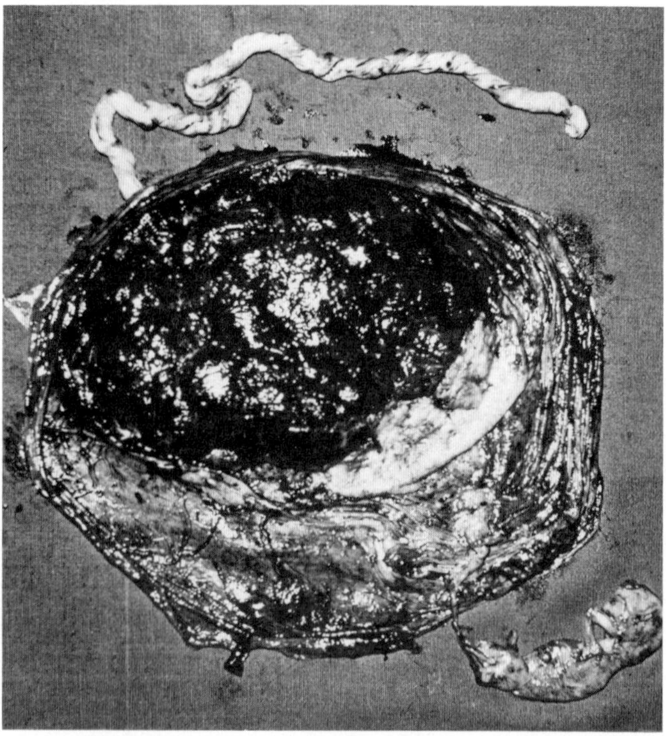

Figure 17.1 Twin pregnancy with fetus papyraceus.

surviving twin—this may have been the result of an early feto-fetal transfusion. If both twins are born alive both may require treatment, blood transfusion for the anaemic twin and removal of blood from the plethoric twin. Blood loss from the placental vessels or cord generally occurs as the result of trauma but abnormal vessels may rupture with minimal injury. Fetal blood loss can again be recognized in the presence of maternal vaginal blood loss by the Kleihauer technique.

POSTNATAL BLOOD LOSS

Following delivery blood loss may be recognizable by direct observation, as when it comes from the cord stump, skin or nose.

Cord blood loss from the cord stump is less frequently seen since the elastic band technique and plastic cord clamps were introduced. Such blood loss can, however, be overlooked in infants who are fully dressed and wrapped up. The cord stump should be the first site inspected when an infant becomes pale and blood loss is suspected.

Gastrointestinal tract. Blood loss from the gastrointestinal tract is simple to recognize when it occurs in the form of vomiting of blood. Melaena is more difficult to recognize when the infant is still passing meconium. By examining the edge of the stool and thinning it out on the napkin the green colour of meconium can be readily distinguished from the reddish brown colour of a melaena.

Swallowed maternal blood. Blood in the stool of an infant does not necessarily come from the infant and may be swallowed maternal blood. Fetal blood can be recognized by its ability to resist denaturation by 1 per cent sodium hydroxide solution. If maternal blood is present the solution turns a brownish yellow colour.

Vaginal blood loss (Fig. 17.2). Vaginal bleeding may occur in female infants on the second to fourth day of life as the withdrawal of transplacental maternal oestrogens produces the equivalent of menstruation. In female infants it is not always clear whether blood on the napkin is coming from the bowel, vagina, urethra or skin. Careful observation after the perineum has been thoroughly cleaned will generally resolve the issue.

INTERNAL HAEMORRHAGE

Haemorrhage into the organs of the infant may prove rapidly fatal and this is more likely to occur where the brain, lungs or adrenal glands are the organs involved. Infants may, however, survive less extensive haemorrhage into any of these organs but are likely to be ill with signs of circulatory collapse, cyanosis and possibly convulsions.

Liver and spleen. Haemorrhage into the liver and spleen tends to occur under the capsule of these organs and may produce a palpable

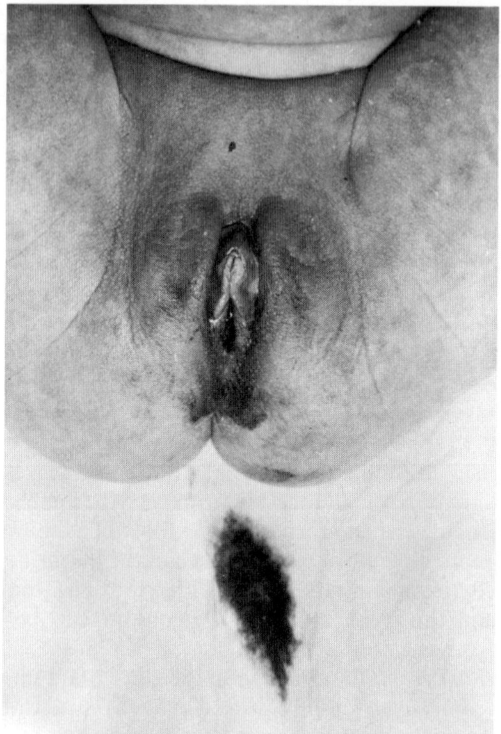

Figure 17.2 Vaginal bleeding.

swelling in the abdomen associated with pallor and collapse. Should the subcapsular haematoma rupture death may occur very rapidly but some infants survive long enough for surgical repair to be undertaken.

Kidneys. Bleeding into the kidneys and muscles is less frequent and generally follows local trauma.

Internal or external haemorrhage will be more marked where there is any failure of coagulation as occurs in any of the group of conditions which can be termed the haemorrhagic disorders of the newborn.

THE HAEMORRHAGIC DISORDERS OF THE NEWBORN

The chief causes of haemorrhagic disorders in the newborn are shown in Table 17.2.

Haemorrhagic Disease of the Newborn

It has been recognized from very early times that some newborn infants were prone to bleed excessively during the first week of life, and the Laws of Moses made allowance for this in their ordinance in relation to circumcision which was to be deferred until the eighth day. It was not until the end of the 19th century that the term haemorrhagic disease of the newborn was coined. This was at one stage thought to be entirely explicable by deficiency of vitamin K. As the limitations of treatment with vitamin K became evident it was clear that more than one condition was involved and secondary haemorrhagic disease was used for a period as a title to cover the non vitamin K dependent bleeding disorders. Further studies have shown that several factors are involved in secondary haemorrhagic disease and this term is no longer used.

Table 17.2 The haemorrhagic disorders of the newborn

Vitamin K deficiency
Thrombocytopenia
Disseminated intravascular coagulation
Deficiency of other clotting factors

VITAMIN K

Vitamin K is essential for the synthesis of four of the factors necessary for the clotting process—factors II (prothrombin), VII, IX and X. These factors are present in the newborn but at lower concentration than in the adult, falling to their lowest level on about the third day of life. The subsequent rise depends upon the provision of vitamin K in the diet or as a result of bacterial action in the bowel producing vitamin K. Cow's milk contains about 6 mg per 100 ml of vitamin K but human breast milk contains only a quarter of this amount.

Breast-fed infants show a more profound fall in prothrombin levels. 'Haemorrhagic disease of the newborn' due to lack of dietary vitamin K is virtually confined to those infants who have been breast-fed or who have been fed on glucose and water feeds. The incidence of vitamin K-dependent haemorrhagic disease therefore varies with the incidence of breast feeding and has become a rarity in most so-called advanced communities.

Bleeding most commonly occurs from the gastrointestinal tract, but bleeding from other sites may occur. The response to treatment with vitamin K is good.

Other haemorrhagic disorders do not respond to treatment with vitamin K.

THROMBOCYTOPENIA is discussed under the heading of purpura.

Disseminated Intravascular Coagulation

Increasing attention is being paid at present to the problem of intravascular coagulation which, by using up clotting factors including platelets, causes a haemorrhagic state by a process of consumptive coagulopathy.

SIGNS

Clinically disseminated intravascular coagulation is evident as widespread bleeding which often involves the brain and lungs as well as the skin and which is frequently fatal. The liver and spleen are often enlarged. The platelet count is low.

Fibrin degradation products. Disseminated intravascular coagulation can only be proven at postmortem examination but in life evidence of raised fibrin degradation products is suggestive that widespread coagulation is taking place in blood vessels. This has been shown in infants with severe birth hypoxia, acidosis, hypothermia and after placental separation. The possible part played by intravascular coagulation in the aetiology of respiratory disease syndrome is discussed elsewhere.

Treatment

The treatment of haemorrhagic disorders in the newborn period must be related to diagnosis of the specific cause of the bleeding tendency. Where bleeding is occurring and a haemorrhagic disorder is suspected it is not generally justifiable to carry out a full clotting screen but a prothrombin time or thrombotest and a platelet count are essential investigations. When specimens have been taken 1 mg of vitamin K should be given intramuscularly. This will prove effective only in haemorrhagic disease of the newborn but will do no harm in other conditions and will not obscure the diagnosis. The management of thrombocytopenia and of disseminated intravascular coagulation are discussed later in this chapter. Investigation of deficiency of other clotting factors will be necessary in the absence of thrombocytopenia and if bleeding continues after vitamin K has been given.

In any situation in which blood loss is of sufficient degree to cause circulatory failure immediate blood transfusion is called for. The site of bleeding, particularly if it is internal, may require direct treatment by the surgeons. Monitoring of central venous pressure by a catheter in one of the venae cavae gives a more accurate assessment of the state of the circulation, but clinical assessment of heart rate peripheral pulse and blood pressure is generally a sufficient guide to the total volume of blood required and the rate at which it should be given.

PURPURA

Purpura in the newly born infant may be produced by:

Thrombocytopenia,
Capillary damage,
(a) Venous obstruction
(b) Hypoxia.

Thrombocytopenia

Thrombocytopenia may occur for the reasons shown in Table 17.3.

Table 17.3 Causes of thrombocytopenia in the newborn

MATERNAL FACTORS INVOLVED
Maternal idiopathic thrombocytopenic purpura
Transplacental infection
Platelet group incompatibilities
Severe rhesus incompatibility
Thiazide diuretics given to mother
Inherited thrombocytopenia
OTHER CAUSES
Infection acquired postnatally
Disseminated intravascular coagulation
Marrow hypoplasia
Giant haemangioma

Maternal idiopathic thrombocytopenia. Purpura, which may be temporary, occurs in about half of the infants of mothers suffering from idiopathic thrombocytopenic purpura at the time of delivery and is apparently due to transplacental transmission of the maternal platelet agglutinins.

Antenatal infection. Syphilis, toxoplasmosis, rubella (Fig. 17.3), cytomegalovirus and herpes virus infection acquired antenatally are frequently accompanied by thrombocytopenic purpura in the infant.

Platelet group incompatibility. Fetal platelets may cross the placenta and initiate the production of platelet antibodies which spare mother's platelets but which agglutinate fetal platelets if they pass back to the fetal circulation. The process is analogous to rhesus blood group isoimmunization, and in severe forms of that condition thrombocytopenia may be present in the infant but not in the mother.

Thiazide diuretics. Thrombocytopenia has been described in a

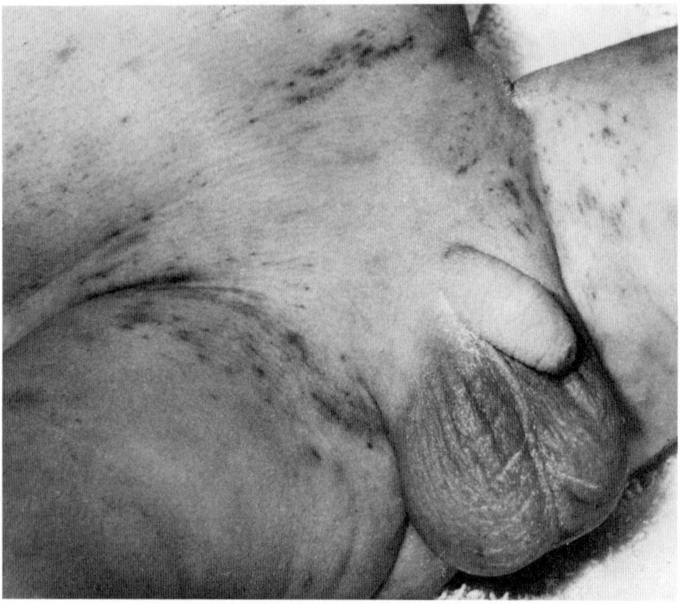

Figure 17.3 Purpura in infant with congenital rubella.

small number of infants of mothers who had been on prolonged courses of thiazide diuretics which may have been given because of pre-eclamptic toxaemia.

The inherited thrombocytopenias are only rarely manifest in the newborn period.

Other causes of thrombocytopenia in the infant do not involve maternal factors. Severe postnatal infection, bacterial or viral, may be accompanied by purpura due to platelet deficiency and this is generally a poor prognostic sign. In such situations thrombocytopenia may be a manifestation of disseminated intravascular coagulation. Marrow depression from any cause such as drugs, congenital leukaemia and bone disorders may present as purpura due to thrombocytopenia. The platelet consumption which occurs in giant haemangiomas (Fig. 17.4) may rarely be a cause of purpura in the newborn period.

NON-THROMBOCYTOPENIC PURPURA

Purpura not associated with thrombocytopenia is frequently due to a local cause such as constriction of the neck veins producing

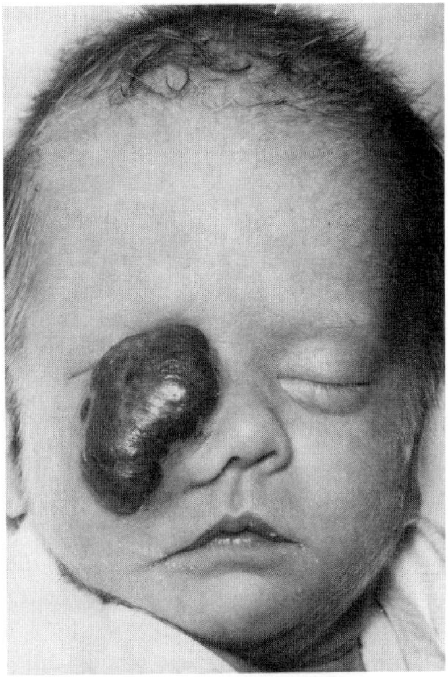

Figure 17.4 Giant haemangioma with thrombocytopenia (Kassabach's syndrome).

purpura over the head and neck. More extensive purpura occurs with persistent hypoxia and as the brain is often involved death is frequent (Chap. 12).

TREATMENT

Treatment of purpura is generally that of the underlying conditions. Steroids are indicated in the isoimmune types of thrombocytopenia purpura. In infants with severe depression of platelets, transfusion of platelets will be required.

The place of heparin and of exchange transfusion in the treatment of disseminated intravascular coagulation has not been firmly established but there are several reports in favour of the controlled use of heparin. This requires very close supervision and should be carried out in an intensive therapy unit to which the infant should be transferred.

FURTHER READING

BOOTHBY, C. B. & DESA, D. J. (1973). Massive pulmonary haemorrhage in the newborn—a changing pattern, *Archives of Disease in Childhood*, **48,** 21–30.

BRITISH MEDICAL JOURNAL (1971). Haemorrhage in the newborn. iv, 1–2.

GILL, F. M. & SCHWARTZ, E. (1972). Anaemia in early infancy. *Pediatric Clinics of North America*, **19,** 841–853.

LASCARI, A. D. (Ed.) (1972). Symposium on Pediatric Hematology. *Pediatric Clinics of North America*, **19,** no. 4.

OSKI, F. A. & NAIMAN, J. L. (1972). *Hematologic Problems in the Newborn*, 2nd edn. Philadelphia & London: Saunders.

18

Weight Loss and Other Important Signs

The more common signs which are found in the neonatal period have already been discussed in the preceding four chapters. This chapter will deal with weight loss and a variety of other different signs which, although some may occur less frequently than others, are all nonetheless of importance.

WEIGHT LOSS

Most babies lose weight for a few days after birth. This drop in weight is normally less than 10 per cent of the weight at birth and may be termed physiological.

Physiological Weight Loss

Physiological weight loss is the result of loss of fluid by evaporation from the skin, and in the course of normal micturition, defaecation and respiratory exchange. The full term baby begins to gain weight about the fourth day of life and the preterm baby between the seventh and tenth days of life. Infants vary greatly in the rate with which they gain weight, and fluctuations in weight progress are consistent with normal growth and development. A weekly gain of 175 to 240 g is usual in healthy babies. Some infants increase in weight more rapidly, but periods of exceptional progress are apt to be followed by phases of relatively slow gain in weight. Too much significance should not be attached to the results of successive weighing carried out at short intervals. After the first week of life weekly weighing provides all the necessary information.

Excessive Weight Loss

Weight loss may be described as excessive when it amounts to more than 10 per cent of the birth weight.

The causes of excessive weight loss are listed in Table 18.1.

Inadequate Intake

UNDERFEEDING

Underfeeding must always be considered in the assessment of the infant with excessive weight loss.

Test weighing. If the baby is breast-fed an estimate should be made of mother's milk production. Weighing the baby before and after a feed gives an indication of the volume of milk taken. It is important that no change of clothing or napkin be made between the two test weighings.

Table 18.1 Causes of excessive weight loss

Inadequate intake
Underfeeding
Difficulty in feeding
Vomiting
Intestinal obstruction
Functional disturbance
Diarrhoea
Excessive surface evaporation
Excessive urine loss

Fluid and calories. In artificially fed infants the qualitative as well as the quantitative adequacy of the feed being offered must be reviewed. The fluid requirements of the very active baby are greater than those of the placid infant of comparable weight and age. The fluid, calorie and other requirements of the newborn infant were considered in Chapter 8.

DIFFICULTY IN FEEDING

Difficulty in feeding may be the cause of underfeeding. The infant may be incapable of taking feeds because of some form of physical handicap such as nasal obstruction or cleft palate. He may be disinclined to accept feeds because of discomfort (e.g. thrush). Infants with cerebral dysfunction due to brain injury, congenital abnormality or infection are poor at sucking and swallowing. The preterm infant may not have the strength to feed from the breast or bottle.

Vomiting

Vomiting may be mechanical and due to obstruction in the gastrointestinal tract, may follow a disturbance of function or be due to overfeeding. The character of the vomitus (Table 18.2) is usually a good guide to the probable diagnosis. Vomiting with severe fluid loss causes elevation of the temperature. Following treatment of the underlying condition and rehydration the temperature rapidly returns to normal.

Alimentary Tract Malformations

Vomiting is an important sign of intestinal obstruction. The timing and character of the vomiting are of importance in diagnosis.

Table 18.2 Types of vomitus

Frothy mucoid
Oesophageal atresia
Bile-stained
High intestinal obstruction
Swallowed meconium
Intracranial injury
Low birth weight
Blood-stained
Swallowed maternal blood
At birth
Cracked nipple
Trauma to pharynx
Haemorrhagic disease
Hiatus hernia
Milk, with or without mucus
Gastritis
Infective
Non-infective
Infections
Enteral
Parenteral
Feeding problems
Low intestinal obstruction
Raised intracranial pressure

EARLY VOMITING

Vomiting within the first day of life usually signifies the presence of a potentially fatal malformation of the alimentary tract which requires immediate surgical intervention.

Oesophageal atresia. Continuous dribbling of frothy mucus coughing, spluttering and cyanosis on feeding and a preceding history of hydramnios are highly suggestive of oesophageal atresia. In 10 per cent of cases there is associated small bowel or anal atresia. Clinical diagnosis should be made before the first feed and confirmed by radiological examination. Pending surgical treatment the baby should be propped up and the upper oesophageal segment sucked out at 15-minute intervals to prevent inhalation pneumonia.

BILE-STAINED VOMITING

Vomiting of bile-stained fluid in the first 24 hours of life is due to high intestinal obstruction, usually duodenal atresia, until proved otherwise. All such babies require immediate investigation and treatment.

Duodenal atresia. A preceding history of hydramnios would suggest the possibility of duodenal atresia which is confirmed by the typical double gas bubble seen on X-ray examination. Surgical treatment consists in duodenoduodenostomy, the mortality rate being low with careful preoperation preparation and expert post-operative care. Duodenal atresia and annular pancreas are often associated with Down's syndrome.

Other surgical causes of bile-stained vomiting after the first 24 hours of life include atresia, stenosis, volvulus or reduplication of the small bowel, meconium ileus and peritonitis and Hirschsprung's disease.

Non-surgical causes. Apart from these surgical causes early bile-stained vomiting may be associated with intracranial injury, is seen in immature preterm babies and frequently follows the ingestion of meconium at birth.

BLOOD-STAINED VOMITING

Maternal blood. The vomiting of blood always causes concern, particularly to parents. Most of the blood vomited on the first day of life is of maternal origin and has been swallowed during delivery. Infants who are breast-fed may swallow blood from cracks in mother's nipple and later vomit the blood. The adult haemoglobin in maternal blood can be differentiated from fetal blood by the alkali denaturation test which was described in Chapter 17.

Infant's blood. Injury to the mouth or pharynx during resuscitation or feeding may lead to bleeding and subsequent vomiting of swallowed blood. Rarely bleeding may take place from a tear of the osesophagus or ulceration of the stomach.

Disturbances of Function

Vomiting may be caused by conditions which disturb gastro-intestinal function such as gastritis, enteral and parenteral infections, ingestion of drugs, raised intracranial pressure and the adreno-genital syndrome.

GASTRITIS

Vomiting due to gastritis may be of infective or non-infective aetiology.

Escherichia coli and *Candida albicans* are causes of infective gastritis while drugs and swallowed meconium are non-infective causes of gastritis leading to vomiting.

Swallowed meconium. Gastric irritation caused by meconium, liquor and swallowed blood is treated by gastric lavage.

INFECTION

Enteral and parenteral infections causing the newly born baby to vomit include gastroenteritis, urinary tract infection, neonatal hepatitis, meningitis and septicaemia.

RAISED INTRACRANIAL PRESSURE

Raised intracranial pressure due to intracranial injury, subdural effusion, hydrocephalus and meningitis is a not uncommon cause of vomiting.

THE ADRENOGENITAL SYNDROME

The adrenogenital syndrome, which was discussed in Chapter 11, may first be evident as vomiting.

OVERFEEDING

Overloading the stomach with a volume of feed greater than the stomach can hold often results in some of the excess being returned in the form of a vomit. Provided that the infant continues to thrive this does not matter.

Frequency of feeds. If such vomiting is associated with poor weight gain or weight loss the volume given at each feed must be reduced. This will involve increasing the frequency of feed by adding additional feeds during the night or reducing the time interval between feeds.

Low birth weight. This problem is most likely to arise in the first two or three weeks of life of preterm infants when, in order to reduce the volume at individual feeds, feeding may have to be at two hourly or hourly intervals. In the smallest infants continuous infusion may be required as described in Chapter 9.

MANAGEMENT

Primary cause. Diagnosis and correction of the primary cause of the vomiting is the basis of management. Where a surgical cause is suspected early consultation with a paediatric surgeon is indicated.

Fluid, electrolyte, calories. The loss of fluid, electrolyte and calories which occurs because of vomiting has to be replaced and this generally implies intravenous therapy. It is not easy to supply sufficient calories by this route without using intravenous fat preparations. As experience with such preparations in the newborn is limited their use should be confined to specialist units.

Gastric lavage. Where vomiting is due to irritation of the gastric mucosa by swallowed foreign material gastric lavage is often the only treatment which will relieve symptoms.

Propping up the infant after feeds may prevent some vomiting.

Diarrhoea

Causes of diarrhoea in the first month of life are shown in Table 18.3. The commonest causes are dietary and infective.

Table 18.3 Causes of diarrhoea in the first month of life

DIETARY
Volume overload
Disaccharide overload
ENTERAL INFECTION
Bacterial
Viral
Necrotizing enterocolitis
PARENTERAL INFECTION
Septicaemia
Pneumonia
Urinary tract infection
Otitis media
Neonatal hepatitis
RARER CAUSES
e.g. Cystic fibrosis

DIETARY

Volume overload. If intake of an excessive volume of feed has not been relieved by vomiting the amount of food passing the pylorus may exceed the digestive capacity of the bowel and diarrhoea follows.

Disaccharide overload. If more disaccharides such as lactose or sucrose are present in the diet than can be split by the intestinal disaccharidases, the sugar-splitting enzymes, undigested sugars remain in the bowel and are fermented by bowel organisms. Water is drawn into the bowel by osmosis and the extra bowel content together with the lactic acid and other breakdown products produce a watery diarrhoea which causes excoriation of the buttocks. The stool fluid contains reducing substances and is acid. Reduction of the disaccharide content of the diet gives relief from symptoms.

Alactasia. Lactase, the enzyme which splits lactose, is relatively deficient in the first few days of life particularly in the preterm infant. Rarely the enzyme is absent because of inherited deficiency. Temporary alactasia may occur after a bowel infection. Where the enzyme is deficient or absent diarrhoea occurs when there is lactose in the diet. Treatment consists of arranging a lactose-free diet. This requires the withdrawal of milk feeds and their substitution by special preparations some of which are based on soya bean flour.

ENTERAL INFECTION

In communities with a high standard of hygiene, bowel infection is now a relatively uncommon cause of diarrhoea in the newborn. Where standards of hygiene are not adequate diarrhoea is a common and serious problem among bottle-fed infants.

Breast feeding protects infants against many of the infections which affect bottle-fed infants. This is probably due to the amount of IgA which is secreted in breast milk. Breast feeding is therefore a prophylactic measure which should be strongly encouraged in any situation where there is doubt about the standard of hygiene.

Epidemics. Outbreaks of diarrhoea and vomiting due to pathogenic *E. coli* do occur from time to time in newborn baby nurseries, the organism being carried by a mother or attendant. The disease is potentially very serious when it affects low birth-weight babies and babies with congenital abnormalities. Less frequently diarrhoea and vomiting may be due to infection with other organisms including viruses.

Clinical signs. Reluctance to feed is the first sign of an enteral infection followed by occasional vomiting and the explosive passage of frequent loose watery stools. Dehydration with loss of skin elasticity, depressed fontanelles, sunken eyes, dryness of the lips, tongue and buccal mucous membranes, and rapid weight loss soon follow. If untreated there is progression to circulatory collapse with tachycardia and generalized grey cyanosis.

Treatment. Isolation is essential to prevent spread to susceptible infants. The newly born infant withstands salt and water loss badly hence replacement of water and electrolytes is an urgent necessity. In most cases scalp vein infusion, starting with 0.45 per cent sodium chloride, changing to 0.18 per cent sodium chloride with added potassium once urine has been passed, is essential. In less severe cases replacement fluid can be given by mouth followed later by the gradual introduction of milk feeds. Antibiotic therapy must be very carefully assessed, taking into account the infant's general condition and the type of organism isolated. Parenteral treatment is indicated if there is evidence of blood-stream spread.

CROSS INFECTION

Only in about 20 per cent of cases will stool culture produce a pathogenic organism, so presumably diarrhoea and vomiting in some cases is of viral aetiology whereas in others it may be due to non-infective causes such as dietary intolerance. If two or more infants develop diarrhoea at the same time, cross infection must be presumed and the babies isolated and barrier-nursed. If infection is proven it is advisable to prescribe an antibiotic such as oral neomycin or gentamycin both to the affected babies and prophylactically to all other babies in the unit to reduce the risk of further spread of infection. Depending on the severity of the symptoms and the number of babies involved it may be necessary to close the ward to new admissions.

NECROTIZING ENTEROCOLITIS

Necrotizing enterocolitis was first discussed in Chapter 9 in relation to low birth-weight infants. No real cause for the condition has been found but the association with the respiratory distress syndrome and pulmonary haemorrhage suggest that hypoxia leads to ischaemic lesions of the gastrointestinal tract. Small preterm babies are principally involved. The condition is characterized by vomiting, abdominal distension, gastrointestinal bleeding, irregular temperature and peritonitis in some cases. The symptoms develop within a few days of birth and treatment is symptomatic consisting of intravenous fluids and antibiotics.

PARENTERAL INFECTIONS

Parenteral infections such as septicaemia, pneumonia, urinary tract infection, otitis media and neonatal hepatitis which are associated with diarrhoea have all been discussed elsewhere.

Cystic fibrosis of the pancreas may present in the first month of life with large, bulky, fatty and offensive stools. Occasionally the stools are numerous and of fluid consistency.

Hirschsprung's disease usually presents with constipation but occasionally diarrhoea may be the earliest manifestation of the condition signifying the presence of a complicating enterocolitis.

Morphine withdrawal in babies whose mothers are morphine addicts is typified by vomiting and diarrhoea. In addition to the diarrhoea and vomiting there is extreme irritability, high-pitched cry, thirst and sometimes convulsions and coma. Treatment consists in sedating the baby with phenobarbitone or diazepam for a few days or weeks.

Adrenal insufficiency, with or without adrenocortical hyperplasia, may be associated with bouts of severe diarrhoea in addition to the more common sign of vomiting.

Hypersensitivity to cow's milk protein may cause diarrhoea in the early days of life.

Excessive Surface Evaporation

Excessive loss of fluid may take place from the respiratory passages if an infant is nursed in an excessively hot, dry atmosphere. Such a situation may occur naturally in certain countries. In temperate climates similar situations may arise if infants are nursed in too hot an incubator, too near to a radiator, in direct sunshine or if they are overclothed. In most instances there will be a rise in central temperature. Treatment is by removing the infant to a cooler environment and giving extra fluid such as a fifth normal saline in dextrose until the infant is back to normal.

Excessive Urine Loss

Polyuria calls for the exclusion of temporary congenital diabetes mellitus and nephrogenic diabetes insipidus. Both conditions are exceedingly rare.

Temporary congenital diabetes mellitus (Fig. 18.1) disappears spontaneously within weeks or months but treatment with insulin may be necessary for a period.

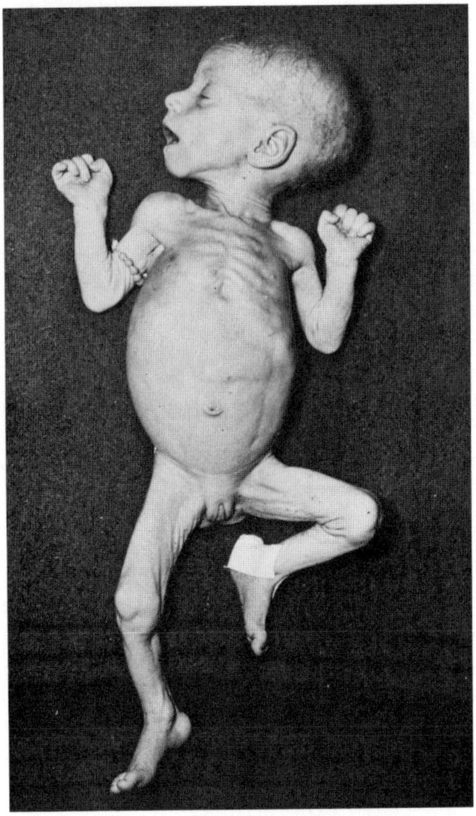

Figure 18.1 Dehydration and weight loss in infant with temporary congenital diabetes mellitus.

Nephrogenic diabetes insipidus is a sex-linked condition in which the infant's brain is damaged by hypernatraemia if water loss is not made good.

Loss of oedema. The oedematous infant who gets rid of his oedema does so by increasing his urine output whether this be done naturally or as the result of medication.

EXCESSIVE WEIGHT GAIN

Excessive weight gain is not a common sign in the newborn period. When rapid excessive weight gain is associated with the retention of fluid it is commonly manifest as oedema and is therefore to be expected in such conditions as heart failure, hypoalbuminaemia and congenital nephrosis.

Oedema

Oedema may be classified into generalized and localized, the causes being listed in Table 18.4. In the presence of oedema the

Table 18.4 Classification of oedema

GENERALIZED
Immaturity
Cardiac failure
Renal disease
Cold injury
Hypoproteinaemia
Protein overload
LOCALIZED
Birth trauma
Limbs
Brain

skin and subcutaneous tissues look and feel spongy or puffy, due to the excess of fluid which they contain. Pitting on pressure is a common but not invariable finding (Fig. 18.2). Oedema should be regarded as potentially serious when it is both gross and generalized, more especially when it develops in generalized form at an interval of some days after birth. In such circumstances possible causes are cardiac failure, kidney disease, cold injury, hypoproteinaemia and sodium overload. The potential seriousness of oedema is increased when there is associated hypothermia.

LOW BIRTH WEIGHT

Many small preterm infants show oedema of the face, limbs, pubis and external genitalia during the first few days of life. Pitting on pressure can be demonstrated in the pubis and legs but not in the face. Oedema of any considerable extent in the very small infant results in the skin having a characteristically shiny appearance. In the absence of renal disease, and provided it begins to disappear gradually within 48 hours of birth, oedema in the newly born preterm infant need not cause undue concern. It should, however, be valued as evidence of the need to prevent heat loss and to record the frequency with which the napkins are stained with urine.

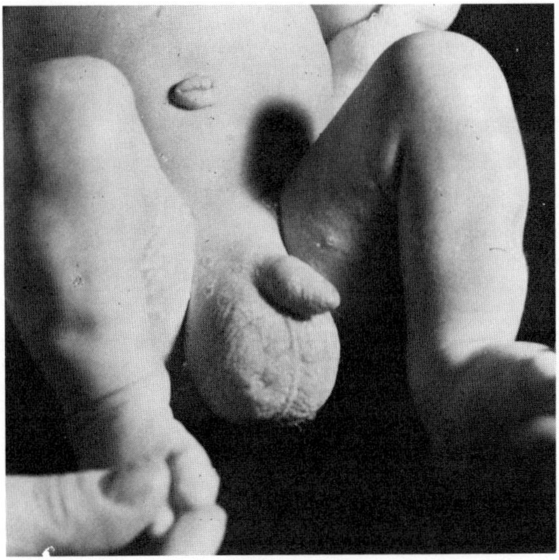

Figure 18.2 Pitting oedema of lower legs.

CARDIAC FAILURE

The infant in cardiac failure from congenital heart disease presents with tachypnoea, tachycardia, hepatomegaly and oedema with unexpected weight gain. Hydrops fetalis is a severe form of heart disease in haemolytic disease. Treatment was dealt with in Chapter 11.

RENAL IMMATURITY

As mentioned in Chapter 9 the presence of oedema in the preterm infant is generally accepted as evidence of immature renal function which is usually associated with sodium retention. It will also be recalled that the immature kidney is unable to deal effectively with urea and phosphate. Apart from these physiological handicaps kidney disease proper, including urinary tract infection, and congenital nephrosis, are both associated with oedema.

Hypoproteinaemia occurs in congenital nephrosis, cystic fibrosis, may be found in immature infants as mentioned above or may result from feeding a protein deficient milk.

Congenital nephrosis may be transmitted as an autosomal recessive condition or be secondary to cytomegalovirus infection, renal vein thrombosis or syphilis. Oedema may be present at birth with albuminuria, hypoalbuminaemia and hypercholesterolaemia. The condition is invariably fatal within the first few months of life, usually as a result of infection.

Mineral overload. Oedema is also associated with the mineral overload which results from use of an overconcentrated feed.

LOCALIZED OEDEMA

The infant born at term rarely shows evidence of oedema other than that occurring locally as a result of trauma. The caput succedaneum is one example, and it should be remembered that oedema of the scalp sometimes changes position under the influence of gravity. Other causes of oedema of the extremities include Turner's syndrome and idiopathic hereditary lymphoedema (Fig. 18.3).

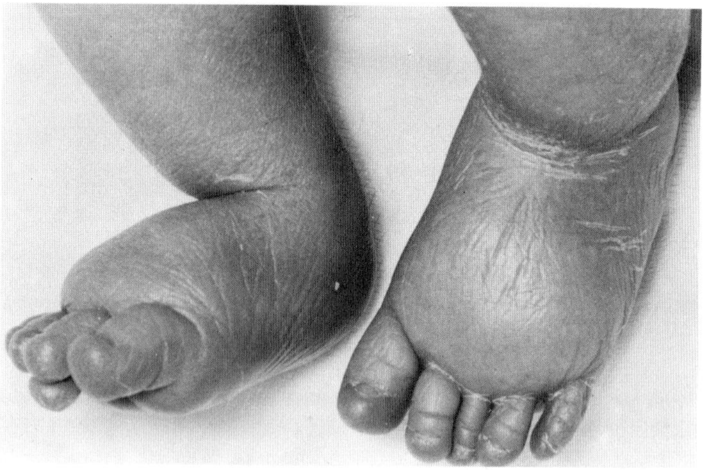

Figure 18.3 Lymphoedema in infant with ovarian dysgenesis (Bonnevie-Ullrich syndrome).

Oedema of the brain was discussed in Chapter 12, which dealt with birth injuries.

PYREXIA

DEFINITION

Pyrexia is present when under normal environmental conditions the rectal temperature exceeds 37.5°C. It may or may not be of serious significance but should it persist for 12 hours an attempt should be made to determine the cause even in the absence of other signs.

Temperature recording. Twice-daily recordings of rectal temperature should be a routine in all maternity hospital nurseries, and the temperature chart of a baby due for discharge should always be carefully scrutinized. Pyrexia may be the first detectable sign of infection and any recent febrile event must be assessed in terms of possible incubating infection which in the event of early discharge could assume serious form within 24 to 48 hours of the baby arriving home. Temperature recording is especially necessary when there is reason to believe that the baby has been in contact with infection, however remote.

A distinction must be made between a fluctuating body temperature, which usually signifies a high environmental temperature, and the permanently elevated body temperature commonly associated with infection. Exposure to the sun, excessive clothing and nursing in an overheated incubator are all factors in promoting a high environmental temperature.

COMMON CAUSES OF PYREXIA

Infection, stress of labour or delivery and dehydration are the commonest causes of an elevated temperature. Infection has been considered in Chapter 13 and birth injury in Chapter 12.

Dehydration fever may result from the baby receiving inadequate fluid. In units where newly born infants are given adequate fluids dehydration fever is rarely encountered.

ABDOMINAL DISTENSION

The common causes of abdominal distension are listed in Table 18.5.

GASEOUS DISTENSION

Air swallowing is a frequent finding in infants who are greedy feeders or who are constantly crying or sucking a dummy. Unless the swallowed air is returned by eructation gaseous distension of the bowel follows.

Bad feeding technique using a teat with too small a hole is another cause of gaseous distension. Gaseous distension is also a complication of overlong feeding of carbohydrate-rich milk preparations.

Infection. Gaseous abdominal distension can complicate serious illness of any kind in the newborn (Fig. 18.4). It is a common complication of septicaemia and of intrathoracic infection, more especially in preterm and light-for-dates infants. The resultant pressure on the diaphragm increases respiratory and cardiac embarrassment and adds to the seriousness of the prognosis.

Table 18.5 Causes of abdominal distension

Gaseous distension
Intestinal obstruction and peritonitis
Enlarged intra-abdominal organ
Absent or weak abdominal muscles
Ascites

Management. Treatment of infection and attention to feeding techniques are necessary. In many situations there is no treatment other than waiting for the gas to be passed from the anus. Trial should be made of keeping the baby supported in his cot in a sitting position. If oral feeds are given they must be small and frequent.

INTESTINAL OBSTRUCTION

Intestinal obstruction is accompanied by distension. The more important causes of intestinal obstruction were discussed earlier in this chapter when dealing with vomiting. In some cases abdominal obstruction may be a complication of hypoglycaemia, hypoxaemia, or hypothermia. Correction of the primary condition relieves the ileus but frequently not without the aid of intravenous therapy.

Milk plug syndrome. In light-for-dates infants receiving large volumes of milk to prevent hypoglycaemia thick curds may obstruct the pylorus or the small bowel—the milk plug syndrome—causing abdominal distension and vomiting. Treatment of the condition consists in gastric lavage with a 5 per cent dextrose solution and substituting clear fluids for milk feeds for a short period.

Peritonitis. In the presence of peritonitis, distension is characterized by limited or absent abdominal movements, shiny tautness of

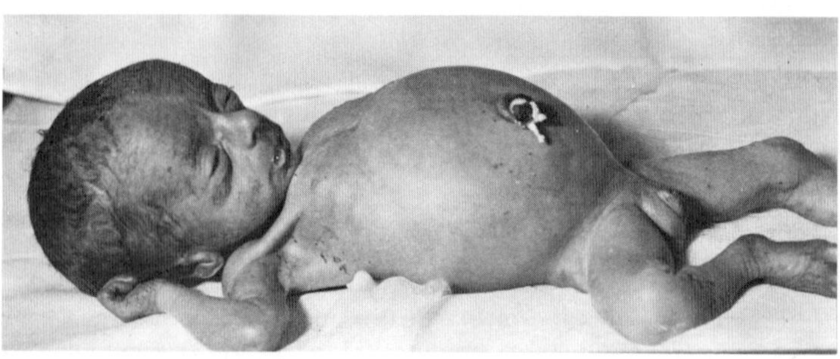

Figure 18.4 Gaseous abdominal distension.

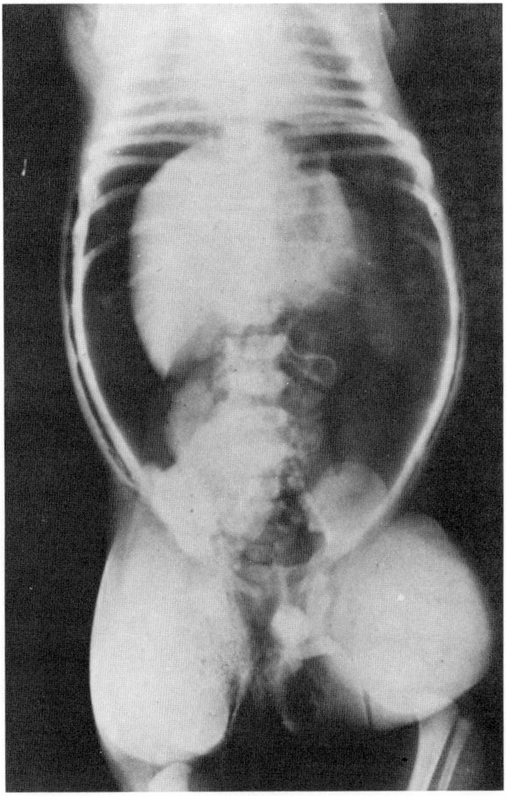

Figure 18.5 Pneumoperitoneum following perforation of the bowel.

the skin and sometimes exaggerated protrusion of the umbilicus. Abdominal distension is a feature also of postnatal perforation due to peptic ulceration or very rarely to appendicitis or Meckel's diverticulum. Bacterial peritonitis supervenes.

Spontaneous perforation of the bowel with peritonitis occurs as a rare but early complication of exchange blood transfusion (Fig. 18.5). There may or may not be signs of intestinal obstruction, and in a significant proportion of cases distension is accompanied by melaena. Treatment consists of immediate laparotomy and broad-spectrum antibiotic therapy. Perforation can occur also after prolonged use of the umbilical vein in the administration of intravenous fluids.

ENLARGEMENT OF AN INTRA-ABDOMINAL ORGAN

Enlargement of an intra-abdominal organ, most commonly the kidney (see later), causes distension of the abdomen. The causes of

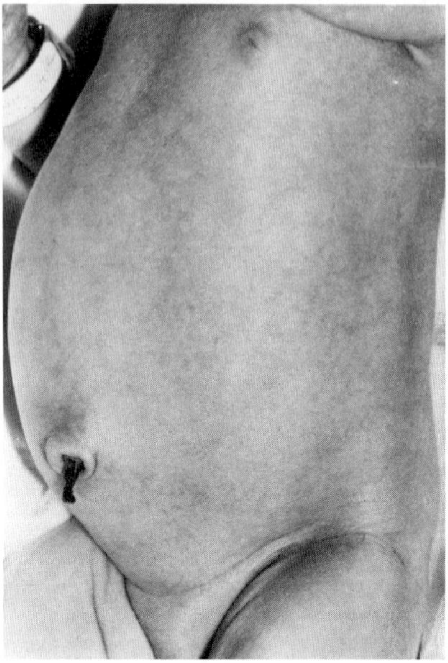

Figure 18.6 Abdominal distension due to chylous ascites.

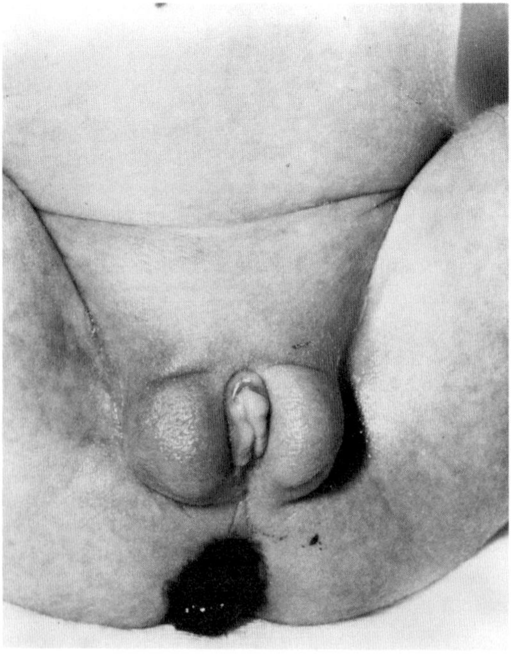

Figure 18.7 Oedema of vulva associated with chylous ascites.

hepatosplenomegaly will be discussed later. Distension of the bladder can also be the cause of an enlarged abdomen.

Stomach. In immature preterm infants temporary distension is a common finding after feeds. The outline or pattern of the stomach or bowel is often easily recognizable and there may be visible peristalsis.

Meconium. Persistent distension in low birth-weight babies may be associated with delay in passing meconium which has been related to the thin abdominal wall and weak abdominal musculature. If delay in passing meconium extends beyond three or four days a gentle low colonic lavage with normal saline (at body temperature) is indicated.

Prune belly syndrome. Congenital absence of the abdominal musculature in association with hydronephrosis, hydroureter and cryptorchidism is a feature of the prune belly syndrome.

Ascites

Ascites is a feature of haemolytic disease (hydrops fetalis), the nephrotic syndrome, cardiac failure and occasionally its presence is unexplained. An even rarer finding consists of chylous ascites (Fig. 18.6 and 7) due to anomalies of the lymph channels. At first clear, the abdominal fluid becomes cream-like in colour and consistency after feeding on human milk or a human milk substitute has been established.

ABDOMINAL MASSES

The majority of abdominal masses are palpable kidneys. During the early days of life it is usually possible to palpate the lower poles of the kidneys. Occasionally the kidney is displaced downwards and it is easily felt in the ectopic position.

Enlarged Kidneys

The causes of an enlarged kidney are listed in Table 18.6. Renal vein thrombosis and renal infarction are the only renal causes likely to make the infant ill.

Renal vein thrombosis occurs as a result of severe perinatal hypoxia and is also related to infections and severe dehydration. Affected infants present with albuminuria and haematuria. The resulting haemorrhagic infarction of the kidney causes palpable enlargement. Bilateral renal vein thrombosis is fatal. Nephrectomy is indicated for unilateral renal vein thrombosis.

Infarction of the kidney. As already mentioned renal vein thrombosis leads to infarction of the kidney. Other causes are severe dehydration, trauma during delivery and as a terminal event in the presence of a failing circulation. Renal infarction is accompanied by haematuria and palpable enlargement of the kidney.

Hydronephrosis. A smoothly enlarged kidney would favour a diagnosis of hydronephrosis (Fig. 18.8).

Polycystic kidneys. An irregular mass is a feature of polycystic kidneys and Wilm's tumour. In the case of Wilm's tumour the mass is firm and hard whereas in polycystic disease the surface of the kidney is finely nodular.

Duplicated and horseshoe kidneys are firm and smooth on examination whilst an adrenal tumour merely displaces a normal kidney downwards thereby rendering it palpable.

Table 18.6 Causes of kidney enlargement

Normally palpable
Downward displacement of a normal kidney
Ectopic
Adrenal haemorrhage
Adrenal tumour
Hydronephrosis
Cystic kidney
Renal vein thrombosis
Renal infarction
Duplicated kidney
Horseshoe kidney
Wilm's tumour

Adrenal haemorrhage. In Chapter 12, when dealing with injury, it will be recalled that severe hypoxia, breech delivery and a combination of these favour massive haemorrhage into the adrenal glands. Death is the usual outcome but should the child survive the glands are subsequently calcified and easily demonstrated on X-ray examination.

Urine examination may be helpful in diagnosis. Gross haematuria is found in renal vein thrombosis although it may occur in renal infarction, hydronephrosis and Wilm's tumour. Albuminuria is a feature of polycystic kidney and renal vein thrombosis. Pus cells and casts are found with infarcted kidneys and are present in the other conditions only in the presence of secondary infection.

The blood urea is elevated in renal vein thrombosis, hydronephrosis and polycystic disease and whenever the renal tract becomes infected.

Intravenous pyelography, cystoscopy and retrograde pyelography usually provide sufficient evidence on which to base a definite diagnosis.

Surgical treatment is carried out where indicated.

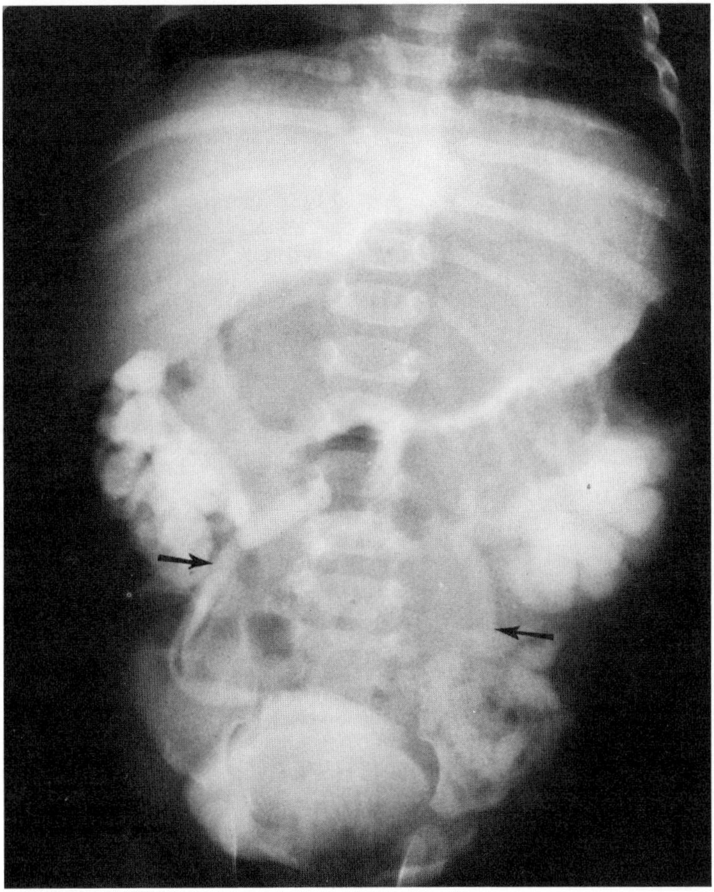

Figure 18.8 Multiple anomalies of kidneys and ureters in a baby with marked abdominal distension at birth.

Hepatosplenomegaly

The liver and spleen may be just palpable in the healthy newborn infant. The thin abdominal wall of the low birth-weight baby makes for easy palpation of the liver and spleen.

CAUSES

Hepatosplenomegaly is a feature of haemolytic disease, septicaemia, congenital syphilis, virus diseases, including rubella, cytomegalovirus disease and hepatitis, and finally toxoplasmosis. Haemolytic disease is usually due to ABO group or rhesus incompatibility. Less commonly incompatibility of the fetus and mother for the Kell or other rare group may be the cause. Other less common causes of haemolytic disease in this country are congenital spherocytosis (acholuric jaundice), sickle cell anaemia, thalassaemia and G6PDH deficiency. Haemolytic disease has been described in Chapter 14.

Delay in Passage of Meconium

The first meconium stool is passed by 95 per cent of normal infants within 24 hours of birth. Failure to pass a stool within the first 24 hours must be regarded with suspicion if meconium has not been passed before or during birth. Delay in passage of meconium (Table 18.7) may be associated with congenital abnormalities of the gut, abnormal consistency of the meconium and weak musculature. Meconium will not be passed when the baby has an anal or rectal atresia and passage will be delayed in Hirschsprung's disease.

Absence of abdominal musculature in the prune belly syndrome and paralysis of these muscles due to spina bifida may account for delay in passage of meconium.

Table 18.7 Causes of delayed passage of meconium

Congenital abnormalities of the gut
Anorectal abnormalities
Hirschsprung's disease
Abnormal consistency of meconium
Meconium ileus
Meconium plug syndrome
Weak, absent or paralysed muscles
Immature preterm infants
Prune belly syndrome
Spina bifida

ANORECTAL ABNORMALITIES

Anal atresia should be recognized at the time of the first examination of the baby after birth (Fig. 18.9). Meconium staining is no assurance of the presence of a normal anus. Absence of the anus and atresia of the anus due to the persistence of a septum are sometimes associated with a rectourethral or retrovaginal fistula. In these circumstances the meconium is voided via the urethra or vagina. Alternatively the fistula may be more in the nature of a sinus and open to the exterior in the perineum of boys or between the fourchette and introitus in girls. Again meconium may be voided via a patent vitellointestinal duct.

HIRSCHSPRUNG'S DISEASE

Hirschsprung's disease occurs when segments of the lower bowel have an incomplete nerve supply. The affected segments do not share

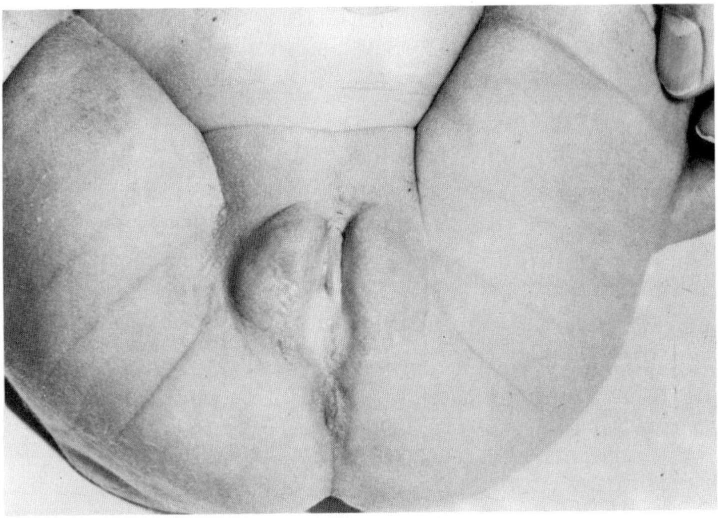

Figure 18.9 Anal atresia.

in the normal peristaltic activity of the gut and remain narrow and collapsed. Segments of the gut proximal to the abnormal bowel are distended as a result of efforts to propel the contents to the colon beyond these abnormal segments. Distension together with diarrhoea and vomiting often first present within days of birth, when the diagnosis should be made. Hirschsprung's disease must always be considered in the differential diagnosis of intestinal obstruction in the newborn. The diagnosis is confirmed by biopsy of the affected bowel and demonstration of the absence of ganglion cells. Definitive surgical treatment, which is the excision of the aganglionic segment, is best postponed until after the age of six months. Emergency treatment consists of making a temporary colostomy.

MECONIUM ILEUS

Infants with cystic fibrosis may present at birth with meconium ileus. In this condition dry, inspissated meconium may cause total intestinal obstruction at or even before birth. Meconium ileus occurring before birth may lead to intestinal perforation and meconium peritonitis. In meconium ileus the failure to pass meconium is absolute. X-ray examination of the abdomen shows tiny bubbles of gas trapped in the meconium contained in the small bowel.

The Albustix test of the meconium is positive. In the absence of proteolytic enzymes the meconium protein content is high and accounts for the positive test. The obstruction may be relieved by repeated enemas and stomach washouts using solutions containing pancreatic enzyme. Where enemas and washouts fail surgical treatment is attempted, but not unexpectedly the mortality is high.

MECONIUM PLUG SYNDROME

Intestinal obstruction due to the meconium plug syndrome occurs in the absence of enzymatic and ganglion cell deficiency. The meconium is unusually thick and hard and rectal examination induces the passage of a firm plug of meconium. Thereafter normal bowel movement supervenes.

Failure or Delay in Passage of Urine

Micturition before delivery. It must be remembered that urine may have been passed unnoticed during delivery and so account for apparent failure to pass urine after birth.

Renal agenesis is a cause of failure to pass urine. Congenital absence of one kidney causes no symptoms but absence of both kidneys is incompatible with life. Lack of passage of urine into the amniotic cavity results in oligohydramnios with amnion nodosum. Fetal compression leads to altered facies (Fig. 18.10), abnormal positioning of the hands and feet and breech presentation. There is frequently pulmonary hypoplasia causing early death. Almost all affected infants are light-for-dates males who possess certain pathognomonic features of the squashed baby syndrome first described by Potter. These include widely separated eyes, prominent epicanthic

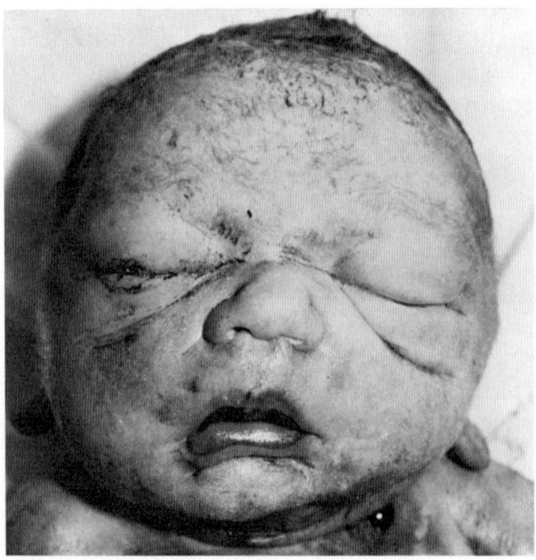

Figure 18.10 The squashed facial appearance of an infant with renal agenesis.

folds which run downward and then laterally below the eyes, flattened bridge of nose, receding chin and large, floppy, low-set ears.

Ureteral obstruction leading to hydronephrosis, hydroureter (but without megacystis) is rare. If bilateral it causes fetal or early postnatal death.

Bladder neck obstruction is evident as an enlargement of the bladder, ureters and kidneys and difficulty in passing urine. It is commonly brought to light by the development of urinary tract infection. Obstruction at the bladder neck may be due to valves of redundant mucosa arising in the region of the verumontanum, stenosis or muscular hypertrophy of the bladder neck. Irrespective of the cause most infants are symptomless until infection develops and the kidneys have been seriously damaged.

CARDIAC MURMURS

AT INITIAL EXAMINATION

Patent ductus arteriosus. A cardiac murmur is frequently heard during the initial routine examination following birth. Despite the murmur the baby is symptom-free and the usual explanation is a ductus arteriosus which is still patent. Normally the ductus arteriosus undergoes spontaneous closure shortly after birth with disappearance of the murmur. The ductus becomes converted gradually into a fibrous cord.

When discussing dyspnoea in Chapter 15 it will be recalled that a ductus arteriosus murmur is a feature of the respiratory distress syndrome which disappears when the baby recovers. In the respiratory distress syndrome there is marked increase in the right to left shunting of blood through the ductus arteriosus.

AT LATER EXAMINATION

Surprisingly cardiac murmurs which signify congenital heart disease (Chap. 11) are not usually heard until after the first few days of life. Such murmurs may be accompanied by other signs and symptoms such as failure to thrive, tiring easily, reluctance to feed, constant or sporadic respiratory embarrassment of varying degree, sudden periods of distress suggestive of pain, and changes of colour which may be characterized by pallor, a grey cyanosis or intense blueness. Any of these signs can occur alone or in combination and may be present at birth or only develop gradually. Additional to the midwife's observations the doctor will note any deformity of the chest, tachypnoea, oedema, enlargement of the liver, position of the apex beat, presence or absence of the femoral pulses, exhaustion following examination and murmurs on auscultation. Such late signs and symptoms occur around the second to third week of life and are found particularly in cases of ventricular septal defect, Fallot's tetralogy and patent ductus arteriosus.

Cyanosis resulting from congenital heart disease has been discussed in Chapter 15. The anatomical and functional abnormalities likely to cause cyanosis were discussed in Chapter 11.

Diagnosis depends principally on the total clinical picture, as murmurs are frequently of little help at this early age. Chest X-ray and ECG often provide important information. Now that surgical treatment is possible in a considerable number of congenital heart lesions an accurate diagnosis is essential at an early age. This will generally involve cardiac catheterization and angiography. For this transfer to a specialist unit is generally indicated.

SKIN RASHES

The skin of the newly born infant is extremely sensitive to rapid changes of environmental temperature, clothing and chemicals, so that rashes are a common finding. It is useful to separate them by cause into non-infective and infective groups (Table 18.8).

Table 18.8 Skin rashes

NON-INFECTIVE
Urticaria neonatorum
Sweat rash
Milia
Seborrhoea of the scalp
Seborrhoeic eczema
Ammoniacal dermatitis
Epidermolysis bullosa
Petechiae
Traumatic cyanosis
Congenital thrombocytopenic purpura
Drug rashes
INFECTIVE
Pustules, infected vesicles and dermatitis
Pemphigus neonatorum
Exfoliative dermatitis
Infected ammoniacal dermatitis
Petechiae
Rubella
Toxoplasmosis
Cytomegalovirus infection
Vesicles
Chickenpox
Smallpox
Granulomata

NON-INFECTIVE

Urticaria neonatorum (also known as erythema toxicum) is an eruption which resembles papular urticaria or nettle rash. It is extremely common and is usually seen in the first week of life. The eruption appears as irregular blotchy red spots, each of which has a pale central papule or wheal. These erythematous spots are not raised above the level of the skin, but the central papules can be readily felt if a finger is drawn gently over the skin. Although the erythema is sometimes extensive, it often consists of only a few isolated spots. Development of the condition may be associated with overheating. Cases of urticaria neonatorum require no treatment. The condition is not infective and does not interfere with the baby's general progress.

Sweat rashes may be erythematous or vesicular.

The erythematous form is usually seen in the flexures after the first week of life and occurs most commonly in babies who have been nursed in a warm atmosphere with excessive clothing and who have not been bathed daily. Prevention and treatment are dependent on cleanliness, efficient drying of the skin and on the provision of clothing which should be light, airy and of suitable texture. Powders and lotions are no substitutes for attention to the infant's personal hygiene.

Vesicular sweat rash appears as collections of very small vesicles on the head and chest of a baby who has been sweating as a result of illness or overheating. Each vesicle is related to a sweat gland, the duct of which has been obstructed and occluded. The vesicular rash differs from milia in that it is more gross in character and lacks the white opacity of the latter. Sweating in small preterm babies is less profuse than in larger infants, but occasionally minute colourless seed-like spots can be seen on the forehead of a premature baby and these correspond to the vesicular rash of other babies.

Milia (Fig. 18.11) is a common finding and is the appearance on the nose and surrounding structures of large numbers of minute yellowish-white opalescent spots. If the tip of a finger is gently passed over these spots they can be felt as extremely small, firmly defined spots. The spots are not pustules but cysts consisting of obstructed sebaceous glands. They disappear without treatment and contrast with a vesicular sweat rash in not being due to excessive sweating.

Seborrhoea of the scalp (cradle cap) (Fig. 18.12) is not uncommon towards the end of the neonatal period and results from lack of attention to local hygiene. The normal secretion of the sebaceous glands of the scalp accumulated as a grey, rather greasy, crusted layer of irregular thickness. Many mothers are hesitant about washing

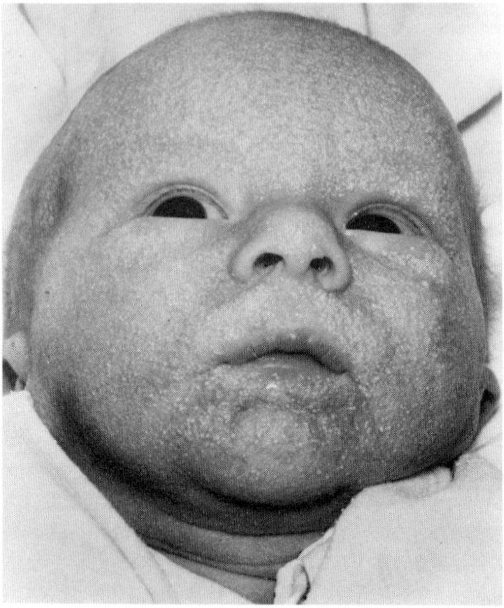

Figure 18.11 Milia.

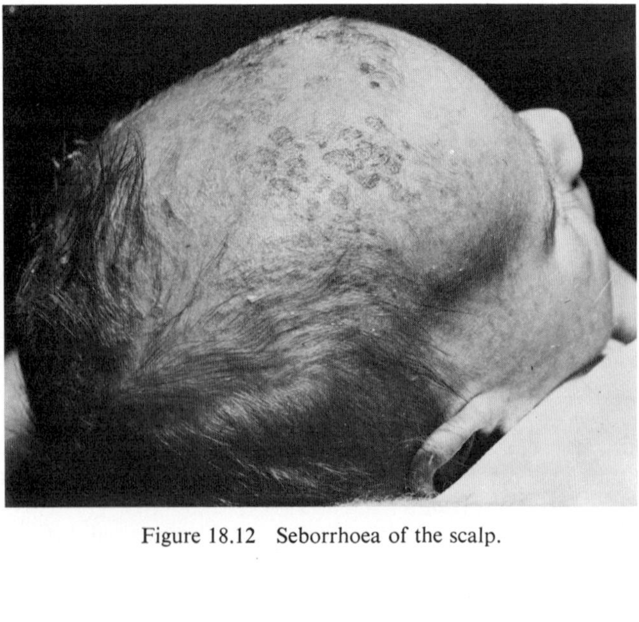

Figure 18.12 Seborrhoea of the scalp.

their baby's scalp because of doubts concerning the risks attached to handling the open fontanelle. Soap and water suffice to remove the crust in most instances. In severe cases cleansing can be facilitated by gently rubbing olive or nut oil into the scalp. This loosens the crust. Where sebaceous secretion is more extensive and persistent than usual and after the crusts have been removed, washing the head with a solution of sodium bicarbonate, 5 ml per 500 ml of warm sterile water is a valuable simple measure. Alternatively Hibitane as a shampoo can be used.

Seborrhoeic dermatitis. Scales of scurf on the scalp and forehead are sometimes accompanied by a seborrhoeic condition behind the ears. This form of seborrhoeic dermatitis is milder than infantile eczema and responds rapidly to treatment. For mild cases bathing with sodium bicarbonate solution is adequate. Where the condition is more pronounced, benefit will result from the use of an ointment containing a steroid after first cleaning the affected areas with liquid paraffin, olive oil or Neutrogena soap.

Ammoniacal dermatitis is not seen so frequently in babies in the first week or two of life as it is in older infants. In its mildest form the dermatitis consists of no more than an erythema. Excoriation and ulceration may occur. Characteristically the skin involved corresponds to the area covered by the napkin, and, where there are folds in the skin, the raised margins are affected while the depressions between are not. The dermatitis results from irritation of the skin by ammonia liberated from the urea of the urine by the action of organisms excreted in the faeces.

Napkin changing. Attention to napkin changing is of first importance in the matter of local treatment. Napkins must be changed as soon as they are wet or soiled. The numbers of changes involved in the 24 hours is considerably in excess of that expected by most mothers. Destructable napkins are valuable but expensive. Ordinary napkins, if used, should be treated with a chemical disinfectant, and if they have been washed with soap or detergents they must be thoroughly rinsed until all the soap or detergent has been removed.

Epidermolysis bullosa is a rare condition which may be mistaken for pemphigus. It is an inherited condition characterized by the appearance of vesicles and bullae in parts of the skin subjected to pressure or trauma. There is sometimes malformation of the nails. Occasionally involvement of the buccal mucous membrane creates a critical feeding problem. Secondary infection is a constant risk. Treatment is limited to evacuation of the bullae, the use of a mild antiseptic ointment and the giving of antibiotics if infection develops. Steroid therapy has been given trial with some benefit.

In traumatic cyanosis petechiae are limited to the head and neck and result from compression during the process of delivery. Usually the cord has been wrapped tightly around the neck or the head has been on the perineum for some considerable time. The petechiae disappear spontaneously and no treatment is necessary.

Drug rashes in the form of bullous eruptions are sometimes found in the newly born infant after the mother has been taking antimitotic or cytotoxic drugs during later pregnancy. When administered in relatively high doses during the first months of pregnancy these drugs may cause fetal death or multiple malformations.

INFECTIVE

Skin infections may present as pustules, secondarily infected vesicles, or dermatitis with or without exfoliation. They may occur in any site, but should be looked for particularly where skin surfaces are normally opposed as in the axillae, the groins, the folds of the neck and the perineum. Any of the lesions may occur singly, in local crops, or simultaneously in a number of situations. They may spread locally, become generalized and diffuse, or assume the form of frank furunculosis. In its most severe forms spread gives rise to cellulitis or deep abscess formation. There may be difficulty in differentiating an early pustule from an uninfected papule or even from urticaria neonatorum.

Pemphigus neonatorum is now a rare condition. Large bullous eruptions with hyperaemic margins and raw moist surfaces after exfoliation are associated with systemic disturbance.

Exfoliative dermatitis. A more severe form of pemphigus is exfoliative dermatitis (Ritter's disease), which constitutes an emergency requiring isolation, antibiotic therapy and frequently intravenous fluids.

Treatment of minor skin lesions consists in the application of spirit and a mild antiseptic powder, having first obtained a swab of the lesion for culture of the organism (Chap. 13). More extensive and more advanced lesions require systemic antibiotic therapy in addition to local treatment.

Secondary infection of an ammoniacal dermatitis by staphylococci *E. coli* and *Candida albicans* is not uncommon. Where infection is due to staphylococci or *E. coli* treatment consists in the application of an antibiotic cream followed by the regular use of a barrier cream. Whenever a napkin rash does not respond to treatment and there is a history of oral thrush, especially if the infant has been in receipt of oral antibiotics, then the possibility of a *Candida albicans* infection must not be forgotten. The affected area is usually intensely red with numerous satellite lesions away from the main area of infection. Treatment consists in giving Nystatin 100 000 units (con-

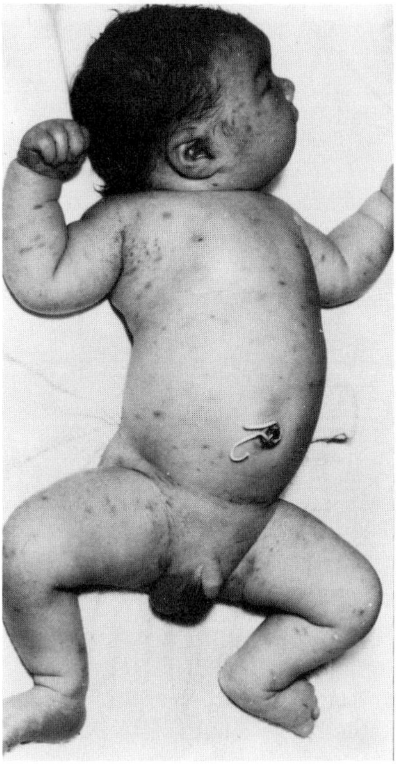

Figure 18.13 Generalized petechiae.

tained in 1 ml) by mouth four times daily after feeds for at least five days, and the local application of a Nystatin-containing cream until the infection has cleared (Chap. 17).

Petechiae (Fig. 18.13) distributed over the whole body are a feature of congenital rubella, toxoplasmosis and cytomegalovirus infection.

Transplacental infections. A baby may show evidence of chickenpox (Fig. 18.14) and smallpox at birth having contracted the disease from his mother *in utero*. Other disease contracted during pregnancy and marked by a rash at birth include syphilis, measles and typhoid fever (Chap. 13).

Granulomata of the skin are a feature of infection with *Listeria monocytogenes* contracted by the baby during delivery. The more usual presentation of *Listeria monocytogenes* infection is meningitis. Treatment consists in the administration of both penicillin and ampicillin when survival is now to be expected.

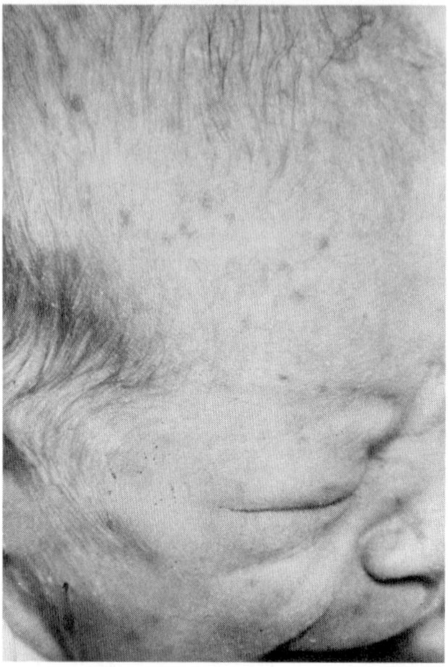

Figure 18.14 Chickenpox in newborn infant.

19

Practical Procedures

Any book on the care of the newborn infant would be incomplete without some guidance on nursing and medical aspects of practical procedures as applied to the newborn. Some procedures such as umbilical artery or vein cannulation will only be of significance at this period but others such as lumbar puncture are essentially similar at all ages but require modification for the newborn. Similarly the general nursing and medical principles of preparation of the necessary materials and of asepsis and antisepsis apply to all ages but may require modification for use at this age.

General Principles

No attempt will be made here to give guidance on those general principles which are taught as part of basic nursing and medical training but attention will be concentrated on those aspects which require particular attention when applied to a small helpless infant. As most hospitals in developed countries have some form of central sterile supply with prepared packs for nursing procedures we shall not give lists of the materials required for each procedure. Some indication of any special instruments likely to be required will, however, be given.

PREVENTION OF HEAT LOSS

The very small size of the newborn infant is the most obvious difficulty to be encountered in undertaking practical procedures at this age. Less obvious is the need to protect the infant against heat loss. This can be done by reducing exposure to the minimum, maintaining a high environmental temperature (above 25°C)—avoiding draughts and moisture on skin surfaces and by the provision of extra warmth from radiant heat sources or by an electrically heated mattress. Precautions must equally be taken to prevent burns. Many procedures can be carried out in incubators if necessary.

IMMOBILIZATION

Whereas the small sick infant may be inactive and immobile healthy mature infants can be surprisingly active and will require immobilization. The success of many procedures is largely dependent on the way the infant is held. We shall describe the immobilization and positioning for each procedure as appropriate.

PROTECTION OF THE INFANT

Gentleness and reasonable speed are requirements common to all procedures.

Inhalation of vomit. Protection of the infant from harmful side effects of all aspects of any procedure must be kept constantly in mind. This includes protection of the infant against the risk of inhalation of vomitus.

Feeds. Although an infant may be quieter after a feed major procedures are safer if left for one hour or more after a feed. If this delay is not justifiable the stomach should be emptied before any procedure, such as lumbar puncture, in which the infant is held with the spine flexed, which might provoke vomiting.

Suction. Facilities for suction of the pharynx and for tracheal intubation should be immediately at hand for the resuscitation of any infant who develops respiratory problems during a procedure.

Equipment. All equipment likely to be required must be checked before the procedure is started.

Training. Because of the potential risks involved no precedure should be carried out by those who have not had full training in the techniques involved.

PREPARATION

It is the responsibility of the senior nursing and medical staff present to make sure that all preparations have been completed and that all the equipment is ready before allowing the procedure to start. If any of the staff have not been present at a similar procedure previously it is essential that instruction be given beforehand about the part that each member of the staff is expected to take particularly any emergency action that might be expected of them.

Records. One member should be given the express duty of keeping a study of what has been done, of any drugs administered and of instructions about further observations or treatment. Such detailed action may seem unnecessary for simple procedures but it is only by being prepared for complications that even simple procedures can be made absolutely safe.

COLLECTION OF SPECIMENS

Of the procedures likely to be carried out on newborn infants collection of specimens for bacteriological or biochemical analysis are the most common and therefore probably the most time consuming. Skill in these minor procedures is just as important as ability to carry out major procedures and attention to detail will save unnecessary disturbance of the infant and avoid wasting the operator's time.

Bacteriological Swabbing of Superficial Sites

As discussed in Chapter 13 knowledge of the organisms acquired by an infant during or after delivery is essential to the management of potential or open infection in the individual infant and in the nursery as a unit.

BACTERIOLOGICAL SAMPLES

Bacteriological samples, should be taken from those sites known to have the highest chance of colonization. These are shown in Table 19.1.

Table 19.1 Sites from which swabs should be taken for bacteriological examination in suspected infections

Nose
Throat
Ear
Umbilicus
Groin

Swabbing. When taking specimens from these sites it is generally most convenient to use a sterile cotton wool pledget on the end of an orange stick in a sterile test tube or some similar type of 'swab'. The swab should come into contact with the area concerned but undue pressure which might cause local injury and promote entry of organisms to deeper tissues must be avoided.

Plating. Special arrangements for the immediate plating of a conjunctival discharge suspected of being due to the gonococcus may be required by the bacteriologists. Similarly special arrangements may be required for viral cultures. Consultation with the laboratory concerned is therefore advisable before taking any specimens requiring special studies.

Labelling. All specimens must be accurately labelled with both the infant's name and the site from which it was taken. It is also useful to record in the infant's notes that the specimens have been taken.

COLLECTION OF BLOOD SAMPLES

Samples of blood are generally only required in healthy infants for routine procedures such as the Guthrie test. Very small and ill infants may, however, require repeated blood samples for biochemical and bacteriological testing.

VOLUME

In some infants the amounts withdrawn, unless strictly controlled, can soon accumulate to surprisingly large volumes, sufficient to require replacement by transfusion.

Micromethods. Infants likely to require repeated investigations should not be treated in units where there are no facilities for biochemical investigations using micro or ultra-micro methods.

Record. Where such methods are available the medical staff must be constantly aware of the volume of blood being taken for investigations and a record should be kept of the volume of all specimens withdrawn. Such a record often has a salutary effect in keeping the number of investigations down to the level necessary to the proper management of the infant involved.

Consultation. An insufficient specimen may prove of no use to the laboratory and a further larger specimen be demanded. Before taking blood the volume required by the laboratory should be checked, bearing in mind the possibility of a high PVC and low plasma volume in the first few days of life and where there is dehydration. Prior discussion with the biochemist will often lead to a more rational and economical form of investigation.

Capillary Samples

Capillary blood is suitable for many biochemical investigations and, except in shocked infants, is easy to obtain.

Sites. Several sites may be used; those most commonly employed being the heel, the finger and the ear lobe. Because of the risk of transfer of infection disposable sterile lancets should be used. The skin must be warm and pink, indicating an adequate peripheral blood flow.

Technique for heel prick. When the heel is used it should be held as shown in Fig. 19.1 the skin is sterilized with surgical spirit and allowed to dry. Smearing the surrounding area with Vaseline helps to prevent dispersion of the blood when it begins to flow. A firm stab with the lancet is preferable to a tentative scratch which may have to be repeated several times. In most infants at least 1.0 ml of capillary blood can be obtained readily.

Specimen tubes. Capillary tubing, heparinized where necessary, is suitable for collecting capillary blood samples but specimens may also be taken into small containers. Wide containers are not in general suitable for small volume specimens.

Control of bleeding. When the specimen has been collected care must be taken to ensure that bleeding has ceased completely and a small protective dressing should be applied to prevent abrasion of the site and possible further bleeding. If blood does not flow freely from the original site another site should be chosen and the procedure repeated or the specimen should be taken by venupuncture.

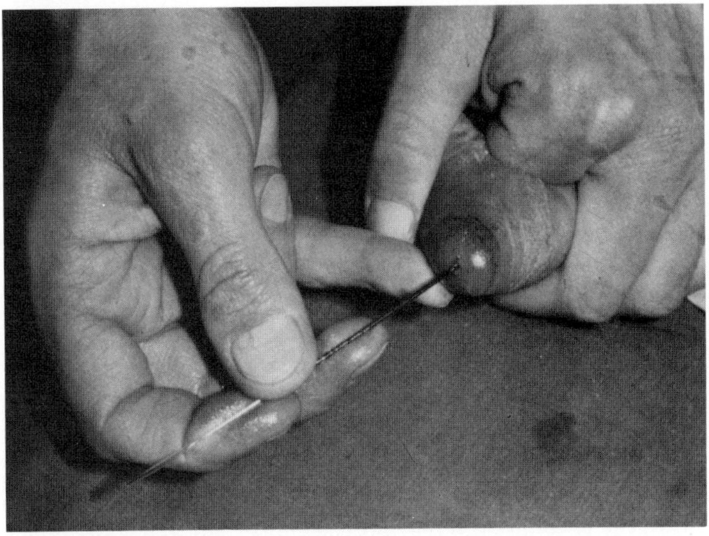

Figure 19.1 Capillary blood being obtained from heel stab.

ARTERIALIZED CAPILLARY BLOOD

The technique for taking 'arterialized capillary blood' for blood gas analysis is as given above. Particular attention must be paid to the state of the local circulation, and unless the skin is thoroughly warm and pink the specimen taken is more likely to represent venous capillary blood.

Venous Blood

When the infant's circulation is too poor to allow adequate capillary samples, or where larger volumes than 1 ml are required, blood should be taken from a vein except in those particular situations where arterial blood is required as discussed below. Individual doctors have their own particular preference as to which vein to try first. Although it is a good thing to acquire expertise in one method it is also advisable to have experience of venupuncture at more than one site.

Hand veins. By using a hypodermic (size 25 g) needle in a small vein on the back of the hand and allowing the blood to drip directly into the specimen tube small volumes of blood, e.g. 2 ml, can often be obtained with minimum disturbance of the infant.

Larger veins are advisable where specimens are to be withdrawn into a syringe and of these the femoral vein, the external jugular vein and the superior sagittal sinus are those most commonly used for percutaneous puncture.

PREPARATION

Position. In each case careful preparation is required with immobilization and accurate positioning of the infant. Such procedures are therefore more likely to distress the infant, and every effort should be made to limit the time of the procedure and to ensure that an adequate specimen is obtained at the first attempt.

Heat loss. As in all procedures precautions should be taken to prevent heat loss.

Two people are required, one to hold the infant and the other to take the specimen.

The skin should be cleaned and treated with a local antiseptic such as 70 per cent spirit.

The syringe should not be larger than is required to hold the specimen.

The needle. For external jugular and femoral veins the needle should not be too small and for all except the smallest infants gauge 21 is generally suitable. Special short shaft and short bevelled needles are required for puncture of the superior sagittal sinus.

EXTERNAL JUGULAR VEIN

The positioning for puncture of the external jugular vein (Fig. 19.2) is not comfortable for the infant and may require the assistance of a third person to hold the head if the infant objects violently.

The external jugular vein can most readily be identified when the infant is crying or the vein has been obstructed by pressure just above the clavicle.

Position. When the most suitable side has been chosen the wrapped infant is held supine with its shoulders at the table edge. The neck is then rotated to look over the opposite shoulder and the head depressed.

Puncture. As the vein is most obvious where it crosses the sternomastoid muscle it is advisable to insert the needle through the skin in the line of the vein but nearer the angle of the mandible. The needle is then advanced to enter the vein as it lies over the sternomastoid muscle and blood is withdrawn. After the procedure local pressure should be applied if there is any bleeding but often all that is required is to sit the baby up.

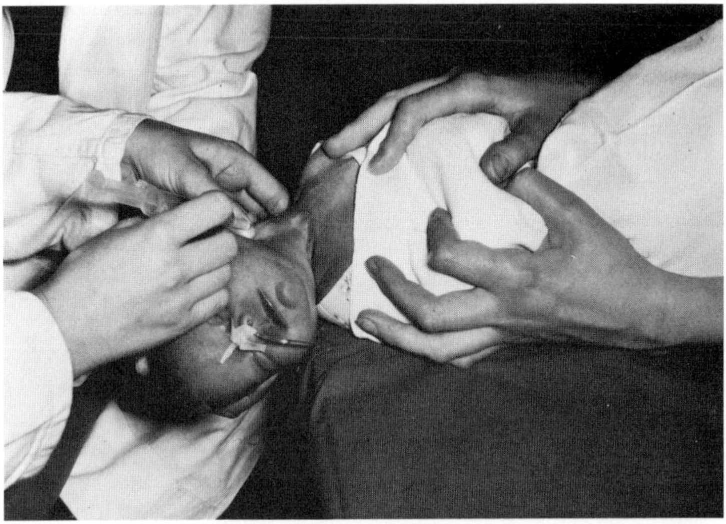

Figure 19.2 Position for external jugular vein puncture.

FEMORAL VEIN

Skin preparation. Because of the probability of bacterial colonization of the skin in the inguinal region particular attention must be taken in cleaning the skin. This site is not ideal for taking blood for culture as contamination by skin organisms is difficult to avoid. Should it be necessary to take a blood culture from a femoral vein a skin swab should be taken for bacteriological examination before the skin is cleansed. If this produces a growth of the same organisms as those found in the blood culture contamination must be suspected.

The femoral vein lies immediately medial to the femoral artery and the femoral artery must be identified before attempting to enter the vein.

Position. For right-handed people it is generally easiest to keep a finger of the left hand on the infant's right femoral artery and to hold the syringe and needle in the right hand. The positioning of the infant therefore is as shown in Figure 19.3. Nurse, or whoever is holding the infant, places the buttocks near the edge of the table and partially abducts the infant's thighs holding them steady with her hands and immobilizing the infant with inward pressure from her forearms. This is made easier if the infant's arms have been immobilized by being wrapped in a small blanket or towel. Having ensured that the infant is comfortably held the inguinal region is carefully sterilized and the femoral artery identified.

Puncture. The puncture is then made vertically slightly medial to the line of the artery and 0.5 to 1.0 cm distal to the inguinal ligament. The fingers of the left hand can now be used to steady the syringe and needle while the right hand is used to withdraw the plunger of the

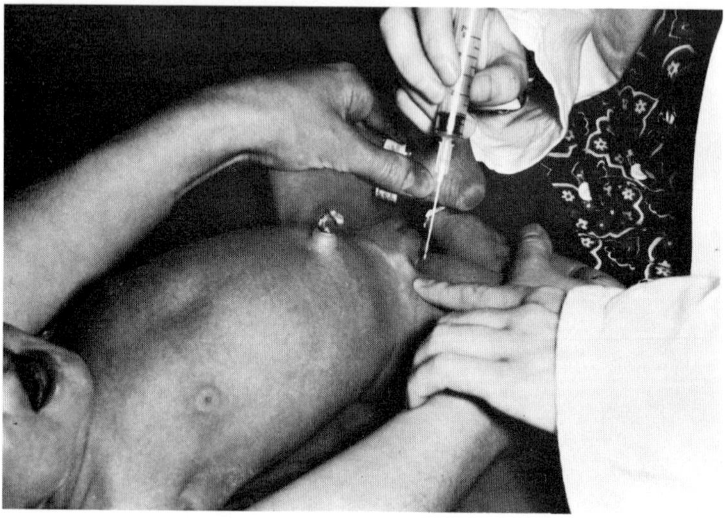

Figure 19.3 Position for femoral vein puncture.

syringe slightly to maintain a small negative pressure in the syringe as the needle is slowly advanced. If blood is not obtained after the needle point has been advanced 1.0 cm the needle should be slowly withdrawn, maintaining a negative pressure. Provided the site has been correctly chosen blood should be obtained readily.

Problems. If blood is not obtained the needle should be withdrawn, the position checked and one further attempt made. If this is also unsuccessful it is advisable to try the left femoral vein or some other vein. After withdrawal of the needle firm pressure should be applied over the vein until it is quite certain that bleeding from the vein whether superficial or subcutaneous has ceased. A sterile occlusive dressing should be applied.

Risks of femoral vein puncture include haemorrhage and thrombosis of the vein. The artery may be entered accidentally. Infection may be introduced. For those reasons the femoral vein should not be the vein of first choice.

SUPERIOR SAGITTAL SINUS

Precautions. Injections of infusions should not be given into the superior sagittal sinus because of the risk of thrombosis or the possibility of the needle moving out of the sinus. There appears to be very little, if any, risk associated with removal of blood from the sinus provided that certain precautions are observed. This method should not be used in dehydrated infants or those with a suspected bleeding problem.

Training. It should only be used by those who have been competently trained in the technique and this applies particularly to the person holding the infant.

Needle. The normal long shaft, long bevelled needle used for other venupunctures must not be used for this procedure. Gauge 22 needles with the shaft cut down to 2 cm length and with a short bevel have to be prepared locally and sterilized. No other special equipment is required.

Fontanelle. As the superior sagittal sinus is larger and has a greater blood flow at the posterior as opposed to the anterior fontanelle, and as the posterior fontanelle is generally open during the first month of life, we shall describe the procedure in relation to the posterior fontanelle.

Position. Before positioning the infant the posterior fontanelle should be palpated to make sure that there is no difficulty in its identification. Both operator and nurse should be sitting on chairs or stools facing one another. The infant is wrapped and placed on nurse's knee in the sitting position with his back towards the operator. Nurse steadies the trunk with her forearms resting her elbows on her knees. With her hands she holds the infant's head with the neck slightly flexed. By applying traction with her palms and fingers she draws the infant's scalp forward and downward so that the area over the posterior fontanelle becomes tense and the sutures are separated to their maximum extent. At the same time nurse must hold the head absolutely steady. The technique of holding the infant is essential to the success and safety of posterior fontanelle tap and should always be rehearsed with each infant before puncture is made.

Technique. When a satisfactory position has been achieved the hair of the infant's scalp is separated and the skin sterilized. The operator should hold the syringe as shown in Fig. 19.4 using the forefinger of the right hand as a guide to the depth to which the needle is inserted. The fingers of the left hand can be used to check on the suture lines and aid in the spreading effect. As the needle is inserted through the skin the syringe should be lowered so that the needle is pointing towards the anterior fontanelle. Resistance will be felt as the external dura matter is entered and a short push will be required to enter the sinus. It is because of the risk of perforating the opposite wall of the sinus during this push that short shaft, short bevelled needles are essential. When the sinus has been entered blood can be easily withdrawn and care must be taken not to exceed the volume required.

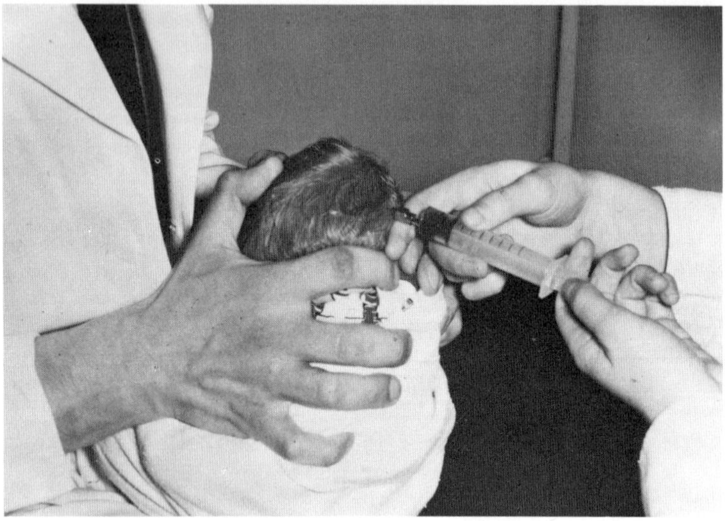

Figure 19.4 Position for sagittal sinus puncture through the posterior fontanelle.

After removal of the needle firm pressure with a circulatory movement over the fontanelle should be maintained until bleeding has stopped.

More space has been spent on describing this method of venupuncture because, if correctly carried out, it is easy and rapid to perform, causes less distress to an active infant and will readily provide larger volumes of blood should these be necessary.

Umbilical Vein Cannulation

In situations where continuous intravenous therapy is required umbilical vein cannulations will provide a route for treatment and venous blood specimens can also be withdrawn from the cannula with suitable precautions to ensure that they are not contaminated by fluid being given.

Equipment. Apart from suitable towels, swabs and antiseptic solution the equipment required is:

1 pair Spencer-Wells forceps
2 mosquito artery forceps
1 pair small dissecting forceps

1 pair small toothed forceps
1 pair dressing scissors
1 pair ophthalmic scissors
Umbilical catheters sizes 4.5 to 9.0 fg.

Preparation. The clamp or ligature used to prevent bleeding from the cord may have to be moved distally or removed to allow about 2 cm of cord to be exposed. The cord over this area and the surrounding skin is prepared with antiseptic and the area draped with a sterile towel.

Incision. It is useful where possible to identify the course of the umbilical vein and an incision is made over the vein about 1 cm from the base of the cord. If the vein can be exposed fully without complete transection of the cord a small distal stump can be left as a lid to help seal the cord when the catheter is withdrawn.

Introduction of catheter. The exposed and transected vein is held by one or two mosquito forceps applied to grip the edges of the vein. With slight traction on these forceps an opening is created into which the catheter can be introduced and advanced (Fig. 19.5). Some

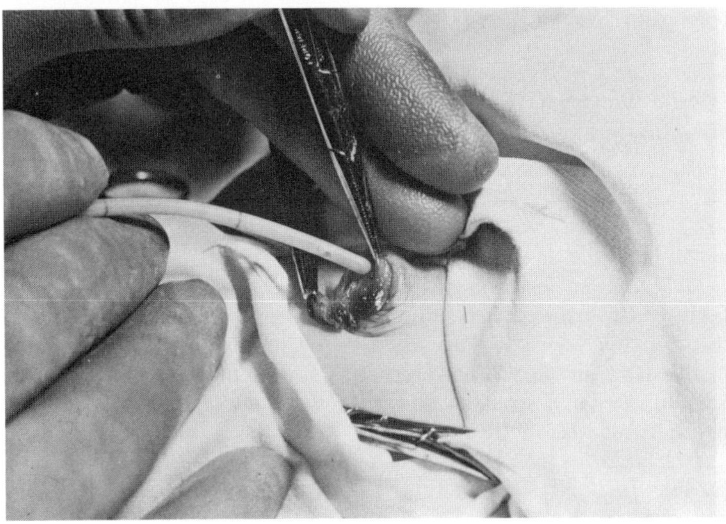

Figure 19.5 Introduction of catheter into umbilical vein.

obstruction may be encountered when the catheter reaches the point at which the vein passes through the abdominal wall. Pressure above the umbilicus may help to overcome this. The catheter is advanced gently to a distance of about 8 to 12 cm according to the infant's size until blood flows back freely. It is useful to note the distance the catheter has been advanced or to mark it.

Management. The catheter is then connected to the giving set or syringe according to the procedure intended. If the catheter is to be left in situ but no immediate transfusion is to be undertaken it should be filled with 0.9 per cent saline containing 10 units heparin per ml to prevent clotting. The forceps are removed. If there is bleeding around the catheter a ligature should be placed around the cord stump but this must not be sufficiently tight to occlude flow through the catheter.

Complications. Umbilical vein catheters provide a possible entry for infection into the portal circulation. Hyperosmolar solutions given by this means may cause thrombosis. These complications must be borne in mind when using this route for intravenous infusions. Other veins may be equally suitable and less open to risk. If the umbilical vein is used the catheter should be left in for as short a time as possible.

Withdrawal of the catheter should be done in stages withdrawing 2 or 3 cm at a time, and leaving a gap of 30 minutes or more before the next stage. This considerably reduces the risk of haemorrhage when the catheter is finally withdrawn and suturing is not then required.

Arterial Blood Specimens

Arterial blood samples are required for accurate measurement of the blood gases and in particular of oxygen (Po_2).

Puncture or cannulation. As specimens are likely to be required on several occasions at relatively short intervals an early decision has to be made as to whether to attempt repeated arterial puncture or to insert an umbilical artery cannula. As these techniques are likely to be required only in infants requiring intensive therapy the decision therefore becomes whether the infant requires transfer to an intensive therapy unit. This book is not intended to cover the work of intensive therapy units and only brief mention will be made of the techniques involved.

Arterial puncture. The radial, temporal and femoral arteries are suitable for arterial puncture. A small gauge needle should be employed.

UMBILICAL ARTERY CANNULATION

Umbilical artery cannulation is essentially similar to cannulation of the umbilical vein (see above) but made more difficult by the contractility and much smaller size of the arteries. These can, however, be dilated by a suitable reamer and a small blunt-ended catheter with side holes (e.g. 4.5 fg) inserted. In order to simplify the subsequent withdrawal of specimens a disposable two way tap should be inserted between the open end of the catheter and the syringe.

Difficulty is sometimes encountered in advancing the catheter more than a few centimetres. This is sometimes overcome by waiting several minutes before attempting to advance the catheter further.

The tip of the catheter will require to be advanced into the internal iliac artery or beyond before an adequate flow of arterial blood can be maintained.

Precautions. Care must be taken to ensure that no air enters the syringe as the specimen is taken, and the nozzle of the syringe must be sealed with a suitable cap before the syringe containing the blood is sent to the laboratory. The catheter must then be filled with heparinized saline (10 units heparin per ml saline) contained in a separate syringe attached to the other arm of the two way tap. The volume of heparinized saline used should be limited to that required to clear the catheter.

Risks. The risk of haemorrhage after arterial puncture or cannulation is greater the larger the needle or catheter used. With small needles, however, bleeding is generally easily controlled by local pressure. Withdrawal of an umbilical arterial catheter should be done progressively, withdrawing not more than 5 cm at a time at intervals of about 30 minutes.

Thrombosis of the internal iliac or other arteries may occur with resulting ischaemia of a lower limb or section of the bowel.

Urine Specimens

COLLECTING BAGS

Urine specimens required for biochemical testing only are most readily collected by using one of the disposable collecting bags (Fig. 19.6) which can be stuck onto the infant's perineum and left until urine has been passed. Such urine specimens are almost certain to be contaminated by skin organisms and even if plated out immediately after urine has been passed often giving a misleading indication of organisms present. Bags are therefore not a suitable method for collecting urine for bacteriological analysis.

CLEAN-CATCH SPECIMENS

Where urinary tract infection is suspected it is essential to obtain an uncontaminated specimen of urine for culture before treatment is considered. 'Clean-catch specimens' are adequate for this purpose if the urine can be caught in a sterile container in mid stream without the urine having dribbled over the perineum. This can be achieved by

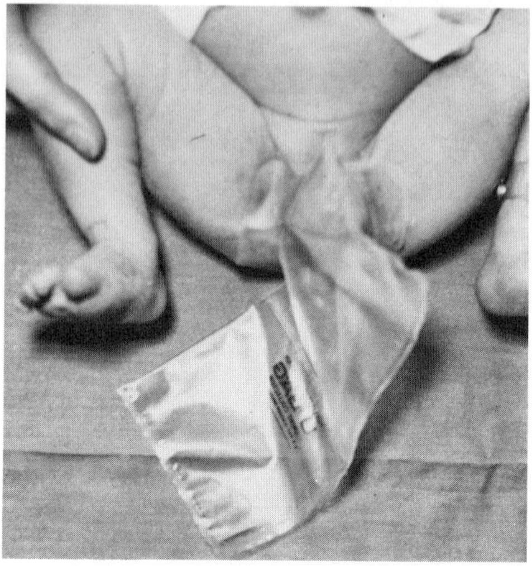

Figure 19.6 Urine collecting bag.

holding the infant in a suitable position according to sex and by being patient (Fig. 19.7). A suitable time is shortly after the completion of a feed. Mothers can be taught the technique. It is essential that the penis or vulva should not come into direct contact with the sterile container. This unfortunately is often allowed to occur and the specimen may be contaminated.

SUPRAPUBIC ASPIRATION

Suprapubic aspiration of urine from the bladder is the only satisfactory method of preventing contamination. Mothers, when given the choice of attempting a 'clean catch' or allowing suprapubic aspiration, generally prefer the latter when they realize how little the infant is upset.

Preparation. If a mother is not aware of the method careful explanation of the advantages and of the safety of the technique must be given beforehand. When a urine specimen is required mother or a nurse should prevent urine being passed by pressure over the distal urethra. In the male the penis can be held and in the female the labia can be displaced laterally.

Position. With the infant lying in the supine position and the legs held in extension the operator then confirms by palpation and percussion that the bladder is easily definable and contains urine.

Puncture. After cleaning the skin in the suprapubic region a gauge 21 needle attached to a 10 ml syringe is advanced through the

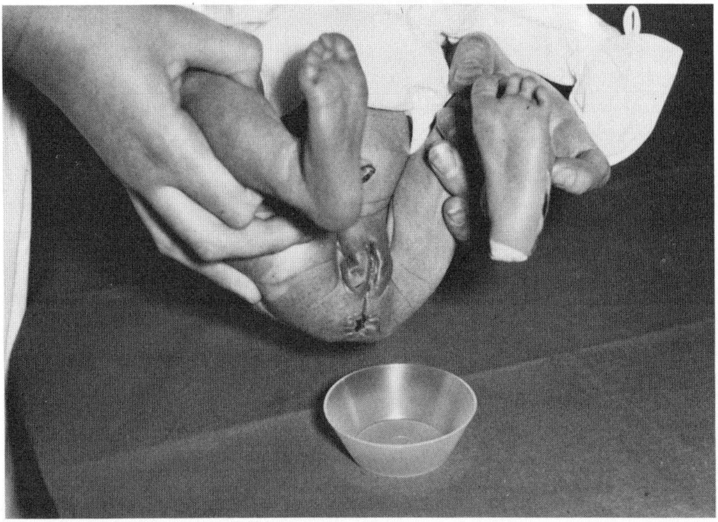

Figure 19.7 Position for collecting 'clean catch' specimen of urine.

skin in the midline about 1.0 cm above the symphysis pubis and over the bladder, which is easily entered (Fig. 19.8). About 5 ml of urine are aspirated gently, the syringe and needle withdrawn and local pressure applied over the puncture site. The needle is removed and the urine transferred to a suitable bacteriological container.

Specimen. It is most important that the bacteriologists are informed that urine has been taken by direct aspiration of the bladder as small growths of organisms which might otherwise be ignored may be of significance in such specimens.

Risks. Experience has shown that the risk of causing haematuria is very small and that if it does occur it is of short duration and self-limiting.

In infants who are ill and who may have infection of the urinary tract suprapubic aspiration of the bladder urine is the method of choice for obtaining the initial bacteriological specimen.

Cerebrospinal Fluid

Cerebrospinal fluid (CSF) may be obtained from the lumbar route, from the lateral ventricles of the brain or, underspecial circumstances, from the cisterna magna.

LUMBAR PUNCTURE

Lumbar puncture is the method of first choice unless local deformity, as in spina bifida, makes this difficult. As the spinal cord ends at a relatively lower level in relation to the lumbar vertebrae during early fetal life and as it still extends to the level of the body of the third lumbar vertebra in a term infant at birth, this difference in anatomy when compared to the older child or adult must be kept in mind.

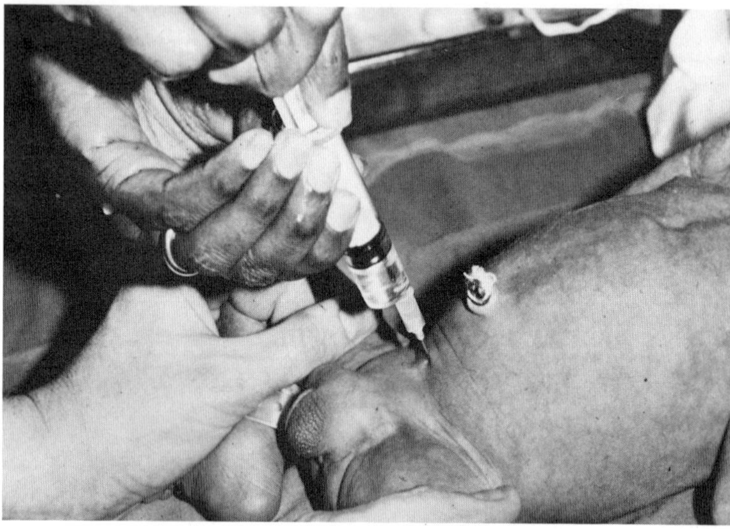

Figure 19.8 Suprapubic aspiration of the bladder.

Preparation. Fine gauge short lumbar puncture needles are advisable. As infants requiring lumbar puncture are generally ill the procedure should be carried out gently but as rapidly as possible and with minimum disturbance to the infant.

Position. The infant should be held by the nurse at the edge of the table, nearest to the operator with the spine as fully flexed as possible and the infant in the true lateral position (Fig. 19.9). Some prefer the infant to be held in the sitting position but this may be difficult to maintain steadily. As the intervertebral spaces are relatively large in the newborn and as the vertebral canal is narrow accurate localization is necessary before the puncture is attempted.

Puncture. Using the junction of the line of the vertebral spines and a line drawn between the highest points of the iliac crests (supracristal plane) the fourth lumbar vertebra can be identified. Lumbar puncture may be carried out between the bodies of the third and fourth lumbar vertebrae, as in the adult, or, in low birth-weight infants, between the fourth and fifth lumbar vertebrae. The needle should be advanced slowly and the stilette withdrawn frequently as it is often

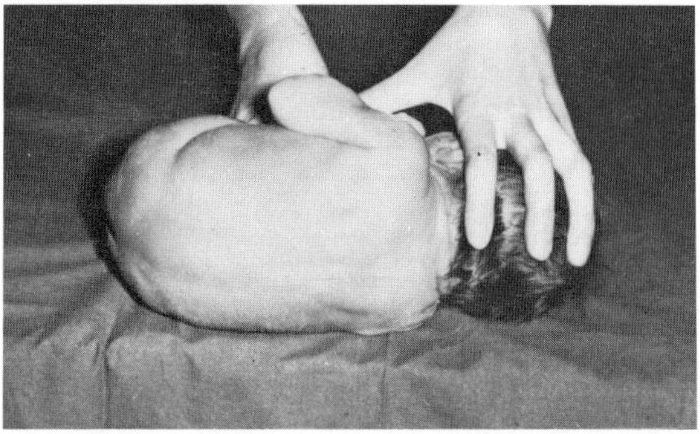

Figure 19.9 Position of infant for lumbar puncture.

difficult to feel when the vertebral canal has been entered. Perforation of the longitudinal vertebral sinuses will result in contamination of the CSF with blood. This occurs readily if the needle is advanced too far. CSF should be allowed to drip slowly into the appropriate container and only the volume required by the laboratory should be removed. The stilette should be replaced before the needle is withdrawn and the puncture site sealed.

VENTRICULAR TAP

Ventricular tap is indicated where it is not possible to use the lumbar route or where it is specifically necessary to obtain ventricular CSF.

Position. The infant is wrapped and held supine with the crown of the head at the edge of the table. After identification of the edges and angles of the anterior fontanelle the skin is prepared and the infant's head draped.

Puncture. A lumbar puncture needle is inserted at the lateral angle of the anterior fontanelle and directed in the plane which would meet the internal canthus of the opposite eye. Once the skin and external dura have been penetrated the stilette should be withdrawn to check on the possibility of a subdural collection of fluid. The shaft of the needle must then be held very steadily within a gauze swab held by the fingers of the operator's left hand so that the plane of advance of the needle remains constant. With the right hand the needle is advanced slowly and the stilette withdrawn frequently while the needle is stationary. If no CSF has been obtained after the tip of the needle has been advanced 3 cm the needle should be withdrawn continuing with frequent withdrawal of the stilette.

Repeated ventricular taps are not advisable.

The risks associated with tapping the cisterna magna are high and this procedure is best left to those with training in neurological techniques.

THERAPEUTIC PROCEDURES

Temperature Control

The commonest problem affecting newborn infants requiring treatment is inadequate control of body temperature. For a discussion of the physiological principles involved readers are referred to Chapter 5. Two lines of therapy are available, the first aimed at controlling heat loss and the second at providing a source of extra warmth or cooling as required. As fall in body temperature is the commonest problem attention will be focused on prevention of heat loss and provision of extra heat.

PREVENTION OF HEAT LOSS

For the healthy term newborn infant, dryness, clothing, a suitable cot and bedding and a room temperature of about 20°C described in Chapter 6 are all that is required. Low birth-weight and ill infants may require to be nursed in an incubator with no or minimal clothing to allow adequate observation. Heat loss, however, still occurs when the infant is nursed naked even in a warm incubator.

Radiation loss can be reduced by covering the infant with a transparent perspex heat shield. If total body observation is not essential an aluminium foil swaddler (Fig. 19.10) serves the same

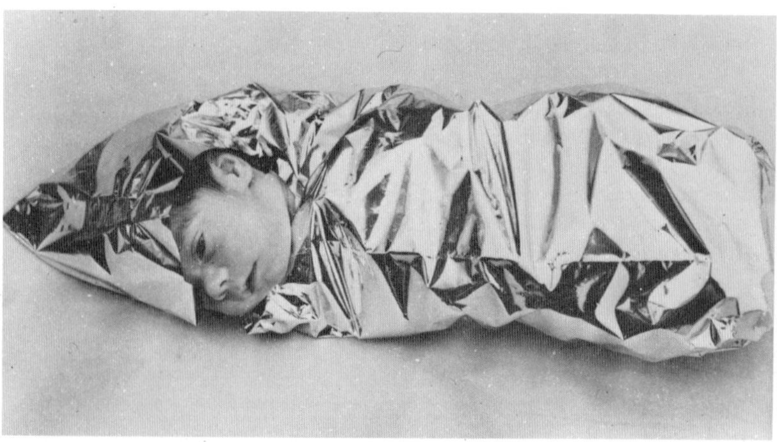

Figure 19.10 Metal foil swaddler. (Photograph by courtesy of Lewis Woolf Griptight Ltd.)

purpose and is particularly suitable if an infant has to be transported through cool areas.

Convection loss can be reduced by limiting opening of the incubator arm-holes and other apertures to an absolute minimum. Oxygen or other gas being given should be warmed before entering the incubator and should not be given by direct mask except for brief periods of crisis.

PROVIDING EXTRA HEAT

Incubators are not entirely satisfactory means of providing heat, relying as most of them do on the circulation of heated and moistened air within the hood.

Overhead heaters. Radiant and conductive heat can be provided from overhead infrared heaters (Fig. 19.11) or from heated mattresses.

Servocontrol mechanisms can be incorporated. The type of

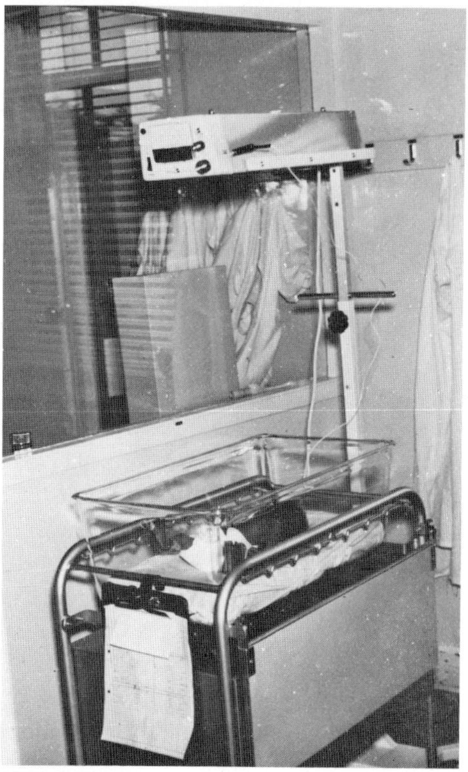

Figure 19.11 Overhead radiant heater with servocontrol mechanism.

apparatus shown in Fig. 19.12 is suitable for carrying out special procedures. Because of its size it is less appropriate for the routine management of low birth-weight infants, for whom incubators

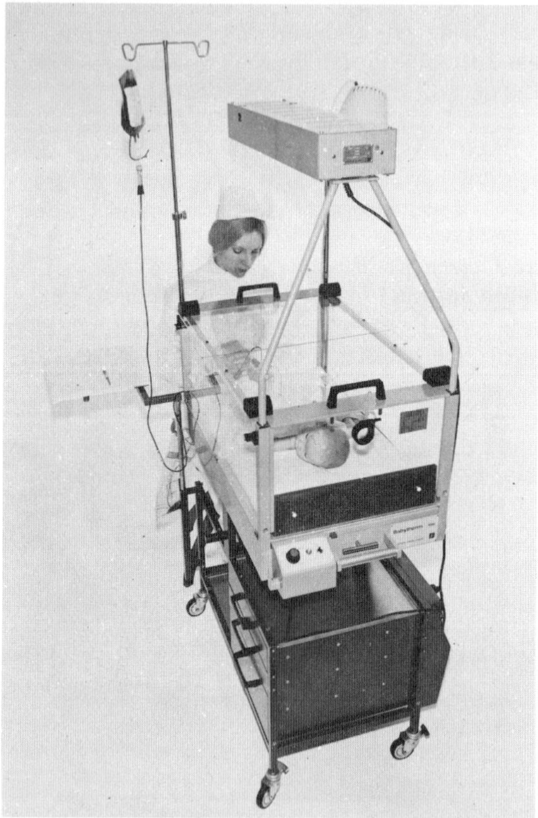

Figure 19.12 Babytherm. (Photograph by courtesy of Draeger Medical Ltd.)

remain the most suitable method for aiding temperature control. Many low birth-weight infants are, however, nursed in incubators longer than is probably necessary or advisable.

Oxygen

CONTROL

Under a number of circumstances in which lowered levels of blood oxygen occur in the infant increased concentrations of inspired oxygen are required.

Arterial $P\text{O}_2$. Ideally oxygen therapy should be controlled by measurement of the infant's arterial Po_2. This is not necessary where oxygen is being given for short periods but is essential when treatment is being given for more than 30 minutes.

The object should be to maintain a satisfactory level of oxygenation (Po_2 of 60 to 90 mmHg) and to prevent higher levels being reached because of the risk of retrolental fibroplasia, cerebral vasoconstriction and possible damage to the lungs.

Clinical assessment of arterial oxygenation can be extremely difficult and at times misleading. Cyanosis is the most obvious clinical sign of hypoxaemia and requires treatment with the minimum added oxygen which will restore a normal colour.

OXYGEN CONCENTRATION

If there is no clinical cyanosis the concentration of inspired oxygen should not be allowed to exceed 40 per cent and preferably should be kept at 30 per cent.

Oxygen analyser. Sampling of the environmental oxygen concentration by an oxygen analyser (Fig. 19.13) is the only satisfactory method of estimating the inspired air concentration of oxygen. The settings given on incubators for oxygen concentrations at a given rate of flow are only guides relating to ideal conditions which are seldom achieved in practice.

High concentrations. If high concentrations of oxygen are required

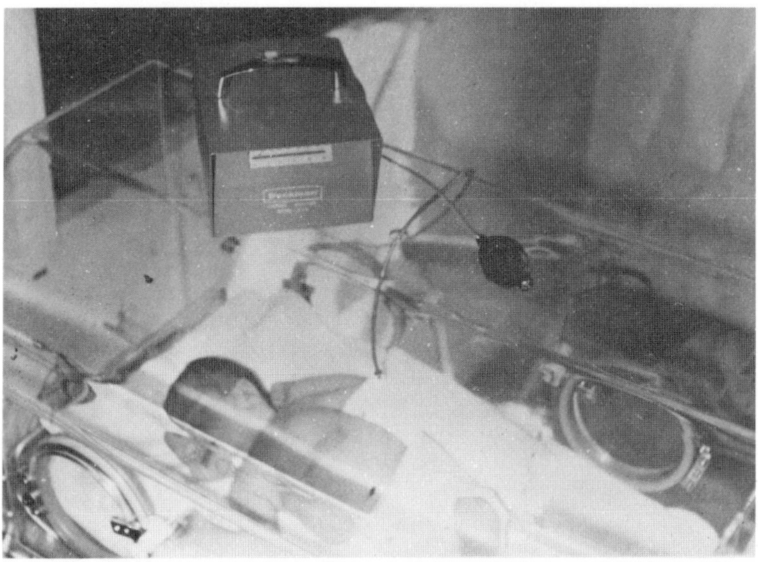

Figure 19.13 Oxygen analyser.

it may be found difficult to achieve these in an incubator unless a small hood is placed over the infant's head (Fig. 19.14).

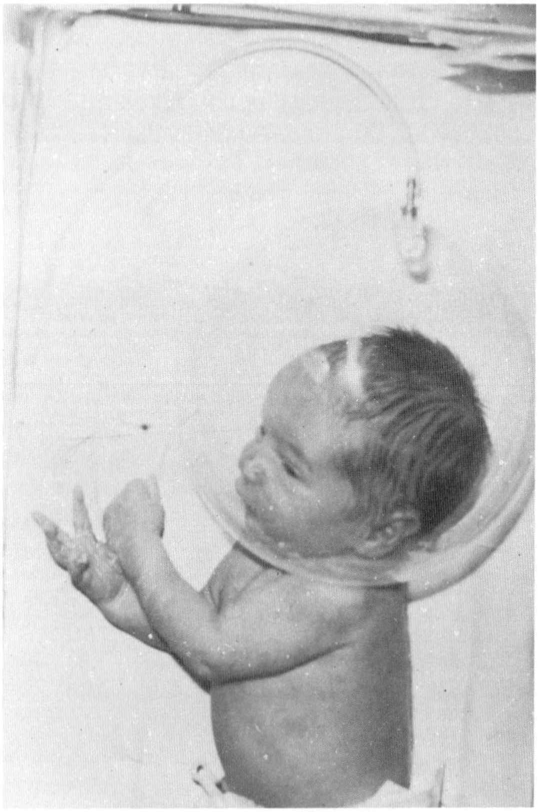

Figure 19.14 Oxygen hood.

Temperature and humidity. The necessity to warm the oxygen and air being given has already been mentioned. Dryness of the oxygen and air should be avoided but there appears to be no advantage in the very high levels of humidity previously recommended. Oxygen and air mixtures given through the mixer valve of incubators are adequately moistened by the incubator humidifier.

Tracheal Intubation

If adequate oxygenation cannot be achieved by spontaneous respiration of an oxygen enriched air some form of artificial respiration will be required. It is not intended in this book to discuss in detail respirator management but all, whether midwives or doctors, who are involved in the care of the newborn should understand and practise the technique of tracheal intubation and intermittent positive-pressure respiration (IPPR).

EQUIPMENT

An infant-type laryngoscope with a Magill infant blade is used.

Endotracheal tubes. For the oral route endotracheal tubes of varying sizes should be available. These may be of the disposable type (Warne's, Fig. 19.15) with a broader section to prevent the tube

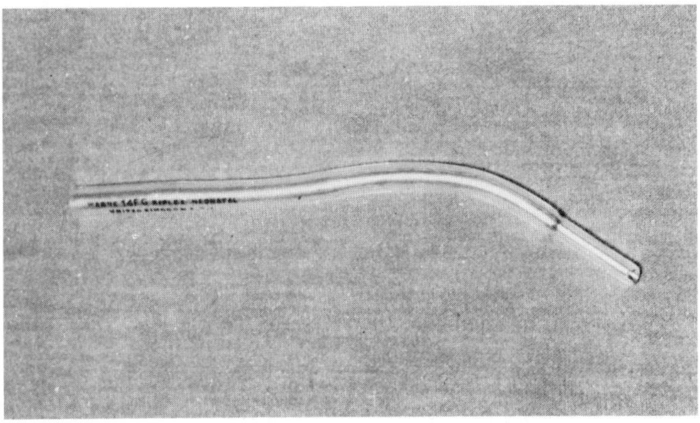

Figure 19.15 Disposable endotracheal tube.

being advanced too far or they may be of the simple anaesthetic type. A soft metal probe or introducer which can be inserted into the tube to aid in positioning is sometimes helpful. For nasopharyngotracheal intubation Jackson-Rees tubes (Fig. 19.16) are required together with special forceps for guiding the catheter from the pharynx into the trachea.

Suction apparatus with a suitable sterile catheter should be held in readiness by an assistant.

A source of air, or oxygen-enriched air, limited to a maximum pressure of 30 cm of water and with a side hole or Y tube to allow expiration must be available together with suitable connectors for attachment to the endotracheal tube. The rate of flow does not need to be higher than that required to ensure a maximum pressure of 30 cm water. This is generally about 1 litre per minute. Intermittent closure of the side hole allows intermittent positive-pressure respiration (IPPR) to be applied.

Resuscitation trolleys. The necessary apparatus is most conveniently available if already assembled and on a mobile trolley with a

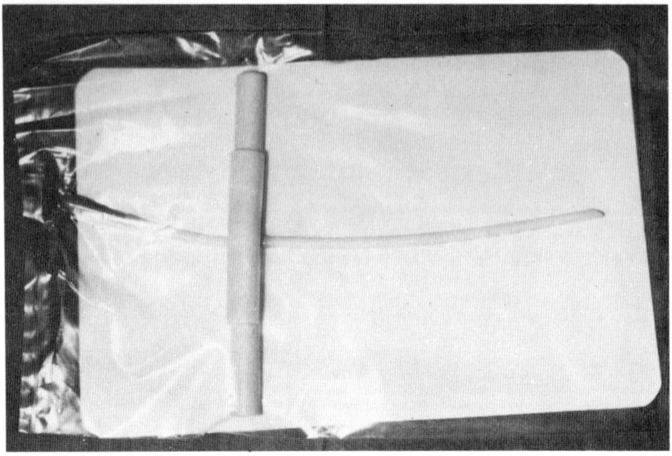

Figure 19.16 Jackson-Rees tube.

suitable area for the infant. Such resuscitation trolleys are available commercially but as many have the disadvantage that no arrangement for providing local heat is available a separate heat source is also required (Fig. 19.17). There is a major risk of fall in superficial temperature followed by fall in central temperature during tracheal intubation unless adequate precautions to prevent heat loss are taken.

TECHNIQUE

Preparation. As the oral route is the easier to perform it will be described. Once the necessary expertise has been acquired this procedure is relatively simple. The beginner should, however, learn the technique required on a stillborn infant or on one of the artificial dolls made for this purpose.

Position. The infant is laid supine with the head partially extended and the neck slightly flexed.

Laryngoscopy. With the handle of the laryngoscope held in the left hand the blade is inserted gently at the left angle of the infant's mouth and passed forward over the infant's tongue (Fig. 19.18). The blade is then used to depress the tongue until the epiglottis comes into view. By sliding the tip of the laryngoscope into the glossoepiglottic fold and pulling the epiglottis forward the vocal cords come into view. Suction is applied as necessary to clear the airway and to allow unimpeded vision. With the right hand holding the proximal end, the endotracheal tube is then passed under direct vision into the larynx and upper trachea making sure that the tip of the tube lies above the

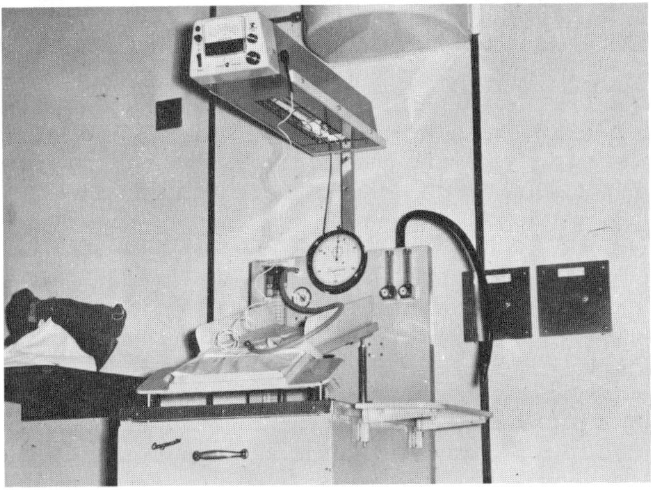

Figure 19.17 Resuscitation trolley with overhead radiant heater unit.

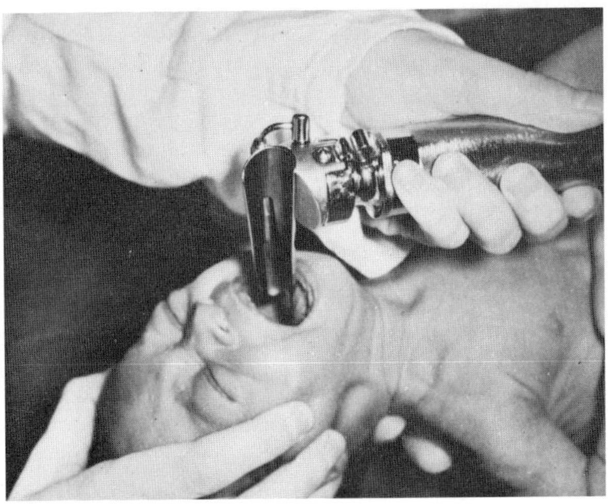

Figure 19.18 Position for inserting laryngoscope.

origin of the main bronchi. Further suction through the tube may then be required.

INTERMITTENT POSITIVE-PRESSURE RESPIRATION

After laryngoscopy and tracheal intubation the proximal end of the endotracheal tube is connected to the IPPR apparatus and air allowed to flow for approximately 1 second followed by a similar period for expiration resulting in about 30 to 40 respiratory cycles per minute. By observing chest movement and listening over both lungs with a stethoscope the operator must check that air is entering both lungs. If not, the situation must be reassessed and, if necessary, laryngoscopy be repeated to make certain that the tube is in the trachea and not in the oesophagus. Should one lung only be adequately ventilated the tip of the endotracheal tube may have passed into a main bronchus and should be withdrawn until both lungs are adequately ventilated. If the tube is in a good position but air entry is poor further suction is required. Once the tube is in a satisfactory position and if further IPPR is required the tube should be strapped to the angle of the mouth to prevent further movement.

Mask and bag. Where apparatus for tracheal intubation is available without a source of air under pressure IPPR can be applied by a mask and bag placed over the tube. If a suitable bag is not available in an emergency situation air can be blown into the tracheal tube from the operator's mouth.

PER NASAL IPPR

Where the apparatus necessary for tracheal intubation is not available IPPR can be given through the infant's nose, using a bag and mask, or by mouth to nose insufflation. For this to be effective the airways must be clear of secretions and the infant's neck should be extended to allow as clear a passage as possible between the nose and the larynx. When available an infant-size Guedel airway placed in the mouth also supplies an oropharyngeal airway. Several suitable masks and bags are available commercially. Some have a pressure limiting valve and most have facilities for connection to an oxygen supply (Fig. 19.19).

For *mouth to nose insufflation* the infant is conveniently supported by the thorax in the palm of the right hand with the fingers palpating the apex beat and chest movement. With the left hand the head is supported and the neck extended. By placing his mouth over the long axis of the infant's nose and across the infant's mouth the operator is now ready to blow small volumes of air from his puffed out cheeks into the infant's lungs. The pressure required can be learned from practice with a water manometer and should not exceed 30 cm of water. This is readily exceeded with a hard puff from the chest which will also be of too large a volume. The fingers of the right hand which are wrapped round the infant's chest give an indication of the respiratory movement being produced and also show whether the heart rate is returning to normal.

Risks. Mouth to nose insufflation and blowing directly into an endotracheal tube naturally carry a risk of virus and bacterial

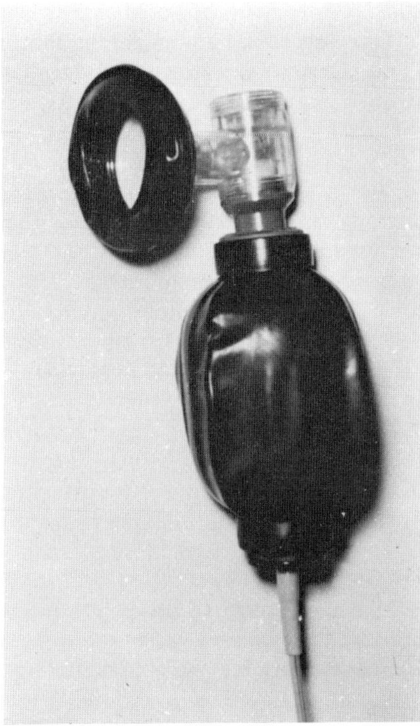

Figure 19.19 Mask and bag for nasal IPPR.

contamination of the infant's respiratory tract. These methods should therefore only be used where no better method is available and they should only be continued as long as they are necessary for the infant's well-being.

INJECTIONS AND INFUSIONS

INTRADERMAL, SUBCUTANEOUS AND INTRAMUSCULAR INJECTIONS

These injections are given to infants by the same technique as apply to older patients. Smaller gauge needles are required and greater care is necessary to ensure that the injection is correctly placed and that no injury is done. Volumes injected must be limited preferably to not more than 0.5 ml in low birth-weight infants. Because of the difficulty in measuring small volumes accurately graduated 1 ml syringes (as used for Mantoux tests) are required for doses less than 1.0 ml.

Risks. Particular care must be taken in choosing the site of the injection in order to avoid important structures such as the sciatic nerve. The margin for error in choice of site is very little in the smallest infants. Too superficial an injection may result in local tissue reaction. Too deep an injection may cause neurological or vascular damage.

Intravenous Infusions

VEINS

Mention has already been made of the use of the umbilical vein for giving intravenous therapy. This route is not generally available after the first week of life, and in the first week is not recommended as the vein of choice if it is not also to be used for obtaining samples of venous blood. Any peripheral vein including those of the hand and forearm may be used but most find that veins of the scalp are the most suitable.

SCALP VEIN TRANSFUSION

Disposable scalp vein needles with a wing attachment for holding the needle and with a length of tubing and adaptor for Luer fitting attached are available in several sizes. Use of such sets has simplified the technique of scalp vein transfusion.

Choice of site. Before starting the procedure the operator should examine the whole scalp to identify several suitable sites. The Y junction of two veins is a useful place to make an attempt as the tributary veins steady the larger vein produced by their junction. The position and size of veins can best be judged after the flow of blood has been temporarily obstructed by pressure over the vein lower down its course (Fig. 19.20). It is advisable to make first attempts near the vertex so that further attempts can be made 'downstream', should the original attempt fail.

Preparation. After the infusion fluid and giving set have been assembled the infant is lightly held in a suitable position and the skin of the scalp prepared. The scalp vein set should then be filled with sterile normal saline or similar clear fluid and the stopper removed from the adaptor.

Puncture. The needle point should be inserted through the skin about 0.5 cm proximal to the Y junction selected. The distal part of the vein is occluded by pressure and the needle passed into the vein at the Y junction. The passage of blood back into the tubing indicates that the vein has been entered. With the needle carefully held in that position the drip set is connected, pressure over the distal vein removed and the flow of infusion fluid checked.

Fixture. When this has been established the wings of the needle are used to fix the needle to the scalp with adhesive strapping (Fig. 19.21) or by a small plaster of Paris protective covering, and the

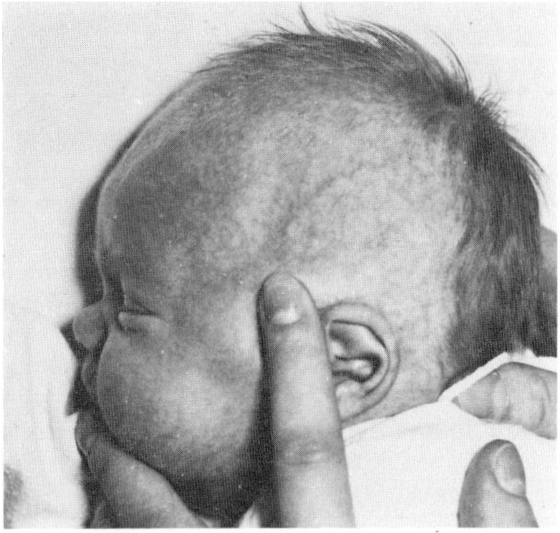

Figure 19.20 Demonstration of scalp veins by occluding flow distally.

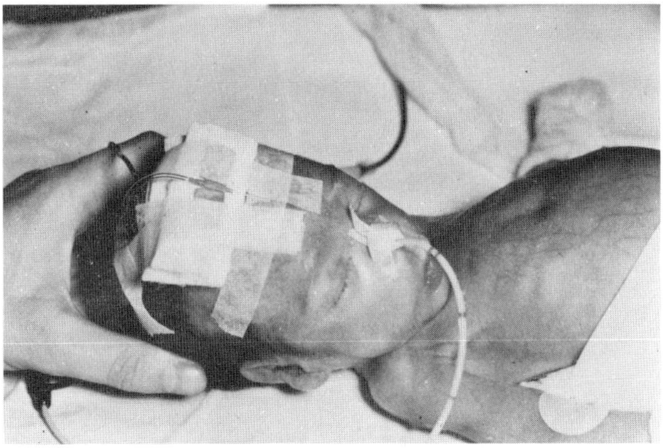

Figure 19.21 Scalp vein infusion.

remainder of the tubing is secured so that accidental movement of the needle is prevented.

Observations. The rate of flow of the infusion is then checked and written instructions given about the total volume to be given and the time to be taken for this. It is important that those attending the infant report immediately if there is swelling of the scalp near the infusion site indicating that the needle has been displaced. The infusion must be stopped and assistance sought. Minor correction of the needle position may restore flow but often a new site has to be chosen and the procedure repeated.

CONTROL OF INFUSIONS

As it is easy to overburden an infant's circulation if excessive volumes of fluid are infused, or if the infusion takes place rapidly, both the rate of flow and the total volume to be given must be carefully regulated.

Giving sets. This is made easier by using giving sets designed for use with infants and containing a subsidiary graduated chamber containing, for example, 30 ml which is filled from the main infusion bottle by a valve which is normally kept closed.

Electronic drop counters with a servomechanism designed to maintain a constant number of drops per minute are available (Fig. 19.22).

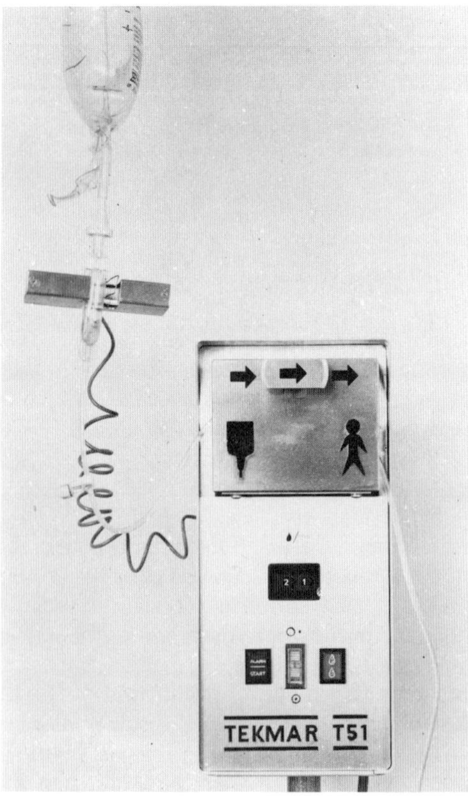

Figure 19.22 Self-regulated infusion pump. (Photograph by courtesy of Tekmar Ltd.)

Roller pumps (Fig. 19.23) which deliver a specified volume of fluid per minute may also be used. Both forms of apparatus are relatively expensive and therefore not universally available.

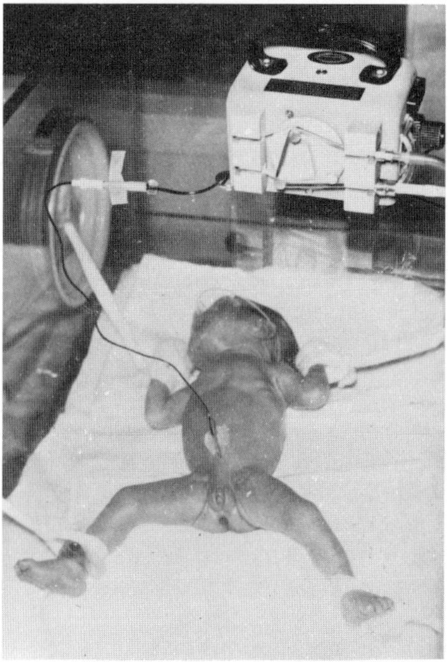

Figure 19.23 Roller pump controlling rate of intraperitoneal blood transfusion.

Regulation. A combination of regulating the drops per minute in the drip chamber combined with repeated observation of the fluid being removed from that graduated chamber provides a sufficient degree of control in most situations.

Rate of flow. As the total volume to be given and the rates of flow required vary so considerably with the condition of the individual infant no absolute figures can be given. Except for the correction of severe blood loss not more than 20 ml per kg of body weight of any plasma expander such as whole blood or reconstituted plasma should be given. Except for shocked infants at least 3 hours should be taken to give this volume. Should the heart rate increase to over 16 per minute the infusion should be stopped temporarily and if the heart rate does not return to normal within 30 minutes no further plasma expander should be given.

Maintenance fluids are given at slower rates and for volumes of the order of 50 to 75 ml per kg per day require rates of 2 to 3 ml per kg per hour. As the size of drop differs with individual giving sets the critical setting of an infusion rate by drops per minute must not be relied upon as a measure of the volume given. This can only be measured accurately by recording the rate of fall of the fluid in the graduated chamber. After a period of observation a suitable number of drops per minute to give the required rate of fall can be calculated. All volume measurements, however, must be measured from the graduated chamber and a careful record kept of the level at quarter hourly or half hourly intervals together with a note of each occasion on which the chamber is filled.

INTRAVENOUS DRUGS

Drugs to be given intravenously at stated intervals can be injected into an intravenous infusion provided that there is no pharmacological contraindication. Some drugs may be added to the infusion fluid in which case it must be made clear whether the drug is to be added to the infusion bottle, bearing in mind the length of time over which this will be administered, or into the graduated drip chamber which will be emptied in a shorter period of time.

Instructions. In either case written instructions should be given and a record made on the donor bottle or graduated chamber of the drug, the dose and the time at which it was added to the infusion fluid. Should the infusion fluid require to be changed further instructions with regard to drugs incorporated with the previous fluid must be sought.

Precautions. Certain preparations given intravenously are irritant to veins and tissues because of their chemical or physical properties. Typical of these are 8.4 per cent sodium bicarbonate and 50 per cent glucose. It is safer to give these only into large veins, but in an emergency situation they may have to be given through smaller peripheral veins in which case the vein should immediately be flushed through with normal saline or 5 per cent glucose, a record being kept of the volume issued.

Exchange Transfusion

The general principles of exchange transfusion have been discussed in Chapter 14. A variety of techniques may be employed some using both an artery and a vein. We shall confine this description to the use of a single catheter in the umbilical vein.

EQUIPMENT

The simplest equipment is that required for cannulation of the umbilical vein plus two two way taps in series (Fig. 19.24) and sterile tubing to connect one side arm with the donor bottle, and the other to lead to a waste blood collecting bucket.

Prepacked sterilized disposable exchange transfusion sets are available but are more expensive than the simple equipment described.

Heparinized saline. Some sets contain three- or four-way taps to allow a bottle of heparinized saline to be connected to the system. A simple system using disposable taps and syringes is not likely to

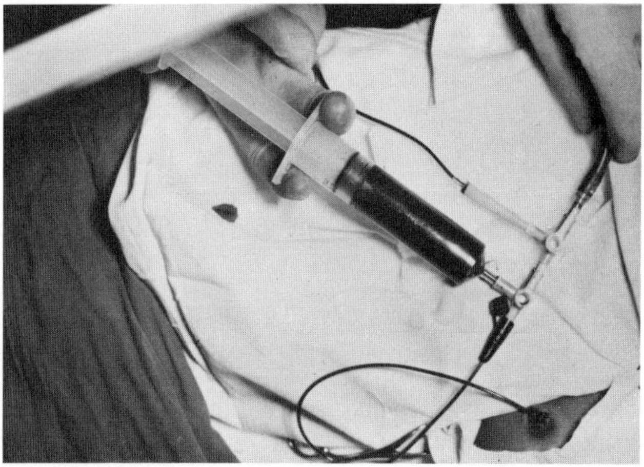

Figure 19.24 Simple apparatus for exchange transfusion.

become obstructed by clot, and it is no longer essential to incorporate heparinized saline into the system. It is useful, however, to prepare a bottle of 0.9 per cent saline with 10 units heparin per ml saline. This can be used to fill the system during any temporary halt during the procedure.

The donor blood should be cross-matched with the infant's blood but in the case of rhesus isoimmunization should be Rh-negative. It is inadvisable to use blood more than 48 hours old as the potassium level begins to rise rapidly over that age. As the haematocrit of acid citrate dextrose donor blood is generally below 40 per cent withdrawal of 100 ml of plasma is often arranged to increase the packed cell volume.

The blood should be warmed slowly to blood heat. Rapid heating causes haemolysis. A water-bath with regulated heater coil is useful.

Time for preparation. Exchange transfusion is only an emergency procedure in infants with severe anaemia from haemolysis of blood loss. In other situations time is better spent ensuring that all preparations are complete and that the donor blood is at appropriate temperature before starting the procedure.

THE INFANT

Some immobilization, particularly for the limbs of an active infant, is desirable during an exchange transfusion. Whatever method is used access to the mouth must be allowed so that the pharynx can be aspirated and the trachea intubated if necessary. A variety of frames or crucifixes have been devised to which the infant can be lightly strapped.

Heat. Extra heat should be available from an electrically-heated mattress or from an overhead infrared heater. Both sources are available in the Baby-therm (Fig. 19.12). Incubators can be used but often present problems of suitable access.

Monitoring. Recording of heart rate is most conveniently made by ECG electrodes on the limbs with the trace visible on an oscilloscope. If apparatus for this is not available a stethoscope should be strapped over the apex so that the heart rate can be monitored constantly. A permanent temperature record is also available and can be combined with a radiant heater controlled by the infant's temperature (Fig. 19.25).

Records of volume of blood exchanged, heart rate, temperature and drugs given should be kept and it is useful to have a prepared sheet on which these observations can be recorded. Containers required for any specimens to be taken should be available.

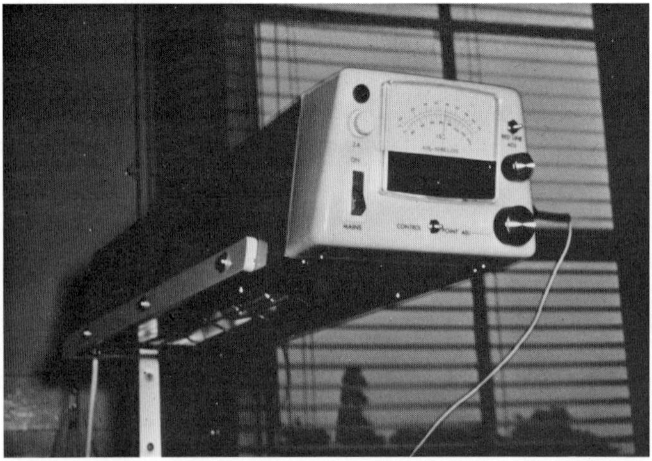

Figure 19.25 Temperature monitoring on overhead servocontrolled radiant heater.

PREPARATION

As will be appreciated from the foregoing remarks preparation for an exchange transfusion takes some time. Where there is a possibility that exchange transfusion will be required rapidly after birth, as in severe haemolytic disease of the newborn (Chapter 14), all the necessary preparations must be completed before delivery is expected. In such circumstances group O, Rh-negative donor blood should be cross-matched against mother's blood and be available suitably warmed so that there is no delay in starting the transfusion should the infant's condition at birth justify immediate treatment.

STAFF

At least two people should be constantly available during an exchange transfusion. The physician who is to carry out the transfusion should scrub up as for a surgical operation and wear sterile gown, cap and gloves. A senior nurse or another doctor is required to supervise the infant's condition and to keep records of the procedure. It is not necessary for them to be in sterile gowns unless they are to assist with the cannulation.

TECHNIQUE

When the equipment has been checked and the infant prepared the area is covered with a sterile towel with a central aperture, and the two way taps and syringe connected to the donor bottle and to the waste tube. Blood is drawn into the syringe from the donor bottle and expelled down the waste tube to check that the apparatus is functioning properly. The infant's umbilical vein is then cannulated with a closed-end side hole tube of gauze 4.5 to 9.0 fg as described earlier. When the blood flows back freely the venous pressure is measured and the catheter connected to the taps.

The exchange may then proceed by withdrawal of a carefully measured quantity of blood, generally 10 ml but varying from 5 ml in very small infants to 20 ml in large infants. As the efficiency of the exchange is reduced by using smaller volumes at each cycle the largest volume which does not upset the infant should be used. By suitable arrangement of the taps this blood is either used for collection of specimens or disposed of. The same volume of blood is withdrawn from the donor bottle into the syringe and then slowly injected into the infant.

Heart rate. The effect on the infant's heart rate of withdrawal of blood or of giving blood should be noted. Heart rates rising to greater than 160 per minute indicate stress. If this occurs only when blood is being given there is probably circulatory overload and the effect of removing an extra 10 or 20 ml of blood should be assessed. Similarly, if tachycardia occurs on withdrawal of blood, extra blood may be required.

Venous pressure. Serial measurements of venous pressure will help in the decision with regard to blood volume adjustments.

An exchange proceeds by repeated cycles of the withdrawal and replacement of blood. Constant supervision is necessary to ensure that no air is injected. The total volume to be exchanged and the time involved were discussed in Chapter 14.

Completion. At the end of an exchange transfusion the umbilical vein catheter should be withdrawn unless required for other purposes. Bleeding from the umbilical stump is generally readily controlled by pressure at the site or immediately above the umbilicus. It is seldom necessary to ligate the vessel. Once bleeding has been controlled the umbilical stump should be sealed with a local application of an agent such as Nobecutane. The area should be inspected regularly for signs of bleeding.

PERITONEAL TRANSFUSION

Occasionally it proves difficult to find suitable peripheral veins for intravenous infusions in low birth-weight infants, particularly when they are a month or more old. At this age blood transfusion for correction of anaemia may be required. Rather than cut down on the internal saphenous vein at the ankle we prefer to give packed cells into the peritoneal cavity from which they are satisfactorily absorbed into the circulation. An infant drip set and scalp vein infusion set are used. After suitable preparation the scalp vein needle is passed vertically through the linea alba about one third of the distance from the umbilicus to the symphysis pubis (Fig. 19.26) making sure beforehand that the bladder is not enlarged to this height. The needle is supported by strapping and the transfusion given as if intravenously.

SUBCUTANEOUS INFUSIONS

Improvements in the equipment available for scalp vein or other venous infusion have made such infusions the method of choice for giving parenteral fluids. Formerly when suitable equipment was not available simple fluids such as normal saline were sometimes given by subcutaneous infusion.

This method can still be used if no better method is available but the lack of control over the speed of absorption and the risk of tissue plane infection make it unsuitable for routine use.

Only non-irritant, isotonic solutions such as 0.9 per cent saline can be used. Hyaluronidase is added to the infusion fluid to aid dispersion and absorption.

Suitable sites are the subscapular fold of skin and the axilla. Rates of flow are adjusted to prevent undue distension of the subcutaneous tissues.

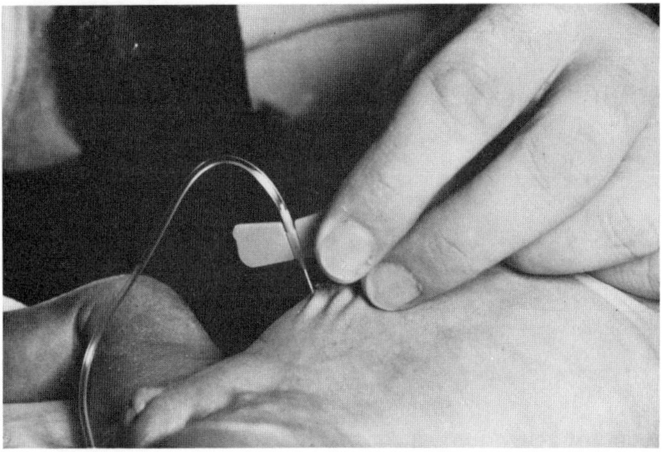

Figure 19.26 Needle inserted for intraperitoneal transfusion.

RELIEF OF TENSION PNEUMOTHORAX

A tension pneumothorax may prove rapidly fatal unless relieved. It is essential therefore that all special care and intensive therapy baby units should have at least one set of apparatus constantly available for the treatment of pneumothorax.

Equipment. The provision of sterile disposable Heimlich valves (Fig. 19.27) has greatly simplified this procedure particularly if combined with a trocar and cannula set of suitable size. For temporary use until more satisfactory drainage can be established the 'Intracath' type of metal needle and inner polythene tubing can be used. If such disposable apparatus is not available a wide gauge needle with facilities for connection to an underwater seal by narrow bore tubing may be used. Such apparatus is, however, cumbersome, and it is generally preferable to request the assistance of paediatric surgeons to establish drainage using a Malecot or similar catheter connected to water seal drainage.

The site at which the cannula is introduced depends upon the clinical and radiological findings. Care must be taken to avoid the internal mammary arteries.

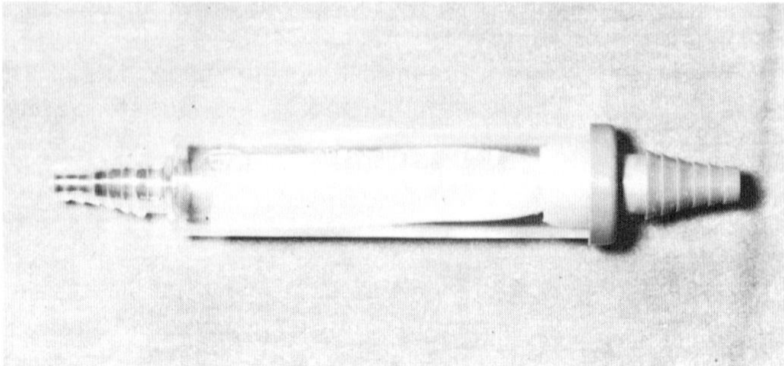

Figure 19.27 Disposable Heimlitz valve.

MARROW ASPIRATION

Site. Marrow is most conveniently taken from an iliac bone or tibia in the newborn period. Suitably small marrow puncture needles are necessary.

Technique. After suitable preparation the infant is placed in the lateral position and held steadily. The needle is inserted into the iliac bone about 1 to 2 cm behind and below the anterior superior iliac spine and with the needle perpendicular to the flat surface of the bone. Less pressure is required than in older children to penetrate the outer table. Once the marrow cavity has been entered marrow is aspirated as in older children or adults. The tibia can be entered at the junction of its upper and middle thirds through its medial subcutaneous surface. In both methods great care must be taken not to pass right through the marrow cavity. Care and gentle persistence are required.

FURTHER READING

BEHRMAN, R. E. (Ed.) (1970). The newborn. *Pediatric Clinics of North America*, **17**, 4.

BLACK, J. A. (1972). *Neonatal Emergencies and Other Problems.* London: Butterworth.

DAVIES, P. A., ROBINSON, R. J., SCOPES, J. W., TIZARD, J. P. M. & WIGGLESWORTH, J. S. (1972). *Medical Care of Newborn Babies.* Spastics International Medical Publications. London: Heinemann.

JONES, R. S. & OWEN-THOMAS, J. B. (1971). *Care of the Critically Ill Child.* London: Arnold.

ROBERTS, K. D. & EDWARDS, J. M. (1971). *Paediatric Intensive Care.* Oxford: Blackwell.

20
Immigrant Families

In certain parts of Great Britain the arrival of immigrant families has faced midwives, nurses and doctors responsible for care of the newly born baby with unusual difficulties.

THE SIZE OF THE PROBLEM

The size of the problem varies throughout the country, but for obvious reasons is greatest in our industrial areas. The district general hospital to which one of the authors is attached serves a mixed urban and rural population of 155 000, and of the 2000 hospital deliveries in 1971 4 per cent were to Pakistani mothers, 1 per cent to Italian mothers, and 0.5 per cent to all other immigrant mothers from China, Holland, Norway, Spain, United States of America, West Indies and Yugoslavia.

LANGUAGE

Inevitably language poses the greatest problems. Mergence in a community takes a long time during which the immigrant is bewildered by the number of medical and social services of which he or she is told.

Terminology. He cannot grasp the difference between a welfare clinic and a hospital outpatient department. Nor can he understand the function of a general practitioner. Mere mention of 'doctor' or 'nurse' conjures up visions of grave disease. Preventive as distinct from curative care is unknown to many immigrants. Much less do they think in terms of the promotion of health.

USE OF SERVICES

Reluctance or even refusal on the part of an immigrant woman to attend an antenatal clinic or to take her newly born baby to a follow-up clinic is explained by her bewilderment and apprehension. Her outlook is determined by her traditionally rigid association of hospital with disease, and of home with health. This same outlook explains the extreme reluctance of many immigrants parent to seek professional advice for an ill baby until his condition is grave.

These are some of the many difficulties encountered daily. Considered from the point of view of the immigrant recently arrived in a strange land they deserve understanding. The problem is how to convey confidence and practical understanding in the face of the language problem. Midwives and health visitors from the emigrant countries and now employed by local and hospital authorities in this country are in a unique position to give invaluable practical help, but even they know perplexity when confronted with a multiplicity of dialects. This same difficulty has limited the effectiveness of teaching Urdu, in particular, to English personnel attending specially organized night classes.

COMMUNITY RELATIONS

Local authorities and voluntary bodies organized to assist community relations have developed new, and partially adapted existing services to meet the situation where it exists. In some areas midwives and health visitors have been advised on means to overcome language difficulties; panels of interpreters enrolled from among immigrants and university students have been developed. Elsewhere lists have been compiled of immigrant doctors, nurses and social workers prepared to help on an entirely voluntary basis in solving language and other problems confronting their fellow countrymen.

Baby Care

In the particular field of baby care the task of midwives and health visitors has been helped by the issue of pamphlets giving advice in various languages for distribution to appropriate immigrants. Additional to local authority issues, a number of valuable leaflets have been produced by the manufacturers of well-known processed cows' milk and other baby food products (Fig. 20.1). Free use is made by midwives of these and of food samples in hospital and in district as effective forms of reinforcing instructions given in sign language. Many immigrant mothers are unable to read and for them illustrated pamphlets intended to instruct by 'pictorial language' have a special value.

ANTENATAL CARE

The response of immigrants to antenatal services varies greatly and is not related to the country of origin of the expectant mother. Perhaps the best results have been obtained in those clinic centres which have assumed a benign all-purpose welfare advisory function and which are staffed by women only.

Neonatal follow-up is best assured by winning the mother's confidence antenatally. Attendance of the father at all sessions—antenatal and neonatal—can be invaluable but allowance must be made for his disinclination to risk dismissal on account of voluntary absence from work. Approach to the employer is always worth while and often gets a sympathetic hearing.

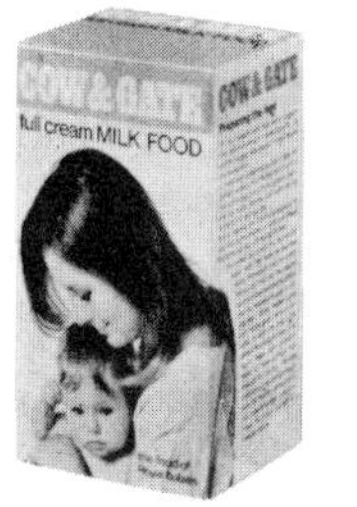

کاؤ اینڈ گیٹ ۔ دُودھ غذا

(پُوری کریم)

دُودھ کی خوراک

نیچے دیئے ہوئے پیمانے اوسط درجے کے بچّے کے لئے ہیں اور انہیں صرف ہدایت کے طور پر سمجھنا چاہیئے ۔ بچے کی اپنی ضرورت کے لحاظ سے اس میں تبدیلی ہو سکتی ہے ۔

یہ خوراکیں پُوری کریم والا دُودھ مہیّا کرنے کے لئے نہیں ہیں ۔

ہر تین گھنٹے کی خوراک :۔

۶ بجے صبح بچے کی عُمر	۹ بجے صبح کاؤ اینڈ گیٹ کا ناپ والا چمچہ	دوپہر بارہ بجے اُبلے ہوئے پانی میں ملا کر کل	شام تین بجے شام ۶ بجے بچے کا اوسط وزن	رات ۹ بجے شکر کے چمچے
ایک ہفتہ	۲½	تین اونس	۷½ پونڈ	ایک
دو ہفتہ	۳	۳½ اونس	۸ پونڈ	ایک
ایک مہینہ	۳½	۴ اونس	۸¾ پونڈ	ایک
دو مہینہ	۴	۴½ اونس	۱۰½ پونڈ	ایک
تین مہینہ	۵	۵½ اونس	۱۲½ پونڈ	ایک

چار گھنٹے کی خوراک :۔

۶ بجے صبح	۱۰ بجے صبح		دو بجے سہ پہر ۶ بجے شام	۱۰ بجے رات
ایک ہفتہ	۳	۳½ اونس	۷½ پونڈ	۱
دو ہفتہ	۳½	۴ اونس	۸ پونڈ	۱
ایک مہینہ	۴	۴½ اونس	۸¾ پونڈ	۱½
دو مہینہ	۵	۵½ اونس	۱۰½ پونڈ	۱½
تین مہینہ	۶	۶½ اونس	۱۲½ پونڈ	۱½
چار مہینہ	۶½	۷ اونس	۱۴ پونڈ	۱½
پانچ مہینہ	۷	۷ اونس	۱۵½ پونڈ	۱½
چھ مہینہ	۷½	۷½ اونس	۱۶¾ پونڈ	۱½
سات مہینہ	۸	۸ اونس	۱۷¾ پونڈ	۱½
آٹھ سے بارہ ماہ	۸½	۸½ سے بارہ اونس	۱۹ سے ۲۳ پونڈ	۱½

دُودھ کی تیاری :۔ ناپ کو دُودھ کے چمچے سے بھر کر اسے ہموار کر لیجئے تاکہ صحیح مقدار آئے (ایک زیادہ بھرا ہُوا چمچہ تقریباً ایک ناپ کے برابر ہوتا ہے ۔)

اگرچہ دُودھ پلانے کے وقت اُسے تیار کرنا چاہیئے لیکن ایک وقت میں ایک سے زیادہ خوراک بنانی ہو تو نیچے بیان کئے ہوئے طریقے سے مقررہ مقدار میں دُودھ کو گرم پانی اور شکر میں کسی صاف کئے ہوئے جار یا ناپ کے برتن میں رکھ کر ملایئے اور فوراً ہی دُودھ پلانے کی صاف کی ہوئی بوتلوں میں جتنی کہ بھرنی ہیں بھر لیجئے ۔ اُنہیں ٹھنڈا کر کے ڈھک کر ریفریجریٹر میں تب تک رکھیں جب تک انکی ضرورت ہو ۔ بچے ہوئے دُودھ کو ہرگز استعمال نہیں کرنا چاہیئے ۔ اور نہ ہی ضرورت سے زیادہ

Figure 20.1 Feeding instruction leaflet in Urdu.

Inevitably problems differ according to the nationality of the immigrants and, to some extent, according to the community into which they seek absorption. Experiences are not alike in any two areas or regions, but the following impressions of midwives and doctors engaged in hospital and domiciliary practice give some idea of the variety of situations encountered. The patience and skill exercised by midwives and nurses in their difficult task cannot be too highly praised.

Indian Families

Difficulty of language can be very great, but reasonably effective interpreter aid within the family is sometimes forthcoming from the father when not at work, or from older children when not at school. Less satisfactory is the need in some households to leave written directions to await the father on his return. This is the more significant as breast feeding is on the decline and a constant need exists for frequent checking of the way in which artificial feeds are prepared, and in which attention is paid to bottle hygiene.

The directions given to the father may have to deal with infant feeding and vitamin supplements. In some homes the 'womenfolk' accept minimal responsibility in which case it is the father who makes the necessary purchases in anticipation of a baby's birth at home, or arrival home from hospital. An impression exists that male infants get more favourable care and attention than baby girls. Understandably, mothers are inclined to wrap their small babies up in too many clothes, and too tightly; and are averse to letting their infants be out of doors even in good weather. Older mothers with newly born babies tend to be rather remote and apparently unhappy and one experienced midwife was prompted to say, 'It is as if they miss support. I often wish I could converse with them about their babies.'

Afro-Asian Families

Until recently these presented few problems, the parents consisting in the main of English-speaking grant-aided students who take full advantage of available medical and social services on their own initiative. The picture has changed with the large-scale immigration of families expelled from Uganda, who no doubt will be faced with the same problems experienced by immigrants from India and Pakistan.

Pakistani Families

In most respects the problems resemble those described in connection with Indian families, but initially at least the difficulties of language and of understanding British customs can give rise to an unintentionally abrupt, apparently defensive suspicion of recommendations concerning their babies. This may show itself in an expectant mother's disinclination to take iron which has been prescribed for her. Tablets and pills are regarded with suspicion and have attributed to them untoward events of whatever kind. There is a high incidence of anaemia secondary to dietary insufficiency and hookworm infestation. A resistant attitude on the part of the father sometimes takes the form, despite satisfactory social, obstetric and medical conditions, of refusing to let his wife be confined at home, or strenuously resisting her early discharge home after confinement in hospital. There is a rooted objection to the services of a home help. Because of the extreme language problem it is difficult adequately to impress upon a Pakistani mother her newly born baby's need for warmth. Unthinkingly, small babies are left in exposed situations and the room temperature allowed to fall significantly. Little use is customarily made of woollen material for clothing or bedding.

In general the Pakistani mother is totally averse to being examined by a male doctor.

West Indian Families

Communication presents no problem: their language is our language. Culturally the West Indian immigrant has much in common with members of the host community, and of all immigrants probably finds least difficulty in adapting himself to his new surroundings. Illegitimacy, which is on the decline, is not associated with moral stigmata. Cohabitation is not uncommon, and the arrival of one or more children not infrequently precedes marriage. Frequently living conditions are extremely poor and many West Indian mothers seek industrial or other employment. Accustomed in their own country to oil stoves for cooking the West Indian immigrant turns naturally to a similar stove for an economical source of heat, regardless of the attendant fire risks.

In the early weeks of life the newly born baby may spend most of his time in bed with his mother. Where there is stable union between father and mother, and the latter does not require to go out to work, the baby is usually fed at the breast. If the mother is living alone, or the union between her and the father is unstable, the future needs of the baby should be anticipated in terms of child-minding or foster care.

OTHER IMMIGRANTS

Immigrants from Cyprus, China and Poland are few in number compared with those from the countries already mentioned. They have in common an inherent desire to preserve the ties and solidarity of the family unit. In many instances the father possesses a shop or small business and he, his wife and family find their pleasures in the home and do not readily develop strong ties with the community. Language is a particular difficulty, the mother in her relative isolation not seeing the need to learn even one word of English. With husband as interpreter, however, she is extremely co-operative.

Derived from personal experience and the experience of a number of doctors and nurses the above observations are made in no spirit of dogmatism, much less criticism. Some of the observations may be unintentionally misrepresented. They are, however, intended only as pointers to a variety of ways in which directly, and indirectly, immigrant problems can impinge on care of the newly born baby. The bewilderment of the doctor or nurse can be as great as that of the apprehensive immigrant.

It is salutary to remember how much more ancient than those of our own are, the culture and histories of some of the countries from which immigrants come.

21

Continuing Care

In Chapters 1 and 2 of this book we looked at the challenge which faces midwives, doctors and all others associated with the care of mother and her child during pregnancy and the newborn period, and in particular we considered perinatal mortality as an index of failure in meeting that challenge. Stillbirth or neonatal death is clearly a failure in that the pregnancy has not resulted in a live healthy child.

GROWING UP

Survival cannot, however, be equated with success unless the child is able to pass through a happy childhood and adolescence to maturity and independence. The title of this book would appear to limit our interest to the newborn period but it is foolish to consider this extremely important but limited period of our lives in isolation. Delivery and adaptation to the external environment are phases in the development of a mature adult. The problems which may arise because of difficulty in the perinatal period are not necessarily confined to infancy or even childhood and may have a profound effect, physical or emotional, on the adult.

Quality of Survival

To the midwife and doctor looking after a low birth-weight infant the immediate problems are so obvious that it is difficult to keep the thought of quality of adult life for that infant in mind. We have now reached the stage of development of maternity and paediatric services where this thought of the future must play a major part in the assessment of our service. It is no longer satisfactory to count survival of the infant as the only criterion of success. Quality of life for the survivor should now be our parameter of success. How does one measure quality of survival?

Quality of life means such different things to different people under different circumstances that no simple quantitative measure can be expected. The severely handicapped child with spina bifida but with understanding and loving parents may have a much happier life than the physically normal child in a broken home.

ENVIRONMENTAL FACTORS

Environmental factors and how they may be improved will not be discussed here beyond the newborn period. It is most important however, to appreciate that the environment in the newborn period may have a profound and possibly life-long effect on the intimate relationship between a mother and her baby and this is a factor well within the control of midwives, doctors, hospital administrators, social workers etc. (Chap. 7). This is not a factor which can be appreciated easily or measured during the newborn period.

The home. The effects are likely to become obvious when mother is trying to look after her baby at home. Unless the midwifery department and newborn nursery staff know of such problems remedial measures cannot be put into effect.

Feedback of information about the subsequent development and happiness of mothers and babies is therefore essential to any assessment of the effectiveness of a maternity department. What has been said about emotional problems applies equally to physical problems. Mothers are perhaps more willing to have their infants re-examined to exclude physical abnormality and it is on this basis that follow-up clinics are generally arranged.

Health Services

The division of the health services into three relatively independent sections at the inception of the National Health Service unfortunately led to some disagreement as to who was to organize such follow-up services. As a result of failure of co-operation between the three branches mothers were sometimes placed in a difficult position and were naturally concerned if conflicting advice was given from different clinics which they attended. It is to be hoped that the reunification of the services will remove this difficulty.

CLINICS

Whether clinics should be run in general practitioners' consulting rooms, in health centres or clinics, or in hospital outpatient departments is of less importance than the standard of competence of those examining the infants, and the ease with which the results of these examinations are transferred to all those who can use that knowledge to benefit the individual or the community. Our present systems of providing a health service to individuals from cradle to the grave are improving but still leave much to be desired.

Acceptability. At present two major problems emerge. The first is that follow-up care tends to be least acceptable to those most in need of it. A disproportionate amount of time and work may therefore be spent with families with little or no problem whereas those most in need may shun offers of help.

Co-ordination of records. Secondly there is at present so little co-ordination of record-keeping and transfer of information that help may be offered from several sources without adequate liaison and co-ordination.

Health education. Better information about services available and the provision of attractive accommodation with well trained staff have proved to be effective in many new housing areas where mothers soon learn to welcome the service provided for them and their children.

Standardization. Co-ordination of records is also being actively discussed and as stated in Chapter 7 it is hoped that the proposed national neonatal record sheet being introduced in Scotland will form the basis of an ongoing health record. Standardization of records should not imply standardization of management. For some purposes, however, standardization of investigational methods, e.g. developmental screening, may be advisable so that the information available in one area can be of significance in another.

The Benefit

The individual infant and child can hope to gain from regular medical examination, including developmental assessment, if illness or minor abnormality is detected at a stage when treatment can be applied with minimal disturbance of normal life and activity.

The community can also gain from such a service. In time it, is to be hoped that the regular feedback of information to maternity units about the progress of children will allow a medical audit of the relative advantages and disadvantages of procedures being employed. This would be the long-term equivalent of the shorter-term assessment of immediate results in the newborn period. Without such information the harmful effects on the fetus of high concentrations of oxygen would not have been recognized.

Reassessment. With more refined methods of serial examination as in developmental screening it could well be that some of our most cherished theories of management in the newborn period will be called into question. We must be prepared to abandon a policy which is shown in the long term to be harmful to the child as readily as most abandon policies which are not in the best short-term interest of the infant.

‘AT RISK’ REGISTER

So far no mention has been made of selectivity in advocating the advantages of long-term supervision of children’s development. The reason for this is that we cannot as yet be certain as to which infants justify being considered as being at risk. By selecting in the newborn period a limited number of infants for follow up and by placing these on an ‘at risk’ register it had been hoped that a higher quality of service could be given to those who were most in need. Experience has shown, however, that not only do many of the children on the present 'at risk' registers prove to have no special requirements but a considerable number of those who do require special facilities or education were not included on the 'at risk' register after assessment in the newborn period. Improving standards of assessment in the first month of life may improve the usefulness of 'at risk' registers. At present, however, we feel that more is to be gained by aiming at periodic assessment of all children. The facilities and staff available will govern the intervals at which this can be carried out.

The first month of life is the basis on which we build the remainder of our physical, emotional and intellectual development. This lays a great responsibility on those who care for us during that formative period. The authors hope that this book has helped to provide some insight into the problems involved and the remedies available.

Index

Index

5/4